AṢṬADAḶA YOGAMĀLĀ

AṢṬADAḶA YOGAMĀLĀ

(COLLECTED WORKS)

B.K.S. IYENGAR

Volume 6

Interviews

ALLIED PUBLISHERS PRIVATE LIMITED
NEW DELHI MUMBAI KOLKATA LUCKNOW CHENNAI
NAGPUR BANGALORE HYDERABAD AHMEDABAD

ALLIED PUBLISHERS PRIVATE LIMITED
1/13-14 Asaf Ali Road, **New Delhi**–110002
Ph.: 011-23239001 • E-mail: delhi.books@alliedpublishers.com
47/9 Prag Narain Road, Near Kalyan Bhawan, **Lucknow**–226001
Ph.: 0522-2209942 • E-mail: lko.books@alliedpublishers.com
17 Chittaranjan Avenue, **Kolkata**–700072
Ph.: 033-22129618 • E-mail: cal.books@alliedpublishers.com
15 J.N. Heredia Marg, Ballard Estate, **Mumbai**–400001
Ph.: 022-42126969 • E-mail: mumbai.books@alliedpublishers.com
60 Shiv Sunder Apartments (Ground Floor), Central Bazar Road,
Bajaj Nagar, **Nagpur**–440010
Ph.: 0712-2234210 • E-mail: ngp.books@alliedpublishers.com
F-1 Sun House (First Floor), C.G. Road, Navrangpura,
Ellisbridge P.O., **Ahmedabad**–380006
Ph.: 079-26465916 • E-mail: ahmbd.books@alliedpublishers.com
751 Anna Salai, **Chennai**–600002
Ph.: 044-28523938 • E-mail: chennai.books@alliedpublishers.com
5th Main Road, Gandhinagar, **Bangalore**–560009
Ph.: 080-22262081 • E-mail: bngl.books@alliedpublishers.com
3-2-844/6 & 7 Kachiguda Station Road, **Hyderabad**–500027
Ph.: 040-24619079 • E-mail: hyd.books@alliedpublishers.com

Website: www.alliedpublishers.com

First published, 2006

Reprinted 2007, 2009, 2012, 2014

ISBN : 81-7764-976-0

Cover design : The Author

Artwork : S.M. Waugh

Published by Sunil Sachdev and printed by Ravi Sachdev at Allied Publishers Private Limited, Printing Division, A-104 Mayapuri Phase II, New Delhi - 110064

Invocatory Prayers

ॐ

Yogena cittasya padena vācāṁ
Malaṁ śarīrasyaca vaidyakena
Yopākarottaṁ pravaraṁ munīnāṁ
Patañjaliṁ prāñjalirānato'smi
Ābāhu puruṣākāraṁ
Śaṅkha cakrāsi dhāriṇaṁ
Sahasra śirasaṁ śvetaṁ
Praṇamāmi Patañjaliṁ

I bow before the noblest of sages Patañjali, who gave yoga for serenity and sanctity of mind, grammar for clarity and purity of speech and medicine for pure, perfect health.

I prostrate before Patañjali who is crowned with a thousand headed cobra, an incarnation of Ādiśeṣa (Anañta) whose upper body has a human form, holding the conch in one arm, disk in the second, a sword of wisdom to vanquish nescience in the third and blessing humanity from the fourth arm, while his lower body is like a coiled snake.

Yastyaktvā rūpamādyaṁ prabhavati jagato'nekadhānugrahāya
Prakṣīṇakleśarāśirviṣamaviṣadharo'nekavaktrāḥ subhogī
Sarvajñānaprasūtirbhujagaparikaraḥ prītaye yasya nityaṁ
Devohīṣaḥ savovyātsitavimalatanuryogado yogayuktaḥ

I prostrate before Lord Ādiśeṣa, who manifested himself on Earth as Patañjali to grace the human race in health and harmony,

I salute Lord Ādiśeṣa of the myriad serpent heads and mouths carrying noxious poisons, discarding which he came to Earth as a single headed Patañjali in order to eradicate ignorance and vanquish sorrow.

I pay my obeisance to him, repository of all knowledge, amidst his attendant retinue.

I pray to the Lord whose primordial form shines with peace and white effulgence, pristine in body, a master of yoga, who bestows on all his yogic light to enable mankind to rest in the house of the immortal Soul.

BY THE AUTHOR

This volume of *Aṣṭadaḷa Yogamālā* published by Allied Publishers, Delhi, is the sixth volume of the second part of the "Collected Works" of Yogācārya B.K.S. Iyengar. Each part comprises several volumes which are arranged according to the following scheme:

Articles
Interviews
Question and Answer Sessions
Techniques of *Āsanas, Prāṇāyāma, Dhyāna* and *Śavāsana*
Therapeutic Applications of Yoga
Garland of Aphorisms and Thoughts
General Index and Analytical Dictionary
Addendum

Also by the Same Author

Light on Yoga
Light on Prāṇāyāma
Concise Light on Yoga
Art of Yoga
Tree of Yoga
Light on the Yoga Sūtras of Patañjali
The Illustrated Light on Yoga
Yoga Dipika (Marathi)
Yoga Ek Kalpataru (Marathi)
Ārogyayoga (Marathi)
Light on Aṣṭāṇga Yoga
Aṣṭadaḷa Yogamālā (Vols 1, 2, 3, 4 & 5)
Yoga: The Path To Holistic Health
Yoga Sarvānasāṭhi (Marathi)
Basic Guidelines for Teachers of Yoga (co-authored with G.S. Iyengar)
Yogacandan (Marathi)
Light on Life

Also on Iyengar Yoga

Body the Shrine, Yoga Thy Light
70 Glorious Years
Iyengar His Life and Work
Yogapushpanjali
Yogadhārā

CONTENTS

PLATES

PREFACE

Aṣṭadaḷa Yogamālā is again presented to you with the incisive and insightful explanations of both the core as well as the content of the yogic path. They have been distilled from a *sādhanā* that spans more than seventy years. There are many explanations that reveal to the reader a depth that penetrates far beyond their original inquiry, leading the reader to further ponder and reflect on this vast subject.

In this volume, a number of interviews are from some of my senior most students, seeking guidance in their inquiry and to quench their thirst for knowledge.

Here I have tried to illumine them in the field of their questions and at the same time indicate the black holes of the body where their minds and intelligence have overlooked or failed to enter and search the deepest caves in the body. In this volume I have given them an intellectual mirror to enter the deepest caves of the body so that they can see and make right use of the directions that are needed to travel on this path of yoga.

At the same time I am showing the steps according to one's understanding so that each one establishes a bridge to further his or her own subjective experience, knowledge and wisdom.

There are several interviews by major international and local publications as well as media representatives. The reader receives a unique perspective of this subject. Each interview offers a rich and vital fund of the content of yoga. What the reader will find revealed in this volume is without doubt unlikely to be paralleled elsewhere.

For one who wishes to know both the depth as well as the breadth of the ocean of yogic knowledge, it is only through the total immersion of the whole self into this ocean. Only then can one know that the true spiritual odour in the whole ocean of yogic philosophy is the one worthy to savour with total attention and awareness.

B. K. S. IYENGAR

THE INTERVIEWS

THE YOGI ON YOGA*

Q.- You have been teaching yoga to thousands of Westerners. How do you explain their interest in yoga when they have such a variety of physical activities and sports?

True, I have been teaching yoga to thousands of Westerners, but I have taught yoga to thousands of Indians as well. Yoga has been established in the West due to their zeal in practice.

No doubt there is a great interest in sports and an almost mind boggling variety of physical activity in the West. It is a reflection of the "zest" and the taste to explore the external world, face the forces of nature, combined with a sense of adventure.

This may be partly attributed to keeping oneself fit in cold climes and the harsh environment. In contrast we in the East have the myriad advantages of the sun and sunlight with respect to physical health and hygiene, and an energising climate that does not invite the "blues" or morose feelings as in the West. Nevertheless the heat induces a great amount of lethargy.

It is also true that Westerners are more health conscious, more outgoing and like to lead and live an active life on all fronts. The ideas of self-denial propounded by our philosophers and saints have not only subdued our spirits but also made us treat our lives as passers-by. So we developed negativity in life. We have not been able to strike a balance between the active householder's life, the physical and emotional planes, and the hard and harsh realities of life, which cannot be wished away by spiritual means. We had distinguished concepts of health and mental culture but were exhausted due to the domination of those who invaded our lands, exploited our resources, made us economically poor and at the same time destroyed much of our cultural and spiritual heritage to thrust on us their cults and religion. Some of us displayed that indomitable spirit that protected our culture, thanks to them we carry on with enthusiasm and can go back to the earliest traces of our civilisation.

The dominant trend in the West is to live and enjoy life fully to the brim, often ignoring the consequences of "excess" or "unbridled" utilisation of body and mind. In a sense, they are

---

* Interview by the students of the *Krishnamacharya Yoga Mandiram-Darśanam*, 1993.

more geared to pleasure – *bhoga*. For me, it seems that they have gone full circle from *bhoga* to *roga* and then to *yoga*; that is from pleasure to diseases and pain and from diseases and pain to the path of yoga, which brings emancipation and freedom.

Pleasures of the world cloud one's mind and of life, and life then can never be an unmixed blessing. It is one thing to be "led" into the process of life; it is another to "lead" a life in the spotlight of full consciousness of our total being, the whole Self. There is a trait of the "individualist" in the East, to seek objective things of the world and we do not have the collective or community approach to bear and share with all. That's why in spite of individual skill and excellence, we get beaten in sports in terms of "team spirit" and collective approach. If the individualistic growth is blended with the sharing of our games in knowledge a new sporting society may come out of it.

Fitness motivation at physical and mental levels is only at the peripheral levels. This was realised when the West was exposed to yoga. *Āsana* and *prāṇāyāma* are not just the culture of body and mind, but essentially they lead one towards spiritual knowledge and culture. The gains experienced in terms of physical health and peace of mind were just the rudimentary side benefits of yoga and one does not strive and struggle for it as an aim but as a means only. Yoga is a spiritual subject. Its total thrust is holistic and universal; its aim is to develop absolute or cosmic consciousness or to have the sight of the soul for looking in towards the interior sheaths of the body, hence the quest of yoga is both within and without.

With sports medicine and modern scientific and technological developments, enthusiasts have taken to sports and allied activities with keen interest both in India as well as outside India. In the West, they were not knowing what they were missing till they discovered it through their exposure to yogic values. Yoga filled the void, approaching the whole being to face, stand and encounter the emotional upheavals that break the personality and reduce the mind to smithereens.

Sports means competition. It has not always been a healthy spirit of competition. Steroids and drugs have become the way of life in Olympic competitions. Yoga caught the West by magic as it cultivates the ethics of fair competition and recognition of excellence in the adversary. It educates the participants to face the opponents without ill will but to exert and get "excellence" out of them. Yoga is practised by people thrown into different circumstances, constitutions and brought up in different environment and has made them to work together with their bodies, minds and souls in concord. A variety of people with differing backgrounds, temperaments, likings, attitudes and aptitudes come and work together in yoga. If sportsmen and athletes take to yoga, their sense of pride and ill feeling in competitive sports will gradually taper off.

Despite glorious achievements in success of modern medicine and allopathy in particular, the latest and the most potent attraction is for dimensions of therapeutic yoga. Healing is wholly a natural phenomenon. After recognition by the western medicine of an "interior milieu", the people yearn to go back to nature. In my small way, I could demonstrate how yoga works incredibly faster than allopathy in a variety of afflictions like hypertension, blood pressure, cardiac troubles, stress, strain, fatigue and tensions, once the focus is turned inwards.

In pursuit of material goods and mundane comforts and blessings, it has been realised that the "external world" had been very much "with the West". Control over the mind, inner poise and calm to face emotional upheavals, the turmoils and vicissitudes of life referred to by Lord Patañjali as *kleśa,* can combat and remove the stress, strain and other anxieties. Yoga helps in ending the inner and outer conflict of apparent "dualities" dissipating the energy or life force. Defusing stress and strain, it fuses the negative and positive polarities releasing new sources and fountains of energy, ushering in the spirit of bliss.

In short, yogic proceses enable man to penetrate from the self to the skin and from the skin to the self playing with conative action and cognitive feeling for the mind to get focussed, which in turn brings its discriminative faculty to play its role so that this faculty bridges the gap between the physical, physiological, mental, intellectual and spiritual sheaths of man to feel and see as one. This I am afraid is missing in physical exercises and sports, hence the point of turning towards yoga.

Q.- Many people are concerned about the wide gap between the interest in yoga in India and the interest in the West. Is this gap real? If so, what is our responsibility to narrow this gap?

This wide gap is not only an astounding situation but also shocking. I too feel it. I sense it as my contacts at home and in the international world bring home the reality of the situation. We should seek the remedy. But before that we should diagnose it.

The cause of the situation is in our genes, our culture. Basically we are highly individualistic, private persons. We are interested in our self-satisfaction, we are self-centred and we are a self-serving lot. We are selfish. So whether in social or spiritual matters, we are for ourselves. This constrains or narrows our outlook, which remains confined to ideas such as "My evolution, my progress, my advancement, my place in the heaven – *svarga* – or hell – *naraka* –, my spiritual advancement, my emancipation – *mokṣa."* In all, the focus is on one's self.

I can clean the house and throw the rubbish in the courtyard of my neighbour. We lack this social sense or collective conscience to ensure that I have a duty to keep not only my house clean, but also my surroundings or the environs.

Suppose I practise yoga and know its benefits, I regard it as my preserve. I am not bothered whether my wife, son, daughter or neighbours will benefit or should benefit from it. The "individualistic" psyche, the product of the centuries, will take time to change. But now, I see the ice melting. People practising yoga are now becoming conscious of a healthy way of life. The wind of yoga is blowing from the West towards the East. The wave of yoga will and shall spread because in the long run it is going to benefit all. This gained benefit makes one go out to keep the community and society healthy at large. This brings social health, congenial environment and a sense of friendly feeling to one and all. It's not a sin to propagate yoga, it's not encroaching on the privacy of the other person.

A beginning has been made by me by taking the message of yoga to the various parts of the globe. Now it is the responsibility of the younger generation as well as yoga journals and periodicals to water the sapling to sprout into a gigantic tree of yoga.

Lord Krishna, who is the only one as *Yogeśvara,* has said that where yoga is, true prosperity grows. I wish for the *Darśanam* to build up a firm foundation for yoga to thrive in the hearts of the East as well.

Q.- In some countries like France and Italy there is a feeling that yoga is a part of the Hindu religion and therefore not acceptable to the Christians. Can you please comment?

I read in the papers that the Pope wanted the Christian community not to do yoga. In what context it was said was not known to me so I cannot talk about it.

A glimpse into the centuries of yoga traditions demonstrates that yoga is not related to any specific religion or even Hinduism. Now, theological reflections of any great religion like Christianity, Islam, Buddhism, Judaism, Zoroastrianism, Hinduism, Sikhism and Jainism are various streams of a single source, God. For example, rituals, namaz or mass, lighting of incense or a candle is common in all religions. All God-made religions are free from conflicts. It is the man-made religions that are causing ill feelings from man to man.

The first founder of yoga is no other than Brahma, the creator. Sage Patañjali, who codified yoga some 2000 years back, refers to *jāti deśa kāla samaya anavacchinnāḥ sārvabhaumāḥ mahāvratam* (*Y.S.* II.31), meaning that the yogic commandments are the great, mighty, universal vows, unconditioned by place, time and class. Any doubting Thomas can make out the universal approach of yoga without the slightest hint or smell of any man-made religion. Yoga has to be taken as a sacred vow and does not dėnote any religious label. That's why I pointed out in my latest book *Light on the Yoga Sūtras of Patañjali* that "I believe this universal approach should be applied to all the other component stages of yoga or *bhakti* or *jñāna* or *karma*, without distinction of time, place or circumstances, to lay down our precepts of our universal heritage." Yoga is an art, science and philosophy. There is no Hindu *dharma*, but it is described as *sanātana dharma* - eternal way of life - or a universal religion for all times. Therefore, I feel yoga is the science of all religions. It begins with a foundation of the ethical disciplines and leads one towards spiritual enlightenment.

In the *Samādhi Pāda* (*Y.S.* I.33), Patañjali says, *maitrī karuṇā muditā upekṣāṇāṁ sukha duḥkha puṇya apuṇya viṣayāṇāṁ bhāvanātaḥ cittaprasādanam.* It means, through cultivation of friendliness, compassion, joy and indifference towards pleasure and pain, virtue and vice respectively, the consciousness becomes favourably disposed, serene and benevolent. What greater hallmark of humanity and universality, compassion and love is required than that which yoga proclaims? Where is the question of any religious denomination through yoga, when yoga aims at culturing the mind and the self; and as far as I know the aim of all religion is in perfecting the divinity in one's self. As the goal or the essence of all religions is in keeping the body healthy, mind clean and self pure, I see that yoga does this only. What yoga proclaims is the concept of *ahiṁsā* and *satya*, non-injury to others and truthfulness to oneself. Yoga ordains the *dharma* in the process of evolution: physically, emotionally, mentally, morally and spiritually.

It is a fact that I have by far the largest following of those who subscribe and practise yoga both in France and Italy. I have been visiting these countries as well as other countries since 1954. I had only two students then and today millions of people are practising in spite of protests and about 200 to 250 Iyengar Yoga centres exist in the world from Alaska to Auckland, and from San Francisco to Tokyo, including Russia. Here, I am delighted to tell you that my books are printed and published in Russian, Ukrainian and Persian languages. Sage Patañjali enumerates the eight stages of yoga namely; *yama, niyama, āsana, prāṇāyāma, pratyāhāra, dhāraṇā, dhyāna* and *samādhi*. In the sixth chapter of the *Bhagavad Gītā*, Śri Krishna explains to Arjuna the essence of yoga stressing the right means.

Yama and *niyama* can be likened to the rules of moral values and codes of behaviour relating to the self and society as a social discipline. They focus on individual discipline as well. Culturing the mind goes with the growth of civilisations. The morals and values of life are also enshrined in the tenets of Christianity, Islam and Buddhism and other great religions of the world. As I said in my book *Light on Yoga*, these commandments are the rules of morality for society and the individual; if not obeyed, it brings chaos, violence, untruth, stealing, dissipation and covetousness. The scenario of violence now is everywhere. The poor, backward impoverished third world countries are in the throes of hunger, malnutrition, disease, ill health and starvation. We are aware of the havoc we are playing with our environment and depleting our mother earth. The principles of *yama* are great universal commandments, which are not limited by birth, place, geographic or regional locations, time and occasion. Non-violence or *ahiṁsā* finally connects us to the concept of total love with no trace of mental thoughts, that is, love without lust. Along with this, yoga wants us to follow *satya* or truthfulness to culture the mental body. Immoderation in sexual enjoyment, accumulation or hoarding far beyond our means is considered as irreligion not only in yoga but in all religions.

If we pause and spare thought by *svādhyāya*, self-introspection, could we not help ourselves individually and the society to cut down the dimensions of the disaster we are inviting? How can we equate yogic practice with "man made religions" which thrive on fear, insecurity, hatred and suspicion? Who can deny to keep oneself physically fit and mentally at peace? Who is not interested in drawing the senses within and to keep the wandering mind under control to set the human mind properly tuned by *pratyāhāra?* Finally who does not want to feel the merging of the individual soul with the cosmic or universal consciousness? This is within the means of humans and the fruit of achievement lies in yoga. How can one develop cosmic or absolute consciousness without knowing the science of yogic discipline that is expressed implicitly or explicitly in all religions?

Our sages have aptly explained religion in such a way that shows no demarcation. It is said that religion is that which upholds, sustains and supports those who have physically, physiologically, mentally, morally and intellectually fallen or those who are falling or in a state of falling. That which lifts them up is religion. This is true divine religion as far as I understand religion.

For your information, I think I am the first yogi to meet Pope Paul VI. It was in 1966. Both of us discussed the subject of yoga and in 1967 I again visited the Vatican. Not only did I have an audience with the Pope, but at his request, I gave a demonstration for the Fathers residing at the Castle Gandolfo. Recently, while I was in London, I was asked to give a lecture on philosophy of yoga at St. James Church, London.

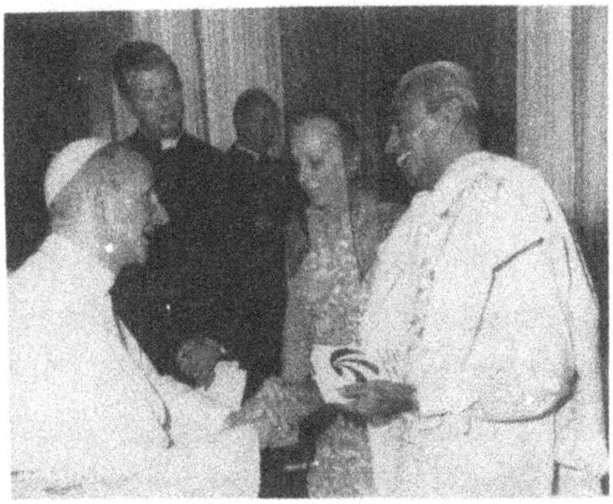

Plate n. 1 – Meeting the Pope

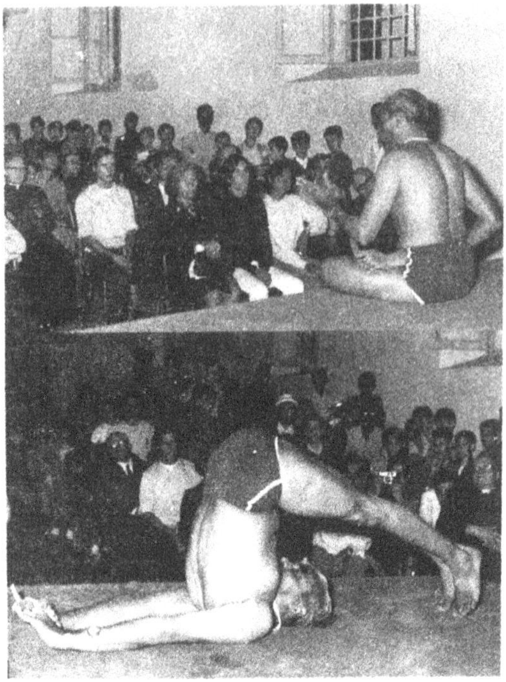

Plate n. 2 – Demonstration at Castle Gandolfo

Besides these, I have taught yoga to many Rev. Fathers and Nuns and one of my pupils, Fr. Joe Perrera, is applying yoga for drug addicts in Bombay and travels abroad to train members for detoxification of drugs through yoga.

Q.- In India people who perform rituals, pray and visit temples are still not free from mental turbulence. They look to yoga for peace of mind. How to explain this anomaly?

True, lots of people are bound by blind belief, the hold of custom and tradition are haunted by want. They find it difficult to sustain themselves physically and economically. They cannot make two ends meet, so they visit temples and perform rituals for solace. But seeking peace of mind is not by knocking down someone's doors but by opening their own heads and hearts. Prayers and rituals are not meant to buy material or physical needs with "spiritual" currency. Because they are done with a motive to earn something in return, the turbulence persists. Love for love's sake, prayer for prayer's sake, rituals for right duty, if done then the mental peace comes.

Also, I see the positive side of it. At least their minds are focused on the divine force though it is of a short duration. With this type of union with the divine, if prolonged, change may take place from the bargaining prayer and transformation might come to pray for the good of all on earth.

Some of our philosophers, frankly speaking were prophets of "gloom". They spread "gloom" instead of cheer and instilling in the common man the will and resolve to "fight" as Śri Krishna says: *tasmād yudhyasva Bhārata*[1], goading Arjuna to fight on. Human life is like a battlefield – *raṇa kṣetra*. It is not for the timid chicken hearted who are daunted by the buffet of misfortune, pain and suffering.

---

[1] Therefore, fight, O descendent of Bhārata (Arjuna) (*B.G.,* II.18).

The self-denial or abnegation of self was like asking a starving or hungry man to tighten his belt. So a large number of people lived in want, poverty, physically, mentally and spiritually weak, with no will or motivation to better their life.

At times the wrong message of the saints who preached tolerance and talked about the virtue of being poor and on suffering, spread fatalism and held promise of better life in the next birth. This inbuilt psyche explains the anomaly of temple going and mental turbulence afflicting millions.

Q.- You have healed many incurable sicknesses. Is it through the special techniques you use or is it through your own spiritual power?

I don't know. It happened earlier and is happening now as well. I don't know whether I have spiritual power or not. So, how can I say when I am not a healer, a Sufi or a saint? I am not aware of whether I have any physical or mental powers to cure sickness. Please know that yoga is not just a technical subject but also it is a healing art. It requires a humane heart to learn and use the art of healing power that yoga has. I am happy that by my touch and adjustment a lot of people get solace, spared of their suffering, physical, mental and psycho-physical.

I am not aware of the special techniques either. But I have the sight to act in an instant to work on the afflicted parts of the suffering people.

I feel however that I may have some "intuitive" faculty because of my devoted yogic practice of precision and dedication of sixty years. I took *āsana* not only as *svādhyāya* but as my *Iṣṭa devatā* – desired deity – and total study and absorption of each *āsana* made me and my self to come in close contact with the Deity[1]. Probably this closeness of me with *āsana* (my deity) is the cause of my success in healing the people who come to me with hope. It seems that I looked into my body for the manifestations of "their afflictions" or disease and worked on my body to get a solution for their suffering. No doubt I used to innovate plenty of things to help people. I constantly think and contemplate them and I can say that it is an "unadulterated" yogic approach. Yoga is not a product from outside. The yogic method and process are natural and not forced or artificial. Nature is inherent in yogic methodology. The cellular body is the instrument. Through the practice of yoga I feed the natural cellular body with defensive energy. My mind possibly works going back to nature gradually, but I don't know how!. Maybe it is the grace of God and *guru*. My insight helps me in diagnosing what goes wrong with those who seek my advice and things at once get planned to help. I don't set a programme of *āsana*, I believe in

---

[1] *Svādhyāyāt iṣṭadevatā saṁprayogaḥ* (Y.S., *II.44*). The desired or a chosen subject, if done with devotion and dedication comes in communion with one's desired deity. *Āsana* is my *Iṣṭadevatā*.

"doing things" on the spot and get results and then leave the rest to the higher powers with a total faith in yoga. Secondly, I wanted to prove to the world the effect of yoga without the introduction of other means. Probably, I am the only one who does not insist on changing food habits, moods or behaviours but insists on making them do the *āsana* with depth to flush, dry and rinse muscles and organs and saturate the affected parts with copious blood supply as well as the supply of vital energy, bringing not only relief but also faith and confidence in them to do more. Through this I learn and know how yoga alone transforms mans habits in food, mood and behaviour changing him towards good health .

Q.- You have been initiated to yoga by Śri Krishnamacharya. What distinguishes him from other masters?

Yes! I was initiated to yoga by Śri T. Krishnamacharya. I revere him, admire him. He was very versatile, endowed with scholarship, mastery in Sanskrit, deep insight in esoteric matters and above all a "practical man", a "doer" in his time.

In one's life, one has only one mother and one father. Similarly, I have only one *guru.* I don't believe in having many *guru,* dozens at a time. I learnt at the feet of my *guru.* I did not have any other *guru* to influence or shape me. I only observed from other masters and *gurus* what they did not practise. I was not trained under anyone except my *guru* Śri T. Krishnamacharya. Śri T. Krishnamacharya was endowed with a fine and strong body. There was lustre in his eyes and lustre on his body. He had a very strong mind. I was too young and immature to study him and his capacities. Being young, I had no choice but to do what he said. The ethos round my *guru,* his learning with deep insight and experience marked him out from other masters and he was in a fine state of preservation and his marvellous practice of all facets of yoga was his strength. He preached what he practised and so I was paying my respects with reverence. The reverence and regard for him did not allow me to distinguish him from other masters.

Q.- What are the characteristics a yoga student should look for in a teacher?

A student of yoga has to look for a teacher with the qualities, which I mention below: as there are three types of teachers explained in our scriptures, students too are of three types. They are compared to a mother cat, mother monkey and fish. The mother cat catches her kittens with her mouth and carries them wherever she goes. The baby monkey sticks to the mother and lastly the fish having no lids, the eyeballs are ever alert and attentive.

Some teachers force their will on their students, like the mother cat, some are soft and make them dependent like the baby monkey holding on to the mother, while the last one is meant for the pupils to keep their eyes and ears wide open for their betterment so that they can follow the teacher. These are the three known methods.

Among these three methods, the last one is very important for the teachers, as it is they who should take the responsibility. The teacher should be filtering and purifying his *sādhanā* to guide the pupil to do, redo, learn, unlearn and relearn so that perfection is attained by both. This technical word "perfection" was known in early days as "divine" practice. This is what the pupils should see in a teacher and the teacher in the pupil. There should be a close interaction between the teacher and the taught.

I have not spoken as an academician on yoga and associated subjects. I have sweated and toiled in my gruelling practice unmindful of the pain and suffering. The taste of a yoga teacher is perhaps the hardest that one may come by. It can be both a blessing and a curse. It depends on whether one looks at it with a positive or negative outlook. The positive outlook will be rewarding. The negative attitude will be frustrating and stunt the growth of a teacher. As a teacher if one is not growing, it is self-defeating. We as teachers have to grow tremendously in stature and outlook if we are sincere teachers working from the bottom of our hearts and shaping the students' minds.

A yoga teacher has to try constantly to be his own critic. I have extensively deliberated and written on this in the article "Teachers and Teaching" in my book *The Tree of Yoga*[1]. The art of yoga is entirely subjective and practical. The yoga teacher has to be aware of the entire functioning of the human body, the varied pattern of behaviour of the people, how they interact and react to the teaching as he shapes them protectively. Not only has the yoga teacher to be strong and positive in his approach and affirm his position and authority, based on his deep practice, but also he has to be willing to be a learner all his life by bringing about reflective contemplation on what he himself is doing and changing. Besides, being Chaste and Calm which come out of integrity and character, he should be Candid, Clear, Clever, Confident, Challenging, Cautious, Constructive, Courageous, Conscientious, Committed and Critical. These attributes must go hand in hand with his caring and daring outlook, which brings cheer to the student boosting their morale. He has to learn to live with a spiritual bent of intellect, then alone can he help the student to go within the "interior" and get a peep into the super consciousness, the soul. Yoga is a spiritual science and philosophy and this requires a fine body and mind, as the rider must have a right attitude to cross over the obstacles on that eternal journey. This alone will help him to achieve clarity of intelligence and cleanliness of mind. Unless the teacher

[1] Published by Harper Collins, London. See also *Aṣṭadala Yogamālā*, vol. 3 – Sect. V – On Teaching.

feels in himself the supreme strength of peace, joy and delight through his *sādhanā*, how can he convince his students of the value of yoga? The teacher has to be a real student and at the same time become a real *guru* who removes darkness and leads one towards light. To quote Rabindranath Tagore, "Light has to be burnt not for the purpose of diminishing it, but giving light to the lamp". I can go on and on about the attributes that transform teacher into a *guru*. As a yoga teacher, I want all teachers to be truthful and teach what they clearly know and accept their limitations instead of trying with others' bodies, minds and souls as "guinea-pigs" while protecting themselves without working on their own selves. This must be the criterion to be a teacher so that the pristine purity of yoga is maintained. A student should look to a teacher who has all the qualities enumerated above with the capital "C".

Q.- What is the overall discipline a yoga practitioner should follow?

Body is the temple of the soul. As one likes to keep his house clean and tidy in order to dwell peacefully in it, so also each student should understand that the body is the dwelling place of the mind and the soul and hence it should be kept tidy.

If the body is afflicted, mind and consciousness too get afflicted. Secondly, for an average intellect, the body is the gross part of the soul. Hence, yoga begins with the body for the *sādhanā* to know and digest the known part of man fully before he wants to move to know the unknown. Yoga helps us to know the known well. When the known is known well, naturally the unknown surfaces and when the unknown surfaces, the known – the finite – merges in the unknown – the infinite. Both finite and infinite become one and both lose their identities. Hence, yoga begins with the cult of the body and then cultures the intelligence to come closer to the Self and then both the intelligence and Self unite as a simple unit without any identification. This is as good as *kaivalya* – Self-emancipation.

This fine question comprehends a very large area for the quest of yoga. We must begin yoga with the first step of the ladder of yoga. Yoga is often considered to be only physical. Understand that yoga is a physico-physiological, physio-psychological and psycho-spiritual subject. It is a science that liberates one's mind from the bondage of the body and leads it towards the soul. I have often said, "If a bird is kept in a cage, it has no movement". When the gates of the cage are opened, the bird flies freely. Similarly, the mind remains thereafter in "peace and beatitude" since it has been freed from the bondage.

I dwelt on this because often, as one practises, one is not aware of the "goal". The practitioners tend to bark up the wrong tree. Now, a very great responsibility rests on the pupils to remain forever genuine yoga practitioners. They have to acquire new experiences by constant practice, search within, and constantly compare as they evolve in their stature and insight. To be a dedicated *sādhaka*, one has to analyse, understand and put it into practice. As one uses a pin to remove a thorn, the *sādhaka* should use his intelligence as a needle to remove the weeds of the mind. The practitioner should be alert, attentive, dedicated, devoted and develop right means of application to tap the hidden knowledge of yoga.

Q.- Your advice to yoga teachers?

Dr. S. Radhakrishnan said, "Yoga is the art of opening the unconscious parts of our being which will enable us to feel the direct touch of cosmic consciousness." This is indeed very well said.

But for a yoga teacher it cannot come all that easily. He must realise that his body – the very shrine of the soul – has a dignity and intelligence of its own as much as the mind or even more than the mind. The body can be the springboard for animal incontinence or divine strength.

If the teacher cannot imbibe the understanding of yoga as a science and philosophy, his approach to teaching will be truncated. Yoga as a science conveys truth. It is a kind of vision, seeing, acting, showing and exhibiting, all combined. The component of yoga also conveys its artistic aspect, its precision and beauty. Art of any kind takes us to the domain of learning, involving imagination, transmission, practice, exhibition and finally revelation. One should know that in any art when accepted and practised, one becomes a fanatic, to some extent, but the yogi does not express it though he is.

The teacher should get involved in his subject whether he is asleep, dreamy or awake. He should get drenched in it. Then only the light of yoga draws by which he should keep himself ethically clean, intellectually clear and pure in consciousness.

The teacher has to strive for this. But this is not the end. The genuine teacher has to be imbued or soaked into the philosophy of yoga, which breathes the ethos. What if the yoga teacher does not breathe the ethos? That means the teacher is on the verge of losing the spiritual path of yoga.

The pole star of our yogic seeker, *sādhaka*, student or a teacher is "divinity". The teacher is not worth his salt if he is not deeply involved in *cintana* – objective thinking. He has to understand yoga objectively to have the frame of it. The next stage is *manana*, which means subjectively contemplating and indulging on ways to apply it.[1]

In the quality of teaching, one should have productive thoughts and experiences that are filtered for seasoned intelligence to develop. Then, to express by combing these two facets is the art of teaching.

[1] Cf. *Aṣṭadaḷa Yogamālā*, vol 2. p. 232.

Mathematically *cintaṇa* plus *manana* is equal to *dhyāna*. So the stage of "reflection" sets in. Reflections alone lead to perfection. The normal connotation of perfection is not acceptable to me. As the fruit fell on the ground, Newton postulated the law of gravity. For him, those were the moments of "divinity" and "creativity" that led to the progress of intellectual evolution. Similarly, *vicāra* or discrimination involves the churning of the thoughts, the thoughts over the pros and cons and the numerous permutations and combinations of things "to be". For me any teacher, however humble, who pines and works for divinity, that is perfection, and he is worth his weight in gold.

My advice to teachers is that they should involve themselves not only in the art of doing but involve themselves totally with the students who come and seek spiritual food. Having embraced toga both teacher and pupil should work together to find the hidden aspects of yoga as yoga becomes the God for both. The seeker and the seer become one and then both lose their identity.

PATAÑJALI'S PATH*

Christian: It must have been a very difficult task to translate the *Yoga Sūtras of Patañjali*. What was your approach to the book?

What can I say? The *Yoga Sūtra* (aphorisms) were by the Sage Patañjali, a top class intellectual of India. Hence, it is very difficult for common men like us to understand the terse subject as he compresses all his ideas in a few words. Unless and until one is intellectually matured and spiritually evolved, it is very difficult to go into his work to understand the depth of his feelings.

I read a lot of books on the *Yoga Sūtra*. They are all academic, like a dictionary, a working thesis on their meanings.

People who have undergone training on the subject have not done justice to this work. Therefore I, as a practitioner, thought that I should think of this book from the average man's intellectual level and how to approach it from the practical point of view for understanding the hidden depth of wisdom to reveal itself for you and me.

In the early days, being below the level of an average intellectual, I could not understand Patañjali's ways and views; but uninterrupted practice guided me in building up knowledge in understanding the essence of yoga as explained in the text and that encouraged me to write a commentary on his *Yoga Sūtra*. As an average individual, I think I have fulfilled the potential for a common man to take to yoga and conveniently follow the philosophy of Patañjali for what to practise and what to renounce. I have done this so that people like you follow, understand and realise Patañjali's way of emancipation and freedom, facing all the turmoils and upheavals of life. I have presented this work to show that it is possible to reach the ultimate without confusion, as often books do confuse. To a great extent I have tried to minimise the confusion and to eradicate doubts. If you take my book as a whole, I think it is more direct, more clear, more straightforward and point by point clears the feelings of the students who have a confused understanding on the *vedānta* of Patañjali. I feel that I have done some service to the practitioners

---

* Interview by Christian Pisano and Claus Grzesch. Recorded at Ramāmaṇi Iyengar Memorial Yoga Institute, Pune, January 1994. Published by *LOYA News*, U.K., issue 19, Winter 1995-96, and reprinted by *Victoria Yoga Centre Newsletter*, February 1996 and *Yoga and Health*, July 1999.

through my expressions, which are mainly based on my experience. I studied Patañjali's words and found the meeting points with my experience. These meeting points helped me to do the job from my heart compared to those who have worked from their heads. As it goes for reprints, I think and feel that people have appreciated my work.

Claus: Can you recommend your book for those who are not practitioners of yoga?

Even if the readers are not practitioners of yoga, this book will help them to understand the background of yogic philosophy. What I have done is that from that angle one who reads this book would be tempted to go in for a trial on the subject. This book is not only for general readers but also for the sensitive intellectuals. They have to think before they criticise my work. Just criticising is a different matter but honestly, sincerely, they have to think.

– *It's such a great help for the yoga practitioner.* –

It not only creates interest for yoga practitioners but also on those who may not be practising. By reading this book they need not just be the lovers of yoga, but may begin to live in yoga.

Christian: This book is like an inner journey for the reader. Could you please explain this inner journey?

My friend, all philosophies are a journey inwards towards the core of the being or the source of life. This text is a two-way path. You can go from the periphery towards the source or you can come from the source towards the periphery by interweaving the intelligence and challenging each and every sheath of the soul, the physical body, physiological body, mental body, intellectual body and the space between the body, mind and soul. When these sheaths of the soul, which are the elements of nature, communicate with each other, externally as well as internally, a new light dawns from that union *(saṁyoga)*.

When the consciousness learns that it is not dependent on the elements of nature, naturally one embraces the cause of that consciousness which is the core. Hence it is a challenge and a counter-challenge. A challenge from the external body to reach the inner body and a counter-challenge from the inner body to reach the outer body, so that these two incoming and outgoing currents interchange and interact. This action brings a new dimension to the practitioner to see a new light in the old practice.

Claus: *Aṣṭāṅga yoga* of Patañjali is divided into *bahiraṅga* and *antaraṅga sādhanā*. How does the practice of *āsana* and *prāṇāyāma* prepare the student for *antaraṅga sādhanā?*

Āsana and *prāṇāyāma* are meant to train the external *aṅga* (namely organs of action, senses of perception and mind) come close with the internal *aṅga*, the intelligence, the 'I' and the consciousness. Once the external *aṅga* reaches the internal *aṅga*, you start integrating the external senses and take both as a means to come in touch with the source – the Self. This is the beauty of yoga. I hope you understand what I mean. When we speak on philosophy we cannot talk on abstract lines. As you and I are practitioners; we have to begin from the base – the body, which acts as a foundation. For us the base is what we can see, what we can feel. Through this feeling and movements, we interpenetrate from the skin towards the flesh, from the flesh towards the circulation, from the circulation towards the sense of vibration or sense of contact or touch, where you get the infrastructure of the elements. These infrastructures are called the *tanmātrā*[1] or the qualitative characteristics hidden in these elements of nature known as vibration, touch, shape, liquidity and solidity. If you can reach these aspects of the elements that can only be felt by *āsana* and *prāṇāyāma*, you have understood nature. As you understand nature, then you channel that energy for the enlightenment of your life, to go and have the sight of the soul. So *āsana* and *prāṇāyāma* constitute the bridge to cross over from the physical body to the spiritual body.

Yama, niyama, āsana and *prāṇāyāma* are *bahiraṅga sādhanā*, the four petals of yoga to channel the outer organs to move inwards towards the internal structure of the soul. *Pratyāhāra* is the bridge that unifies *bahiraṅga* and *antaraṅga*, then to have the taste of *antarātmā* through *dhāraṇā, dhyāna* and *samādhi*, as they are the subtlest aspects of yoga. The first four are within the mind, the fifth is the threshold and the last three are beyond the mind. The mind being the bridge between the physical and spiritual bodies, the moment you cross over, naturally the mind takes you to the understanding of the other side, the other bank of the body that is *antaraṅga*, which engulfs *buddhi* and *ahaṁkāra*. When the word *bahiraṅga* is used, it means that you have to use external sheaths to understand the inner sheaths of our existence. Without them it is impossible to learn.

Patañjali's *Yoga Sūtra* are not meant only for the elite but for the average intellect as well as the undeveloped one. This is the wholeness of Patañjali. In order to uplift a common, or an undeveloped, or an average person, he shows them how to understand what is the visible body from *yama* to *pratyāhāra*, and what is the invisible body when he speaks of *dhāraṇā*,

---

[1] See *Aṣṭadala Yogamālā*, vol. 2, "Practice of *Prāṇāyāma*" and "From *Moha* to *Mokṣa*"

dhyāna and *samādhi*. From here, he directly makes us touch the core. This division is for the sake of understanding but one has to take it as a whole. You have to go from the external towards the internal or you can come from the internal to the external with unison of harmony, balance and rhythm between the physical body, physiological body, mental body and spiritual body. This earning of rhythm and balance between body, mind and soul is taught by Patañjali.

Some may reach the highest state like Ramana Maharshi; but we are neither Ramana nor Jesus Christ. We are just ordinary human beings gripped in the turmoils of the world. I feel that Patañjali is the only person who shows the way and the means, without confusing us, to evolve from our present position to reach the highest and subtlest intellectual growth. Through *yama* and *niyama* he begins from the visible organs *(karmendriya)* of the body. *Yama* helps in controlling the organs of action – *karmendriya*, and *niyama* in controlling the senses of perception – *jñānendriya*. When the organs of action and senses of perception are controlled, disciplined and fused, naturally you get access to the inner body, or the physiological body. This body is filled with the circulatory and nervous systems. In order to bring concord between these systems, the *āsana* are taught so that they are kept free from impurities. The organs of action and senses of perception are the gates to see and act in the outer world. When the control on them is achieved, they make the practitioner to look and see inwards to understand the flow of circulation, the flow of the nerves and their usage. Through *prāṇāyāma* the practitioner develops the energy called *śakti*. *Śakti* is power. *Śakti* is vital power. The moment *śakti* is under control, *puruṣa* also is under control. Wherever there is power there is attention: where there is attention there is energy. They are like twins. By this realisation the practitioner understands the flow of energy and the ways to control the flow of energy through *prāṇāyāma* wherein the senses are naturally made to become quiet. When they become quiet, the mind is free from the outgoing world as if you are in a desert. It is a peaceful desert wherein you reach a desert without the mind.

Claus: Is that *dhāraṇā*, *dhyāna* and *samādhi*?

No, I don't say that. I said desert. This means a vast place of emptiness, Sufis and others have talked about the emptiness of the mind. You reach the emptiness of the mind because the mind – which is always active with the senses of perception and the organs of action – is automatically released from this contact. Then it becomes empty, in a peaceful desert. I do not think it is the end. From here on one has to move positively towards *dhāraṇā*, *dhyāna* and *samādhi* so that he moves towards the fullness of consciousness: this is how yoga begins from the base towards the zenith. For those who are at the zenith, it is essential to maintain that state without losing their practice. Those who have reached that state and continue practising, the final impressions *(saṁskāra)*, give a fresh birth so as to be born geniuses in the next life. They are geniuses because they have maintained virtuousness in their *sādhanā* in their previous lives and when they get new life they are considered to be a genius. We call it *saṁskāra*: latent, hidden *karma* that are brought to fruitfulness in this life. They can be counted as one in a century. Hence, Patañjali wrote the *Yoga Sūtra* not only for them but for the whole of humanity. He has touched the subject not only for those who come once in two or three centuries, but also for the common man by using the terminologies, *bahiraṅga* to *antaraṅga*, and from *antaraṅga* to *bahiraṅga* to reach the *antarātmā* – the soul.

Christian: Could you explain the *sūtra, vitarkabādhane pratipakṣabhāvanam?*

Bādhana means pain or *kleśa*. Pain, suffering, greed, obstruction, obstacles are not only *kleśa* but *vṛtti* also. Similarly *bhāvana* means conception, perception, reflection, contemplation and so forth. Afflictions *(bādhana)* and *bhāvana (vṛtti)* are terms that express bad feelings or good feelings. Transforming the afflictive feelings *(bādhana)* into good feelings is *bhāvana*. The word *pratipakṣa* conveys analysing the pain, greed and sorrow, which is simply the counter study of that which is free from pain, greed or sorrow. Suppose you are doing *Utthita Trikoṇāsana*, there is a pain on the right side and you change from right to left and you don't get pain on the left side. This feeling of pain of one side and feeling of non-pain on the other side, has to be studied and analysed by yourself. Study the feelings of pressure and pain on one side and serenity, calmness and harmony on the other. What wrong am I doing between the right and left side? Study the pain and non-pain, the action and the counter-action in the necessary way.

Many give the academic meaning that if you are violent, think of non-violence. When you are violent, can you think of non-violence? You may think of non-violence afterwards. Similarly, you steal something and at the time of stealing can you think of the opposite? As such it is easy to say think of the opposite, but being a student of yoga, I analyse *bādhana* and *bhāvana*. *Bādhana* means pain, *bhāvana* means the feel, when I am feeling good on one side and bad on the other side. I have to understand why it is paining on one side and not on the other side. I have to go back to re-study how am I doing. This way, I compare the non-painful positioning of the body in an *āsana* to the other side, where it is paining. I watch the mistakes I am committing, and what is the sensation I am getting. Then I correlate the feeling of goodness to the side that is giving grief. By re-adjusting I break that obstacle. I take this as a guide to study on either side to find out the feelings and the obstacles. If there is grief, then like me, you should know from the *pratipakṣa* of the grief that you are doing wrong on that side. This is why *haṭha yoga* speaks of right and left which is nothing but *pakṣa* and *pratipakṣa* (right and left).

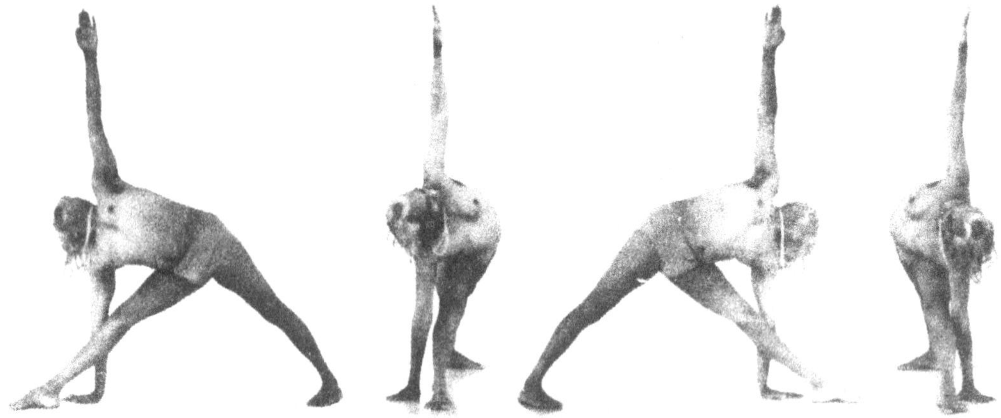

Plate n. 3 – *Utthita Trikoṇāsana* – right side / left side

Think on *pakṣa* and *pratipakṣa*. If the right side is *pakṣa* (current flowing according to motion), and left side is *pratipakṣa* (making the current to flow in the opposite direction), this rectifies the obstacles which come in the way. When you come to the conclusion that the feelings are even on both sides, then know that that is the effect of the *āsana* and that is the effect of *prāṇāyāma*. If you can inhale from the right side well and not on the left, you have to question why you cannot inhale from the left well. If I am exhaling well from the left and not from the right, then I have to question how my inner membranes are blocking on the side where I cannot inhale or exhale. Find out on either side, how the membranes are behaving, what is the quality of the membranes, what is the textural quality of the skin of the fingers, the positioning of the fingers, the placement of the fingers, the spacing of the fingers, the spacing between the membranes and the fingers observing the passage of the breath and learn to adjust them to find the right means. The passages on the right and the left may not be the same. You may keep the fingers mechanically on the same side, which is not correct. You have to search where the breath is in contact inside the nostrils and whether it is flowing roughly or smoothly, interruptedly or otherwise. Observing all these intricate points learn to adjust and change the fingers to trace the exact spot from where the sense of the breath is felt. This is how I read *pakṣa* and *pratipakṣa*. To understand their meaning, you have to learn the skill of re-adjustment.

- So unless there is balance between right and left, it is not yoga. -

That is what the *Haṭhayoga Pradīpikā* says. The energy of *iḍā* moves on the left, and the energy of *piṅgalā* moves on the right and they intermingle in between feeding each other. It is clearly said that they crisscross at each *cakra* and supply energy to each other for equal distribution.

Here the *pakṣa* and *pratipakṣa bhāvana* and *bādhana* convey identically the same meaning but on a mental level. There it is spoken of on a bio-energy level because *cakra* and *nāḍī* are not on the physical level, nor on a physiological level. Today everybody compares the *cakra* to the glands, the plexus and all, but they are beyond them. Actually *cakra* are spoken of on a spiritual level, but here it is a mental action.

Patañjali explains *pakṣa* and *pratipakṣa* not only on the mental level but also on the emotional level. If you have mental obstruction on one side and not on the other while practising yoga, then how do you work? You remove that mental obstruction that is obstructing on the other side so that the flow of energy as well as the movement of the mind is smooth and equal to that of the non-obstructing side. This is the essence of this *sūtra*.

Christian: What about *sthira sukham āsanam*?

Patañjali is very clear. When he speaks of *sthira sukham āsanam* (*Y.S.*, II.46), to understand it you have to read the next *sūtra*, *prayatna śaithilya ananta samāpattibhyām* (*Y.S.*, II.47). He speaks in three *sūtra* of the four dimensions of an *āsana*, which we are not able to understand due to the calibre of his intelligence and the calibre of his spiritual capabilities.

Sthira and *sukha* means stable and comfortable. Suppose you are sitting in *Padmāsana* for some time. What happens to your leg after some time? Stability goes. You feel pain and discomfort. The moment discomfort sets in, what happens to that *sthiratā* and *sukhatā*? I hope you get the correct meaning of the *sūtra* now. Whether you stay in an *āsana* for one minute or for hours, you should be thorough in both comfort and in stability and this is the meaning of the third *sūtra* on *āsana*, *tataḥ dvandvāḥ anabhighātaḥ* (*Y.S.*, II.48). *Dvandva* means dualities. What are these dualities? Think. Do not go just with the academic translation. *Sthira* means stability: the stability may become unstable. You may be doing first class *Śīrṣāsana* for one minute; after one minute what happens? You re-adjust. Then where is the stability? It means, according to the *sūtra*, stability may become unstable, comfort may become discomfort. Your effort may fade. The moment effort fades you lose the quality; when you lose the quality you have to exert again. These three are the three dimensions: *sthira*, *sukha* and *prayatna*: *sthira* has the opposite *asthira*, *sukha* has the opposite *duḥkha*, opposite of *prayatna* is *śaithilya*. So, one who practises *āsana* should cross these three aspects to go to the fourth dimension where all dualities in work and thought culminate. This is the meaning of the mastery of the *āsana*.

Actually *sthira sukham āsanam* is experienced only when the *sādhaka* loses the differences between body, mind and self. Till then *sthira* and *sukha* of an *āsana* remain a fantasy.

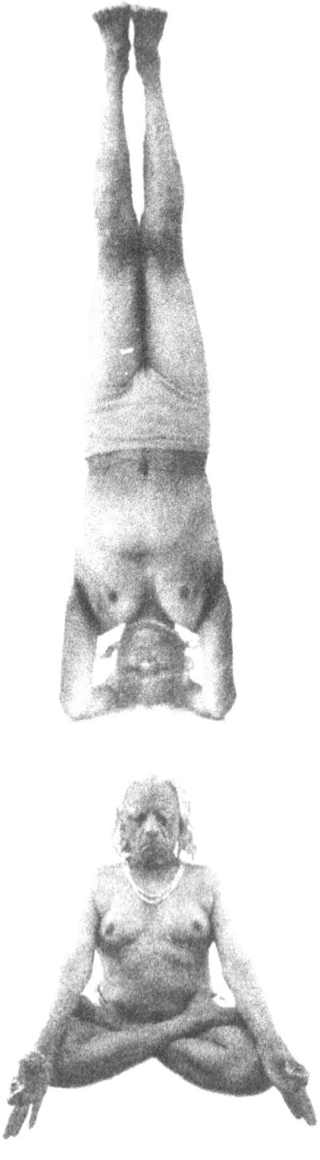

Plate n. 4 - *Padmāsana* and *Sālamba Śīrṣāsana*

Similarly it is interesting to know that Patañjali explains *prāṇāyāma* in three *sūtra*. 1) *Tasmin sati śvāsa praśvāsayoḥ gativicchedaḥ prāṇāyāmaḥ* (II.49). 2) *Bāhya ābhyantara stambha vṛttiḥ deśa kāla saṁkhyābhiḥ paridṛṣṭaḥ dīrgha sūkṣmaḥ* (II.50). And 3) *Bāhya ābhyantara viṣaya ākṣepī caturthaḥ* (II.51). Why did he use the word *caturthaḥ*, means the fourth type? There are only three *sūtra* on *prāṇāyāma*. Is this not puzzling us? In *āsana krama* (*āsana* sequence) he says the difference between body, mind and Self fades away, *tataḥ dvandvāḥ anabhighātaḥ* (II.48). People say that the dualities such as honour - dishonour, heat - cold, *sukha* - *duḥkha* and so on fade. They are objectively explained to us. For me the meaning is all-subjective as body, mind and self are subjective dualities. That is, stable consciousness may become unstable, stable physical posture may become an unstable physical posture, effort may expand, reduce, extend, and distend. That's why he gives the fourth dimension on *āsana*. When these dualities are removed, he considers then that is the mastery of *āsana*. Here, in *prāṇāyāma*, how do you count? Here the third *sūtra* speaks of the fourth type: Then, which is the third one? The two *sūtra* on *prāṇāyāma*, are like the first two on *āsana*. The first *sūtra* speaks of the rhythmic channelling of the in-breath and the out-breath, which he defines as *prāṇāyāma*. The second *sūtra* is the most complex and many people misread it: *bāhya ābhyantara stambha vṛttiḥ deśa kāla saṁkhyābhiḥ paridṛṣṭaḥ dīrgha sūkṣmaḥ* (II.50) - it means inhalation-retention and exhalation-retention. In the previous *sūtra* he speaks only on the regulation of inhalation and exhalation. The second *sūtra* is a compound *sūtra*. In my understanding, this *sūtra* has different dimensions. He speaks of the first dimension as in-breath, out-breath and retention. In the second dimension he explains *deśa*, *kāla* and *saṁkhyā* in *prāṇāyāma*. *Deśa* is the body, *kāla* is time and *saṁkhyā* is precision, while the third part or dimension is *dīrgha* (expansion) and *sūkṣmaḥ* (subtleness) (II.50).

You can take a deep inhalation *(showed by example of taking a forceful inhalation).* Here he shows the depth but not the subtleness or *sūkṣma.* For me *prāṇāyāma* is not only deep but also subtle. This subtleness of drawing in and releasing is the third dimension. Normally, you are carried away by *sthūla prāṇāyāma,* where you inhale too long, making it gross by a heavy sound. Patañjali says that it should not only be long, but should be subtle. Everybody takes gross deep breaths *(sthūla prāṇāyāma).* Patañjali wants us to move from *sthūla* to *sūkṣma.* Your length of inhalation, length of exhalation or length of retention may be unknowingly gross in your practice. He wants this gross practice to be converted into subtle practice. This is the third dimension of *prāṇāyāma.* He says the fourth dimension is where neither the mind nor the energy work. Both energy and mind become silent. That's the highest type of *prāṇāyāma* according to Patañjali.

Here, the technique of *prāṇāyāma* ends with the awareness of the self. At the end of the book he completes, "It's all in the power of the soul, beyond that I can't tell you – *citiśaktiḥ iti"* (IV.34) After *citiśakti,* what is next? Though this is puzzling, he has guided before that the end is *Īśvarapraṇidhāna,* or total surrender to God as the ultimate. No doubt, he ends the book with the quality of the seer. After explaining the quality of the seer, he wants one to move from Self-realisation towards God-realisation, though he doesn't touch God-realisation at the end of the book. How difficult it is to understand this great man! No doubt the book is complete, but as it ends by explaining the quality of the seer, it may give a wrong reading that the sight of the soul is the end. But one should carefully re-read, which explains that *ātma-darśana* is the threshold for *Īśvara darśana.* As he says after *prāṇāyāma,* the mind is fit for meditation;[1] here too you have to understand that when the seer is known, the Self is fit to surrender to God. As this development has to come from each *sādhaka,* he ends the book with *ātma-sākṣātkāra.*

Many think that Patañjali speaks of monism or of qualified monism. Remember, these ideas came later. The translations and the commentaries have been done according to the background of philosophical thoughts of Shankaracharya and Rāmānujācārya. He only ends it with *citiśaktiḥ iti* – quality of the Seer. Then why did he speak of surrendering to God in the beginning? He left it there, knowing very well that when you know the quality of the Seer, the next step is *Īśvara praṇidhāna.* Because there is no *ahaṁkāra* at that moment one automatically surrenders to the Supreme in a true *bhakti* form. Thus he implicitly ends the *Yoga Sūtra* with the thought of *bhakti.*

Citta vṛtti nirodhaḥ is said to be yoga. What is *citta vṛtti?* Everybody says, waves of thoughts. Stop the waves of thoughts and that is yoga. Consciousness is caught up not only with waves of thoughts but also with afflictions. So afflictions and movement of thoughts are all

---

[1] *Dhāraṇāsu ca yogyatā manasaḥ,* (*Y.S.,* II.53), the mind becomes fit for concentration.

part of *citta vṛtti.* When you are free from afflictions, when you are free from waves, and not wandering, then where is *vṛtti?* There is no movement at all. This is the fourth dimension. When there is no movement of the flow of energy, no flow of mind, no afflictions and no wandering in the mind, where is *śakti* and where is consciousness? Both dissolve. The seer surfaces who is untouched by thoughts – *vṛtti,* untouched by afflictions – *kleśa.* He leaves it to us to decide what we have to do next. It dawns on the seer that it is the time to surrender. He has the character of God who is free from all types of afflictions. The ripe time for the seer to surrender to God dawns. That is how I conclude the text, though he does not conclude explicitly this way.

Claus: Why does he not conclude?

This is not for me to comment on, as I do not know what he had in mind. When he explained the quality of the Seer probably he did not want to explain from the state of consciousness. As he has taken one beyond the state of consciousness, how can he take one back to *citta?* He wanted one to have experienced the *citi (ātman)* and its *śakti* (power). That might have made him silent and that is why he did not express it. There lies the beauty of his greatness as an aphorist. He did not want to bring that state to the verbal level. Living is not on a verbal level. Living is a factual, experiencing state.

The *ātman* is part and parcel of God. The *ātman* is a parcel of the Universal Spirit. The Universal Spirit is here and there and between you and me. I don't know how many individual spirits there are without bodies. So these are all bodies of God. As we have the body of the soul, all of us put together form the body of God. When you have reached the free state, you cannot become God, but you become godly. Though you are equal, you cannot destroy, you cannot create, that power is God's. Therefore Self-realisation has to end in surrendering one's Self to God.

Many people may refute me; it does not matter because when somebody has to refute, I also say that his knowledge has to be thoroughly ripe before he comes to any conclusion. I am living in it. Yoga is not an objective science or art for me. Every cell is ringing with the bell of yoga in me. I am subjective, but when you put me a question, I have to explain objectively. Yoga is my subject and I am yoga. Yoga is me, so it is in me. It does not speak. I live in yoga; each moment of me is yoga. See how difficult it is for me to explain! That is why I struggle. Someone mayask, "Why do you write?" I write in order to make you also tread that path without fear.

Christian: You say that you want to give your students the taste of the present life in your lessons. As you shout at them to straighten their legs, they cannot be wondering what is for dinner or whether they will be promoted or demoted at work.

It is correct. My shout brings instant alertness in the students. What I have said is a fact. When I am teaching in classes, as you say, I shout for two hours or three hours or five hours, but can anybody know what time it is at that moment? Don't you feel that you are living moment to moment? Is this feeling of not knowing the time at that moment spiritual or not?

– *Yes! Spiritual.* –

At that time, you are free from the dependence of past and future. So are you not divine at that entire moment?

– *Yes! Divine.* –

At other times one may not be divine. Even those who work with me, do I not treat them as divine for such a long time with this hard work? So that is the quality I impart in yoga. I make it possible for you to live in that moment which is divine and pure, where the mind is not allowed to play with the past or the future. When I am teaching, does memory, which is dependent on the past and the future work, or does intellect work?

– *Intellect works.* –

That is right. The moment you work with memory, I lose my temper shouting at you. "Why do you do it that way? Why do you want to go to your old thoughts?" This shouting is to keep your intelligence ever fresh. That's what it brings. As I have experienced, I want everybody to experience the same. So I try to take you towards the conquest of time. While I am teaching, there is no known time. So you have conquered time. Your mind is not on the past or the future, and it is neither in the present, you don't know what present is at that moment. So I bring divinity. I have to express that divinity through the vehicle of the body to reach the soul. Not speaking or keeping quiet does not make one divine. Just keeping quiet may be a ploy. I do not want to do so. With my shouts I make you be with yourself moment to moment.

Honesty, integrity and oneness between the pupil and the master, is the only pendulum to live actively in the state of divinity doing one's day-to-day jobs. That is my experience and that is what I give to others. Those who have this type of interpenetration experience what I experience. Those who just practise for the sake of practising, for them it is just a "keep-fit-exercise" programme. If such people treat *āsana* as an exercise, it ends as an exercise. Treat *āsana* as a posture where you compose and recompose the posture to feel the sensation of totality, of oneness and precision where all further recomposing comes to an end. Then you experience that it is not the body that did the *āsana*, it is the very core, which appears in the extremities of your body. That brings oneness between you and the *āsana* and that is divinity.

Claus: What is your final message?

I trained myself only to show where *āsana* leads to. No doubt, when I began I practised from the external level. My teacher did not give me any philosophical background but only the presentation of *āsana*. It took me several years to purge myself, purge my body and my intelligence. I read books, which confused me a great deal. Fortunately I did not stop my practice. That is God's grace on me. I made up my mind to write the book when I achieved maturity on these two aspects of yoga, namely *āsana* and *prāṇāyāma*. I read the *Yoga Sūtra*, keeping my experience and studying his words to find out where they meet. It helped me to realise that my practice is almost closer to the *sūtra* of Patañjali. My practice must have become ripe to reach that level.

In the beginning I used to read and close the book saying it was not for me as it was hard to grasp and understand. Through years of *sādhanā*, it became possible for me to bring out the most difficult *sūtra* for all to read and understand with ease. Of course if you read with attention new ideas may strike. I have tried my best to make the reader understand the philosophy even sitting in the drawing room, so that he gets ignited to make an effort to feel what he reads. From this angle I think I have done a service to the students of yoga to learn from the base to go towards the zenith of yoga. I started step by step from the base and I can say that students who are interested in the philosophy of yoga cannot get confused as I have minimised the doubts to a great extent and created enthusiasm for them to make a beginning. Probably it is the only practical book on the *Yoga Sūtra*. I may not know the reactions; but those who are interested, and study *Light on the Yoga Sūtras of Patañjali*, along with *Light on Yoga, Light on Prāṇāyāma, Tree of Yoga, The 70 Glorious Years of Yogachārya B.K.S. Iyengar*, they will reach the goal faster than me. I consider with humility that in presenting this most terse philosophy in a simple language I have served the average intellectuals to understand the background of life and the utility of yoga for themselves.

I have spoken that by the practice of various *āsana* how the five elements and the five qualities of the elements are controlled, creating rhythm and balance in the body. When one conquers the elements of nature, then what is left? Patañjali ends the text by saying that everything merges in the One, that is the seer. This is all I can explain to you and now you have to find out yourself where it leads you from the state you are.

HOW YOGA CREATES JOY IN LIFE*

Q.- How did you take to yogic practice and then to teach yoga?

I was born in 1918 at Bellur during the world influenza epidemic. I was constantly weak and in bad health, and I could not even stand upright or walk. Then I caught tuberculosis. A parasitic life at that young age of fourteen disturbed me. As no one could care for me, I was on the verge of committing suicide.

One day, my brother-in-law, a master of yoga, asked me to visit Mysore and learn some *yogāsana* under his direction. He taught me just a few simple *āsana*. As my body was poker stiff, I could hardly bend forward or backward. Though I did not feel any improvement in my health, I kept on and on and a few years later, I felt that I could at least live.

In 1936 my *gurujī* took me as baggage carrier on his tours and to look after his comforts. While other pupils accompanied him to give demonstrations, I was taken as a servant. One day he asked me to present a few simple *āsana*. As I began presenting, the womenfolk got interested and expressed their desire to my *gurujī* to learn *āsana* only from me, being the youngest of the group.

Especially in 30's and 40's, women in India were very reserved and shy. The pupils of my *gurujī* were adults. I being young in age, he asked me to take the classes for ladies as per their desire. Though I did not know much of yoga or the art of teaching, I took this chance to teach as God sent. Fortunately, in 1937 I was invited to teach in Pune for six months. I was thin, with a narrow chest, and I had to teach pupils broader and elder than me. It was really a great challenge for me and I accepted it. As I could not do the *āsana* correctly, I began working ten hours a day. This is how yoga entered into my blood. Then destiny made me take to yoga and teach as well.

---

* Interview by Dominique Umbert, published in *Terre du Ciel*, n. 27 – December 94 – January 95.

Q.- What is the best way to learn the postures or *āsana* correctly?

When we are doing an *āsana*, it is possible to feel a certain discomfort due to our incorrect habits in our sitting or standing positions. At the start, we have to learn to bear with the *āsana*, and make an effort to observe and understand each *āsana*. You have to question, "Why does it hurt at one place, why doesn't it hurt at other places, in one or the other movement? What should we do with this particular painful part of our body? How can we make the pain go away? Why do we feel such pressures? Why does one side hurt? How do the muscles function on one side and how do they react on the other?"

I began to put such questions to myself to analyse. This way self-inquiry began in me. Similarly, I like you to analyse in this same way, repeatedly so that your analysis and experimentation go together. In yoga practice, these two approaches are necessary in order to comprehend. This comprehension should be a guideline for the next day's practice. Once again think "Am I repeating the *āsana* the old way, or am I re-posing for a finer feeling? Am I doing the *āsana* with habitual repetition or am I getting new thoughts and ideas for a progressive experience?" Analysis in action is a guide that proceeds with trial and error.

Secondly, when you are doing a yogic *āsana*, can you find the delicate balance that exists between the position of its finest stretch, and then think of going beyond your present state of the *sādhanā*?. At this point tension is created due to further effort.

If the tension gives a bad taste, you have to re-think. For example, when you stretch one part of the body to get the optimum stretch, you have to observe how at the same time giving the same attention to the other parts of the body. This upsets the rhythm and makes the body tremble. Suppose you are doing *Sālamba Śīrṣāsana*,[1] you stretch your legs to get a good position but at the same time you may let loose your neck muscles. This non-attention in the neck muscles or shoulders brings fear of falling and you sway from side to side. The strong muscles help to control the balance but the weak muscles cannot. In this *āsana* you must keep the stretch from the ground to the top without letting any part to go loose. When you stretch your legs, you must at once alert your arms, trunk, chest, back and so on and so forth, and vice versa. "I am stretching my legs, let me not allow the shoulders to drop or the mind to go blank!" That is awareness in attention. You might have the attention but it remains at one place or in one area. This is how one fails in getting stability. Learn to spread your awareness evenly all over while doing the *āsana*, that is how you understand the correctness of the *āsana*.

You need to have constant awareness on your attentiveness. When you are not consciously attentive, your attention becomes partial and you don't know whether you are doing the *āsana* correctly or not.

---

[1] See plate n. 4.

While trying to improve the *āsana*, you lose the benefit of what you are doing when you give too much attention to one part of your body. If you are not aware of that, you are neither reflecting nor meditating in the *āsana*: you do the *āsana* but you don't reflect on it. You want to do the utmost, you concentrate to do, but you do in a lop-sided way. You do your best only on that area where you concentrate. It is concentration and not meditation. If you attend and extend the span of concentration from the stretched part to all the parts of the body without neglecting any part, then it becomes meditation. Let me put it in another way, if you spread the light of your attention from one side of your body to the other, in such a way that it reaches both the sides evenly and lights the whole body, then you do not lose either the internal action, nor the external expression of the *āsana*. This process teaches you meditation. Concentration is on a single point; meditation is on all points without deviation. This is the secret of meditation.

Being consciously aware of your entire existence, act as a witness. Seek to explore further the movements in the body. Trace where and when the attention is, or is not. Do not be greedy or possessive, remaining attentive on one part is like possession. Keep the mind open to observe each part. See what you can learn and see what's happening to the body, circulation, mind and intelligence together, and spread the awareness absolutely in the body. The water running over the ground spreads evenly finding its level. Similarly, let the awareness spread evenly everywhere, then it becomes meditation. Connect the body's energy with the energy of the intelligence and vice versa in such a way that the comprehension emerges. Feel the link between the consciousness and the flow of energy with the movements of the body.

Q.- What do you mean by alignment?

If I have to do *Tāḍāsana*, just standing straight, it often happens that one leg is strong, attentive, steady and straight whereas the other leg remains inattentive. One can feel that one leg is in a non-violent state and the other is in a violent state. Hence, it becomes necessary to balance the two legs evenly so that one will not be able to differentiate between violence and non-violence. Secondly, if you keep the legs unevenly, the mind remains unstable. Establish alignment in the body; align the muscles, joints and intelligence, energy and attention. The intelligence is placed in such a way that there is no tension between the motor nerves and the sensory nerves. Create room between these two nerve centres to bring perfect alignment in body, mind and soul. This alignment in body, mind and soul leads to enlightenment.

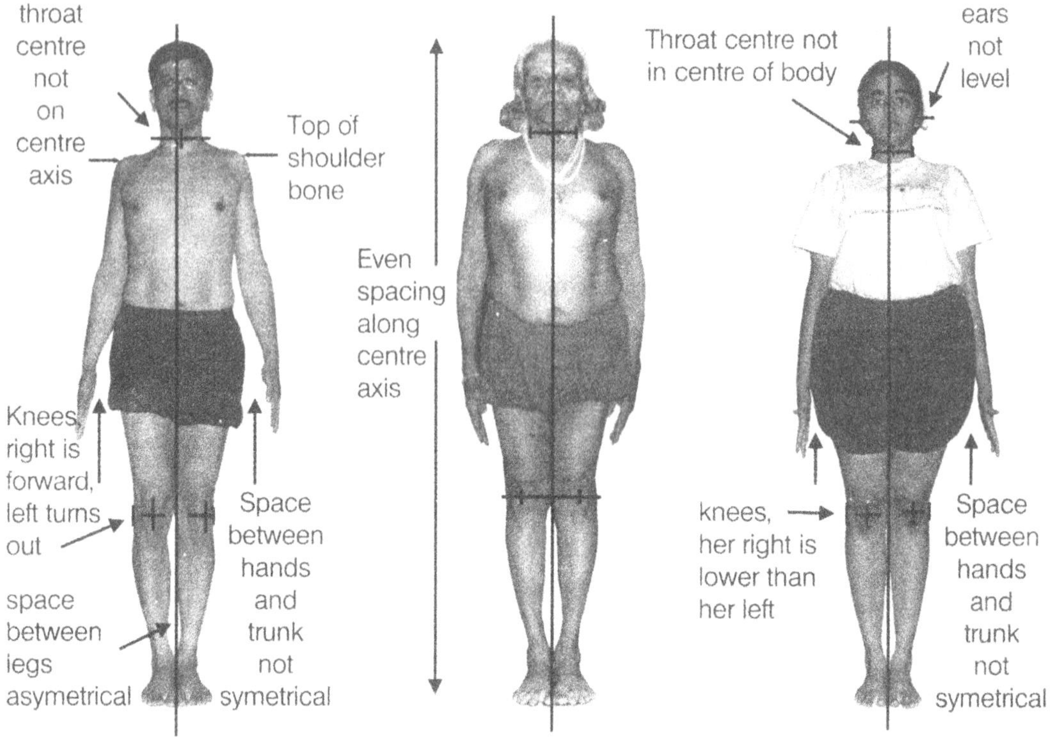

Plate n. 5 – *Tāḍāsana* – stable/non-violent & unstable/violent

Awareness is like a flame. Awareness is the first principle that creates action and movement. It's like a button: when you press it, it works; if it is not pressed it remains in the dormant state. Now you are listening to me, your awareness is in your head, is it in your big toe?

- No, it is not there. -

It was inattentive and I have woken it. When I said "big toe", it began to vibrate.

- Yes. -

The vibration became conscious, which means that consciousness listens when energy reaches these places. Energy and consciousness cannot be separated. These are two sides of a coin. That is how we work in *āsana*. Through the movement of energy we learn the movement of awareness. Awareness is cosmic intelligence. The moment I spoke of the toe, your intelligence sprouted there and it woke you up. Try to keep this awareness awake the whole day through. The practice of *āsana* helps to keep this awareness awake.

Q.- You emphasise the continual improvement of *āsana*.

I emphasise the continual improvement of *āsana*. The body is the means through which we perceive and act. Therefore, a healthy, firm body is an incomparable basis for a yogic *sādhanā*. The *āsana* reinforce and purify each fibre, each cell of the body. In this sense, the effect of *āsana* is infinite.

I define *āsana* as firmness of body, attention and calmness of intelligence, delight in the heart. Whatever *āsana* one is trying, it ought to be done in this spirit. In *āsana*, when body, mind and soul are balanced with harmony, we feel nourished and enlightened.

To be more precise, the practice of *āsana* gives us the understanding of the very path of yoga, preparing us at every level to reach the goal. The body, senses, mind, intelligence, consciousness and conscience seem to be far from us or at a loose end. The practice of *āsana* brings us closer to all these aspects of ours.

Yoga is a discipline, which sweeps away dualities and divisions. It works with the structure of the body, with proper functioning of the muscles, with perfect blood circulation. It brings an equal distribution of vital energy and channels the mind to integrate the body with the breath, the breath with the mind and the mind with the soul.

Q.- To sum up, yoga has the function of both uniting and purifying.

Yes, first it begins in purifying the body: each joint must be cleansed within. We use soap to remove dirt from a garment: when we want to wash the body, we take a bath. Yoga is an inner bath. Blood gives us a bath inside the body. To do this, the blood has to circulate extremely well, and with a constant, even power or force. Think of a waterfall, how much energy it generates. By the practice of yoga, we have to generate energy in our blood to nourish every part. Then the cells sense comfort and freedom, and send the message: "I am happy". It's not me thinking "I feel relaxed", it's the body's knowledge that tells this. I want each part of my body: cells, joints, and muscles to tell this.

So purify the body and purge the intelligence. It is not a question of purifying the mind but of purging the intelligence of its pride.

The self cannot express itself, it needs an instrument. I use my body as a painter uses his canvas, a musician his instrument, a singer his voice. Our body must go at the speed of our selves. Then, there is no division, no deviation. We use *āsana* and *prāṇāyāma* to feel the Being. This internal vibration and serenity is only felt through the body expression. If the body is the mirror of the mind, the *āsana* reflects back this depth of clarity, awareness and intelligence.

Q.- How can we practise yoga in our daily lives?

Without consciously cultivating discipline, one cannot expect to keep up the liveliness, intelligence and maturity for progression towards the ultimate goal. We can reach infinity by using the finite means, which are at our disposal and utility. Certainly even in irregular practice some effects would be there, but it does not develop the sensitive quality of intelligence and awareness. Therefore, it is preferable to work judiciously and regularly each day. Once we have integrated a canvas of regular practice into the structure of our daily life for the divine grace to play on its own, continue to work. When the grace comes, it comes. If it doesn't come today, it may come twenty years later. Even if it never comes, at least one will have good health and happiness. If health and happiness come, that's a divine grace in itself!

Moderation in life is equally essential. That is why yoga teaches a code of conduct which each one of us should develop. Spiritual life is a grace of God, but to stick to ethics is our duty, it is a part of our responsibility. We are children of God. When we follow certain principles in life, God takes care of us all the time and makes the way easier.

Most of the time our mind is on the surface. When I practise *āsana* and *prāṇāyāma,* I make up my mind to penetrate deep inside. Unless we have a moral discipline, physical well-being and an undisturbed smooth flow of energy, we cannot proceed in spiritual life. Good bodily health, a clear mind and a clean heart constitute the foundation, which brings us automatically to think of the higher eternal aspects of life.

There is an important balance to find between the philosophical ideas and practical living. We should study our daily lives in the background of philosophy so that life with its difficulties, sorrows and joys does not block us towards higher thinking. Can we remain faithful to our own development and to our own evolution keeping our individual path, living successfully in society, with a happy married life, loving our partner with all our heart? Religious life does not consist of retiring from ordinary living: on the contrary, we ought to find the harmony, which is in the heart of our lives. The circumstances of our lives are not there for our destruction but for our evolution.

All these years, despite all my family obligations, I never stopped practising yoga. I express my sense of gratitude to my family members and friends who brought me to this level. My regular practice of *āsana* raised me to the level at which I find myself today. Yogic discipline threw out the sub-human level of my childhood mind and made me a conscientious man. Yoga helped me to surmount all the obstacles of my life that came in my way, whether it was physical, mental or spiritual. Today I rejoice in life and taste the yogic nectar.

A SUBJECT OF THE HEART*

Q.- You have students throughout the world spreading your teachings. How do you envisage the *guru-śiṣya* relationship under these conditions, where meetings with you are rare?

You know, this question is very simple, straightforward and clear, yet there is, in between the lines, something else, which I can read.

The subject of yoga and the method as taught by me grew at a speed faster than my expectation. Naturally, it is hard for me to guess or know how the teaching is going on, and how the students are imparting it.

On my part it is a question of trust. The trust is that I have given my knowledge and experience wholeheartedly to those who came in contact with me to learn or to teach. From them I would expect they carry the message of yoga with honesty, integrity, sincerity, devotion and dedication. At the same time, I expect that the teaching would be with the touch of feeling of the heart to heart contact to help humanity for its physical, mental and spiritual well being. Having given a good foundation on the subject of yoga with this humane touch, if my pupils teach the same way, I think it is possible for the subject to get well established with majesty, purity, clarity and precision.

It may be your misconception that meeting me has become rare. I am always available for all in the Library.[1] I might be teaching less but it does not mean that meeting me has become rare. It is possible that without direct contact with me, there are chances that the subject may be twisted or diluted and digressed, due to the interpretations of second or third generations. The mind, being very clever and tricky, believes that it is innovating, manipulates in such a way that one gets carried away without giving any thought to the correctness, clarity and divineness. If the teacher does not lose the integrity and honesty in the art of teaching, I am sure, this subject will spread holistically everywhere and become a household subject.

---

* Interview by Cathy Boyer, Johanna Heckmann and Anne-Catherine Leter, August 1995.

1 Every afternoon the *Yogāchārya* can be met in the library of the Ramāmaṇi Iyengar Memorial Yoga Institute, where he goes to attend to correspondance, write and to meet and discuss with teachers and students from all over the world.

The groups that have learnt from me directly and the group that has not met me, but learned through my pupils, should reflect and question themselves what they did teach and did not, or how far they were honest and how far they reflect with correctness or without. Then I feel, without doubt in myself that the quality of teaching can be maintained. It is not that a lot of talk is necessary, but they should learn to have self-introspection and find out the right way. Whether they have known me or not, met me or not, if they impart the knowledge maintaining the same lineage, then *guru-śiṣya paramparā* remains intact.

Times have changed. As the times change, so too the methods. Traditional methods, which were the links throughout, are called *paramparā*, which means coming from the teacher to the pupil. In this modern world, it has become hard to maintain the link to keep it up. It is the first generation teachers' responsibility to maintain this link with those who are not in contact with me. This way the link is maintained. If a good link is maintained, then I don't think there is any chance of going wrong subject-wise, or method-wise, while teaching and practising. If this link ceases, then it may find its natural death, and this should not be a point of worry to anyone. Having learnt from me, you have taught many students. These students may say that they are the students of Cathy, or Johanna or some other teacher. But do they know the *paramparā* or the source of what you teach? Do they realise that your teaching is linked to me, mine to my *guru* and my *guru's* to his *guru?* Do they appreciate the lineage that has brought the teaching to them? If they can know the source, that it was taught by such and such a person, even though they are following other teachers, then they will know the link. If they can keep up the link, the subject will never die, and that is known as *guru-śiṣya paramparā*.

When the mind has accepted the source, what wrong is there in accepting tradition? You all remember men who make history. Do you not? A traditional man is the one who makes such history, because he imparts the traditional method with a little adaptation according to the needs of the day. "Tradition" is the source. If we keep close to it, we can culture and build faster. Tradition is a foundation, which is maintained through the pupils. My teacher gave me the basic knowledge, which I protected according to his guidance and within my capacity tried to build on further, carrying the thread of tradition. Similarly, the pupils have to continue the thread. Our ancestors have shown the path and we are following it. Tradition is not imitation. Lineage saves time. You need not scratch from zero. If tradition is only copied or imitated, it becomes meaningless and dead. Any sort of imitation is superficial. One can imitate only the external appearances. Reality cannot be imitated. Tradition has to be followed and repeated meaningfully; so that the depth of the tradition is understood. Tradition is to carry the skill of the source, the skill of the very core of teaching. So you teachers, who have come in contact with me, must carry that very core of the teaching to pupils, but do not carry sediment.

– The problem in the West is that people are not accepting the guru-śiṣya *relationship. –*

If the West does not accept *guru-śiṣya* relationship, it is not my concern. But do they accept the teacher or not? If they accept, is it not a matter of lineage? This is *guru-śiṣya* or teacher-student relationship. I do not know whether to respect a teacher is taboo. Recently, in Canada, the same question was asked. I think Shirley Daventry-French wrote[1] a very good letter saying that after all we have learned from Mr. Iyengar, so naturally what is wrong in saying that we are Iyengar's pupils. She says – "Without Iyengar we wouldn't have imparted knowledge to you all. We were able to impart this knowledge only because we learnt first from him. So there is nothing wrong in calling yourselves 'Iyengar' students". I think I too would say the same thing.

Is this not a form of pride in people where they do not allow themselves to accept the source? The Eastern way of thinking is opposite to this. Traditionally, from time immemorial, we were commanded to recite names of the teachers. We are proud to say that we are the pupils of so and so.

The question is not merely of the relationship, but of the origin. Are you not proud to say that you are from France? Are you not proud to say that you got your degree from a particular university? Are you not proud to say that a particular honey is from your hometown, so on and so forth? You cannot deny the source, deny the seed, and deny the origin. You cannot deny your parents, can you?

The relationship depends on your attitude. You may or may not accept it, but the source remains the source. The knowledge does not fall as if from heaven.

Sometimes those who have not learnt from me say proudly that they are my pupils. Then there are pupils who have learnt from me, and yet avoid using my name? This is sheer arrogance. Then let them give up my method, my way of teaching. It requires the intelligence of heart to accept the *guru.*

– In the West it is the pride, and individuality, which has developed more. –

Exactly! That is the unintelligence of the heart. I do agree. It is the modern way of thinking. Not only in the West, but even in India this new style of thinking has come. It happens because pride and ego are part of human nature. Our ego is such that we all want to show that we are the masters. Yoga has become popular and egoistic people quickly take the opportunity from its popularity. These people are opportunists. How far can such people progress spiritually is the question. This makes the pupils to lose the touch or the link with the source. If the touch is gone, naturally a fall is certain. If the link disappears, *guru-śiṣya paramparā* also vanishes.

[1] See *Victoria Yoga Centre Newsletter,* February, 1995, p. 4

All these waves of mind are inevitable. One has to accept these things since human nature is like that. There is no remedy for the disease called "ego-pride". Ego develops out of intellectual arrogance and spiritual ignorance. True knowledge is the only answer. Knowledge comes to those who are humble. Pride and individuality are not the same. Pride restricts knowledge. Individuality is a branch of that restricted knowledge, the branch of ignorance – *avidyā*. If one has to gain or acquire further knowledge, then one has to leave this pride. A practitioner has to decide whether he wants to embrace arrogance or humbleness to progress towards knowledge.

Q.- Could you explain the evolution of your teaching since the publication of *Light on Yoga*,[1] and give the principal reasons for your changes?

You know, knowledge has no end. It is like a beacon of light. As you go on practising judiciously, which involves thinking, rethinking, adjusting, readjusting, the subtle things that are hidden surfaces. This is known as evolution. Evolution takes place if one practises judiciously. If one practises without any judicious feeling, then I don't think that evolution will happen. Judiciousness opens new horizons of the mind.

When I wrote *Light on Yoga*, it was thirty years ago. Naturally, at that time, I thought that I was at the zenith of knowledge. But now I say *Light on Yoga* is a base and not the zenith. As time went on and my practice became finer and finer, I reached a new horizon as the wisdom of heart opened more than the wisdom of the head. You saw the 1975 film. I think that I have performed *āsana* in that film better than in my book *Light on Yoga*. Even today, though the body has grown old, many new things and ideas strike on one I do better than before.

As the river flows towards the ocean, knowledge also flows towards the infinite. Knowledge does not flow in a reverse way. It does not flow backward, but only flows forward. If we get stale, then naturally, the growth comes to an end. As growth comes to an end, evolution stops. As intellectual stagnation has taken root we don't know the end. Sometimes our pride may say that we have reached the zenith. But who decides the zenith? We certainly have to laugh at ourselves. I thought that *Light on Yoga* was the zenith. It was my pride. Today, I say that it is a base which helps as a stepping-stone for further growth. This humility and humbleness built up in me due to my continuous practice. Similarly, I advise you all to practise judiciously so that the darkness, which covers the light, is uncovered for the light of wisdom to shine. I say

---

[1] Harper Collins, London. First published in 1966.

often, "Practice makes one perfect". What is that perfection? As you continue to practise, the hidden facet begins to surface and the unknown begins to reveal itself;. This revelation of the unknown shines out from the heart and not from the brain.

From the time of *Light on Yoga* to now, I have experienced tremendous change. I have transformed to such an extent not only in my intelligence, but even in the culturing of my cells. Like a diamond, the more you cut the better it shines. Similarly, I think I have cut and sharpened each facet of the diamond, i.e., the body, mind and intelligence, for them to shine better and better. So the knowledge is growing but I cannot say that this is the end. I only can say that it has grown farther than what it was before.

– Even now, the way you teach in the classes, a lot of things have changed. Johanna too feels the same. –

Previously, I could not give the basics, but I could give the techniques. Nobody would have accepted the basics in the beginning. When a tree grows and gives beautiful flowers and tasty fruits, then you question the gardener about the type of seed that was used, the fertilisers and minerals that were used. You inquire about how care was taken so that it could yield such a quality of flower and fruit. So, I too began imparting techniques to attract people and soon began appreciating the method and liked yoga. First I gave some understanding of the technique of *āsana* and *prāṇāyāma*. Now I ask that they find the hidden power of the seed, the source. This is the way, I followed in educating people towards yoga.

Techniques are different from the fundamentals, the basics. Techniques can be as many as the branches of the trees, but the root, the base is one. Today, my way of explanation of the techniques is to search the fundamentals so that you know the results. I begin there so that you understand the reason, the cause, why we have to practise *āsana* in a particular way. Previously, it was just an evolution of techniques. First, one has to know how to practice, and then one has to know why to do so in a particular way. The first step is technical and the second is fundamental. While evolving the technique, I could think which is better than the other for my students to adopt. Now, I see the principle behind the technique. The principles do not change. Now, I know the fundamentals of the techniques are very difficult to know. You may know the techniques, but you may not understand the fundamentals of the techniques. Fundamentals are the original basics, and techniques are superimposed on the fundamentals. At the same time the techniques are meant to approach, to reach, the fundamentals. So my teaching at present is at the fundamental level. That is why I am closer now to the root-nature than before. I am not only closer to the root-nature; I am also closer to the Self. The root-nature and spirit are very close to each other. You may demarcate them philosophically, but not practically. The philosophical analysis is verbal intellectualisation, but the practical analysis is experiencing intellectualisation, filtered very often.

Let me explain it a bit more elaborately. Nature means *prakṛti.* It has as its agents, the body, the organs of action, senses of perception, mind, ego and intellect for evolution. These agents project themselves always as separate entities with little co-ordination or understanding between each other. There is a distance, a space between them, as though each one is separate from the other. All of you have taught beginners. Often, when you give an explanation, can they co-ordinate the action between the right leg and the left leg?

- *No.* -

How long does it take for a person to turn one foot in and one foot out?

- *It takes quite a long time to understand.* -

This is only about the feet but what about the entire body and the mind, the mind and the ego, the ego and the intelligence? It takes a long time for this kind of intelligence to develop in order to lessen the gap.

In the beginning it was like that for me too, but today it is very different for me to differentiate between nature and spirit. When I practise, nature follows the spirit. At this stage of practice the soul is silent. The fundamental nature is also silent; there is no turbulence in the nature. The body and the self - *prakṛti* and *puruṣa* - meet in my practice. This is what yoga has given me now, and that is why my method of teaching has transformed from the gross to the subtle.

Today a greater understanding exists than before. People then used to say that it is very difficult to understand. Today they cannot say that it is very difficult to understand, because they too experience the same state as I do. I simplify the complex way of explanation so that even the high aspects could be explained in simple sentences for a simple mind to practise and experience.

Q.- Your teachings are based on an intensive practice of *āsana* and *prāṇāyāma*. This necessitates constancy and regularity. What is your advice for maintaining this practice?

First of all, understand clearly the word "intensity". Intensity is not understood properly. Intensity is a mental attitude more than a physical attitude. Many people misunderstand what intensity means. They think it means straining and sweating. No! That is a wrong meaning of the word! Intensity is to get totally involved, fully immersed and absorbed in what one is doing. Intense practice means a fast and keen mode in adjusting, correcting and progressively proceeding. When I say that I practise intensely, it means that my mental attitude and my mental disposition to the posture in *āsana* and the breath in *prāṇāyāma* is definitely deep inside. This I cannot express in words. Now, you say that you practise with an intensity of feeling. For me, *āsana* and *prāṇāyāma* blend my physical flow, emotional flow, intellectual flow and the feel of the core evenly in my existence.

- Emotional? -

Yes! Emotional. For me, emotional means a mental flow of equipoise, emotional equipoise. The mind is not focused on one thing, but exists everywhere, even in the corner of the fingernail. I have to feel that I am there, and that is known as intensity. When I say emotion, do not attribute emotions like love and sorrow to this state. What I mean to say is that when the mind is charged with an emotion like love, the whole mind is passionate and devoted to the subject. The mind undergoes certain qualitative changes when charged with such an emotional urge. Similarly, to me, the mind undergoes a qualitative change when I am doing *āsana* as well as *prāṇāyāma*.

I don't think anyone can understand the meaning of intensity so clearly unless and until there is devotion. The devotional practice is one thing and mental disposition is another, which changes from position to position in each *āsana*. The mind is not the same in each *āsana*, because the positioning being different, approach too becomes different; the way of thinking differs; the way of action differs; the feel also differs. As each *āsana* varies in its presentation, so too the thinking and feeling process varies. As thinking varies, action varies. This totality of action and reflection changes the attitude of mind instantly from one *āsana* to other. It is a kind of mental and intellectual involvement. In your case, when you start, you are in the past and the moment you finish you are already in the future. You are never in the present. As emotion keeps the present moment lively, my mind remains alive with the moment seeing its movements in that *āsana*. So one has to see the way of thinking, the way of approach, and how it changes in a split second to come to the present moment. This observation teaches us to feel the freshness of mind, freshness of action, freshness of thought. And that is what I consider very important in the art of intense practice.

Please, do not be carried away by the word intensity. Intensity means attentive involvement, it's not merely the physical strain but intellectual strain also. Though we use the word 100% perspiration, and 100% inspiration, it refers equally to the body, mind and intelligence.

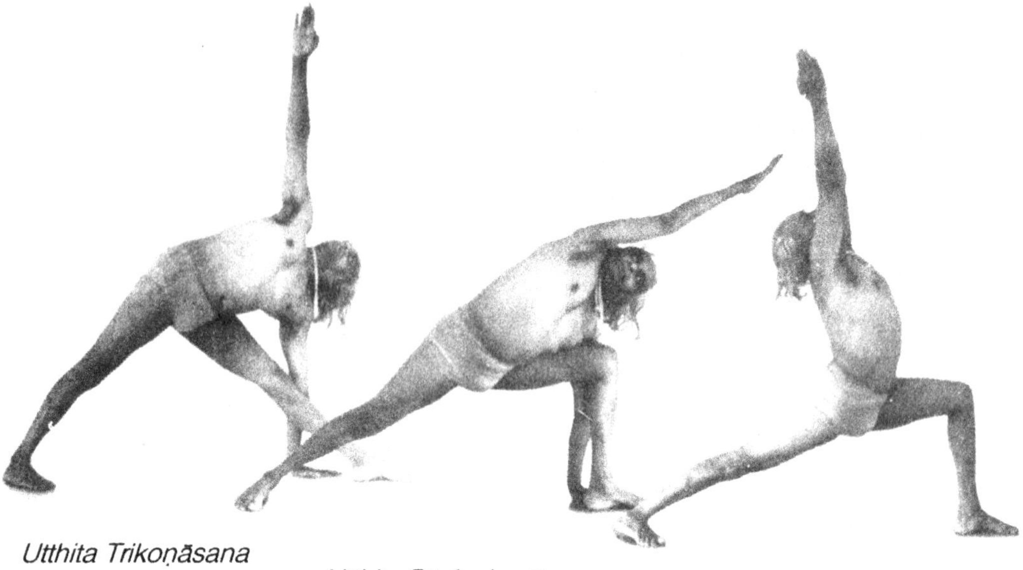

Utthita Trikoṇāsana *Utthita Pārśvakonāsana* *Vīrabhadrāsana I*

Plate n. 6 – Different *āsana* for involvement and disposition of the mind

Intensity is the total attitude of the mind and total attitude of the cellular system of the body. That is why it's called 100%. So you can't measure that by percentages, but it is a commonly used word. Total involvement and total disposition of mind in the *āsana* is intensity. *Utthita Trikoṇāsana* is different, *Utthita Pārśvakoṇāsana* is different, *Vīrabhadrāsana* is different. You cannot do all these *āsana* with the same attitude that you had in *Utthita Trikoṇāsana*. *Utthita Trikoṇāsana* is a different realm for the mind. Just as India is a different world, France a different world, England a different world. Similarly, each *āsana* is a different world. Each *āsana* has its own features, its own characteristics, its own representations, as well as its own attitudes. The behavioural pattern in the cells, the fibres, the tendons, the joints, as well as the mind differs from *āsana* to *āsana*. If we can gather these things, then the true meaning of intensity will set into your heart. Then you don't use the word intensity, you use the word absorption or oneness in what you are doing. So the difference between the performer and the performing art disappears. Art and you, or art and I, become one, and that is intensity. The art is the expression of the heart and not merely the head. I hope you understand. As I said, people mistake physical exertion for intensity. That is not right. It is total absorption, total reflection, and a total ministering of the mind. I use the word ministering of the mind so that the order goes directly to the body. Also the other way round, the body ministers to the mind. In other words there is oneness between the head and the tail, what you call, between the body and the mind. That co-ordination is intensity.

– But we become so carried away by the circumstances in our lives that sometimes the mind is not ready to do this. –

My friend, when the mind is not ready, then let us forget about it. But when you are practising, why don't you keep your mind wholly in that? The nature of mind is to carry you away from one thought to the other. But there is an inner mind that is beyond the habitual mind, and you have to learn to approach that inner mind. The habitual mind wants to remain engaged in its incessant, habitual, worldly thoughts. This mind regularly involves itself in just picking up the same thoughts over and over. It cannot see anything beyond the fence. The mind that is superior to this habitual mind breaks the fence and goes beyond. It administers the body. That is why I say that mind is the minister of the body, but the body should also act as a minister of the mind. That is what *āsana* and *prāṇāyāma* teach.

For many, the breath acts as the master of the mind. Hold the breath a little longer than you usually do and feel what happens to the mind. It shakes you, does it not? This you have to understand that the mind wants to shake the breath and breath wants to shake the mind. The zigzag habitual breath resists the body and mind. You have to change the pattern of the breath, tame it so that the mind is quietened. Since the mind wants to hold on to its own habitual thoughts and feelings, naturally the distraction is more. Before going into *prāṇāyāma*, *āsana* help one to go closer to the inner mind from the outer mind or habitual mind.

In today's world, it is impossible for people to devote the necessary time to any art, unless somebody supports them. Still, one has to know that whatever time is available, if one becomes totally involved and absorbed in the art, it keeps out all distractions.

By this freedom from distractions, one finds time and energy; the mind saves time for constructive development. Naturally you say, why waste time? The habitual mind engaged in thoughts consumes time and saps the energy. Instead of sapping energy through unnecessary thoughts, restrain them, then the time factor doesn't arise. You find enough time exists at any moment.

Q.- We find that this "intense involvement" is very hard when we practise yoga. The other arts we can learn. Why can't we penetrate when it comes to yoga?

Intense involvement is not hard. It does not require hard thinking but skilful intelligence to act in the right direction. No doubt, yoga is the most challenging subject in the world to a *sādhaka*. It is one's own counter-challenge from within. Music is not challenging. Dance is not challenging. There is a challenge in these arts, but the challenge is objective, whereas in yoga it is subjective.

Do you understand? In these arts the presentation is such that you want to win applause from the public. These arts have exhibitive attractions. You exhibit and win a prize. Yogic practice is not a show for public attraction. Hence, it is a hard *sādhanā* on one's own self. You are a dancer, aren't you?

– *Yes.* –

Does it challenge you?

– *Not so much.* –

Was it a challenge as much as in yoga?

– *No, certainly not!* –

Why not?

– *Because in yoga I have to penetrate more and reach deeper.* –

No other art in the world can proclaim this in-depth challenge on one's own body, mind, will power and sensitive intelligence. I dare say that the beauty of yoga is that it challenges the very core of the practitioner.

Even when you demonstrate the *āsana* and *prāṇāyāma* as an exhibitive art, there is a limitation. Yoga is filled with dynamic silent action whereas other arts are filled with dynamic motion, vibration, emotion and sound. All other arts are a feast for perception. However, yoga is an art that is inapprehensible by the senses. You can't show the intensity of involvement in yoga externally. You can't exhibit the role of your mind, your heart, your intelligence and your consciousness. This is a challenge that differs from other challenges.

In yogic practice there is a deep inter-penetration. In other arts you may exhibit and succeed. As you said, you have to get involved in the art of yoga, you have to go inwards, and the expressions have to come from within. You have to tackle the mind, the intelligence, the ego and the consciousness. In other arts you are carried away by motion or expression. Here there is no motion, no expression, so you are caught up in action. Hence, it is an inhibitive art. In dance you move from place to place, even if you make a mistake nobody notices it. The audience is carried away by the rhythm, but you still feel something is wanting, something is missing, though you do rhythmically. Here, you act, you observe, you challenge and you control. That is why it is more challenging to the practitioner as yoga challenges the practitioner. For me, this is a devotional art. Other arts don't challenge. They may play devotionally. They may sing devotionally. In yoga, you have to get involved devotionally and totally. While dancing or singing, you do not have to restrain yourself. Yoga has to come from the intelligence of the heart. If you don't restrain yourself, you fail in yoga. To present yoga in public, one needs perfection and restraint. Read what Patañjali says, *abhyāsa vairāgyābhyāṁ tannirodhaḥ* (*Y.S.*, I.12), meaning, practice and detachment are the means to still the movements of consciousness.

Q.- You speak often of the way of approaching *abhyāsa*. Could you speak about the way to approach *vairāgya* in everyday life?

Suppose you are doing *Śīrṣāsana* accurately, does your mind waver or wander anywhere? Are you not free from the other attachments at that moment? So *abhyāsa* – the practice – leads to *vairāgya* – the restraint – and *vairāgya* compliments *abhyāsa*. As far as my understanding goes, they go hand in hand. Without one, the other is ineffective. Without one, the other is blind or lame. I have already dealt with this in the very beginning, without the use of terminology.

When you are in *Dwi Pāda Viparīta Daṇḍāsana* or *Setu Bandha Sarvāṅgāsana*, does anything come to your mind? Don't you keep your mind engaged within the body and free from all the outer entanglements? Probably if you make your body a little lazy, your mind may wander, otherwise the moment you extend your inner awareness, breaking the laziness in your body, you know and feel what happens. Suppose you are relaxing, but suddenly you stretch or adjust your hip; what happens to the mind at that moment?

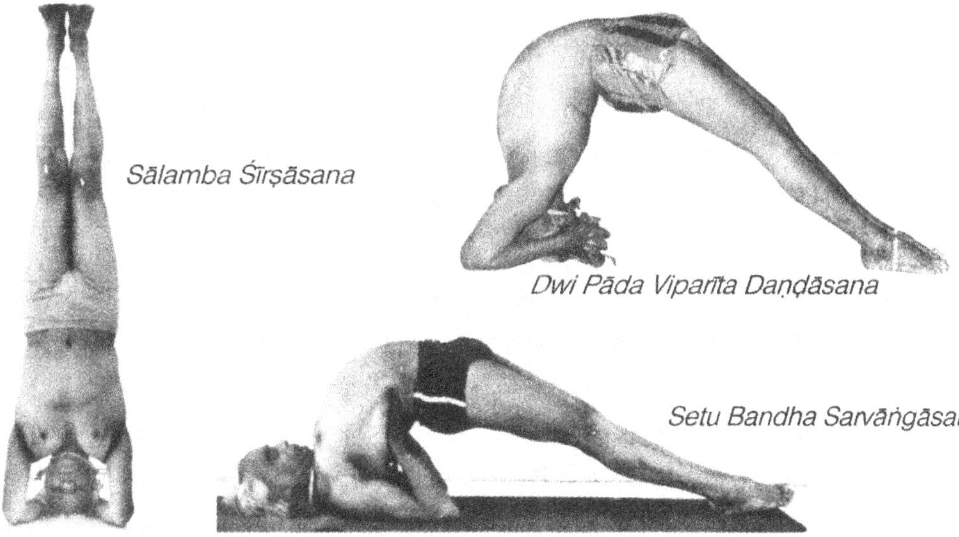
Sālamba Śīrṣāsana
Dwi Pāda Viparīta Daṇḍāsana
Setu Bandha Sarvāṅgāsana

Plate n. 7 – *Abhyāsa* for *vairāgya, vairāgya* for *abhyāsa*

- Gets oriented. -

Oriented, concentrated, right? Then when it is channelled, what is the meaning of it?

- We are free from thoughts, we become stable. -

Yes, you're free from emotions. It means the conquest of emotions has already begun. This is *abhyāsa* in *vairāgya* and *vairāgya* in *abhyāsa*.

Vairāgya develops slowly, step by step. It's very difficult to feel the change and understand. If you say that you have to get complete *vairāgya*, then you are to be totally God-minded. How can you at once restrain everything? How can you conquer *vairāgya* at once? For *abhyāsa*, Patañjali has already said that it takes a long time for a firm foundation to be laid. Does it not apply to *vairāgya* also?

This morning, for example, I was doing 108 *Viparīta Chakrāsana*[1]. You saw it. Did my mind wander? Tell me. Did I look here or there? Is it not a part of *vairāgya?* Hope you catch what I am saying and understand the way of renunciation. To renounce, one should have great determination. Is not self-determination an *abhyāsa?* Without determination there can be no *abhyāsa*. Similarly, *vairāgya* also needs *abhyāsa* –practice. Without practice, can one renounce anything? In order to get rid of attachments, one has to practise. In fact, we all have to practise with keen consciousness to move into the field of restraint. Please understand that practice is *vairāgya* and the practice of *vairāgya* is *abhyāsa*. They are co-related. Don't we toss the coin asking for head or tail to come up on top?

- Yes, we ask for either heads or tails. -

It is the same in yoga. You may call *abhyāsa* the head, and *vairāgya* the tail; or tail as *abhyāsa* and head as *vairāgya*. It doesn't matter. But the head and the tail are two faces of the same coin. So also if yoga is the coin, *abhyāsa* may be the head and *vairāgya* may be the tail, or vice versa. I hope now you understand *abhyāsa* and *vairāgya* clearly. When you are thoroughly involved in action, you are cut off from attachment and also the rest of your thoughts. As there is no movement of thought, it is *vairāgya*. Do you not experience this state?

- Emotions. -

---

[1] See *Aṣṭadaḷa Yogamālā*, vol. 4, plate n. 29.

It is stability, not only on emotional thoughts but non-oscillation of the intelligence. Yes, in one sense emotion is attachment or *rāga*. When you are free from *rāga*, it is *vairāgya*. When you do perfect *Śīrṣāsana* can your mind wander?[1] Yesterday, I put you in *Śīrṣāsana*, making the small end of the tailbone vertical. Did you allow your mind to wander when adjusted?

– *No.* –

Hence, these subtle adjustments help you to be free from thoughts, that is *vairāgya.*

Q.- You said that Patañjali is the first one to introduce God. Can you elaborate?

Correct! All orthodox systems of philosophy, known as *darśana,* are dependent on *Veda.* Some of the *darśana*, such as *Cārvāka,* did not accept *Veda* or God. *Yoga darśana* has accepted God. Patañjali, as a genius, was the first person to explain God in a brilliant conception in *sūtra* I.24.[2] He introduced "God" to the practitioners to surrender to the Supreme Force. He explained precisely and distinctly, defining God as one who remains free from cause and effect.(1) Realising that this surrender of oneself to God(2) is hard for most people, he shows the other avenue in the form of yoga with eight petals.

With all of our intense efforts, there is an invisible force upon which one has to depend and seek the support of. Patañjali in the first chapter assures the students of yoga that by acquiring qualities such as faith, vigour, memory, awareness and profound meditation, they succeed. This means that all of us should be enthusiastic, intense and energetic in our application and dedication. With all these efforts, a human being may fail, either due to feeble will power or on account of ego and pride. If one expression is of a negative and inferiority complex, the other is of a positive superiority complex. Some may practise with a low profile and others may be absolutely the opposite. Whether one is an intense or a mild practitioner, one still needs a seed(3) as support. Whenever one has to take support, the supporter or the supporting seed has to be stronger or superior to the one who seeks the support. Patañjali introduces "God" exactly at the threshold when one is realising that with all efforts he needs strong support. To take a support, one can't be aggressive. One has to be humble. One needs humility. We, as

---

[1] See plate n. 8.

[2] (1) *Kleśa karma vipāka āśayaiḥ aparāmṛṣṭaḥ puruṣaviśeṣaḥ Īśvaraḥ* (I.24). God is that Supreme Being who is free from afflictions, unaffected by actions and their reactions and untouched by cause and effect.

(2) *Īśvara praṇidhānāt vā* (I.23). Surrender of one's everything to God with profound meditation.

(3) *Tatra niratiśayaṁ sarvajñabījam* (I.25). He is the seed or source of all knowledge.

human beings, have less potential than God. God is omnipotent. Patañjali is not asking us to know God with some "make believe" process. He wants his followers to know God and surrender to God after putting in all the individual efforts.

In the succeeding *sūtra*[1] Patañjali also clears *'paramparā',* wherein he says that "God is the first, foremost absolute *guru,* unconditioned by time". Hence, you see, *guru-śiṣya paramparā* begins from God.

As one begins to know more and more, one realises how much the unknown is. What is known today, why was it unknown yesterday, or in yesteryears? Why do certain things remain in the dark? If so much was unknown in the past, then how much unknown lies in the future! This understanding brings about a gradual subjugation of our ego, our pride, and makes us realise that there is an "omniscient" Universal Soul. We are taken towards this state as the veil of ego gets removed.

Patañjali introduces God to us for the purpose of surrendering of our *ahaṁkāra* – the individual pride, and this keeps one from holding on to anything. This state is nothing but *vairāgya,* i.e., freedom from *rāga,* freedom from attachments. Patañjali says, *Īśvara praṇidhāna. Praṇidhāna* is devoted contemplation and the art of surrender to God. Desires create movement and action. Desirelessness keeps one passive, steady and stable. When one is contemplating God, there is no desire and there is no movement. One experiences a pure mind.

This highest state of *vairāgya,* or desirelessness, is called *guṇavaitṛṣṇyam*[2], i.e. free from the clutches of the *guṇa* of nature, and the sublimation of nature. One may say that *prakṛti* (nature) is different and *puruṣa* is different. But at this stage, when one is desireless, one is not touched by the *guṇa* of *prakṛti.* This desireless state is the state of the present. Patañjali says that God is omnipresent i.e., ever present, He has no beginning and no end. *Vairāgya* takes one to experience the state where there is no beginning, no end, as one is free from attachment.

God will not be known without *abhyāsa* and *vairāgya.*

- When we practise we forget completely about the world outside. -

That's right. The more we practise, the more we become absorbed in the subject and we get non-attached. We are cut off from the external world. *Vairāgya* is to take the mind away from the pleasures of sensual or temporal objects and direct one's mind towards God. *Vairāgya* has detachment as well as attachment. It is detachment to the worldly objects and attachment

---

[1] *Sa eṣaḥ pūrveṣām api guruḥ kālena anavacchedāt* (I.26).

[2] *tatparaṁ puruṣakhyāteḥ guṇavaitṛṣṇyam Y.S.,* I.16 – when one transcends the qualities of nature, the renunciation sets in and he perceives the soul.

to God.[1] In *abhyāsa* also there is attachment as well as detachment. When we are attached to practice, we are unattached to worldly matters, and when we are not attending to the practice, we are attached to other things.[2] This is like the balance of scale tilting to a gentle wind. As it is steady when windless, we have to learn to keep the mind wavering, away from emotional disturbances and intellectual fluctuations.

- Tricky. -

Yes, it may appear tricky for you and me, but not for a man of wisdom. *Abhyāsa* solidifies the attachment to the soul and detaches one from the clutches of the external world. *Vairāgya* solidifies the detachment to the external world and the sensual objects; establishes non-attachment, un-attachment and desirelessness. Stability comes only to a real yogi. When stability comes, *vairāgya* is further consolidated.

- It can take a long time for this also... -

My friend, everything takes its own time. Nothing can come except to one who is graced and gifted by God. Even the gift of God is a result of one's previous life's effort. God is not there to distribute the gifts. One has to earn it.

If you are a violinist, can you all play like Mr. Menuhin or like Mr. Heifetz?

- Impossible! -

They are considered geniuses at the violin. Each one of them develops special qualities of their own. These qualities later turn their playing into a spiritual art. One has to develop ripeness for these things to happen.

You can sow two seeds in the same place on earth. One will give fruit very fast, and the other may take a long time. You may have sown the seeds on the same day. The care you have taken of these plants also might be the same. But one grows fast, and the other doesn't. One gives fruit, the other doesn't. Why does this happen? That means the *karma* was there for those seeds too. So, you may have to take a special care, to give more attention to that plant which does not grow fast.

---

[1] *Tadā draṣṭuḥ svarūpe avasthānam* – then the seer dwells in his own true splendour.

[2] *Vṛtti sārūpyam itaratra* – at other times, the seer identifies with the fluctuating consciousness.

Similarly, for all of us, lots of obstacles come, but we must not stop our practice. Unfortunately, if the obstacles come to you, you say "good-bye" to your efforts. To give up practice is also a sort of *karma*. I faced all obstacles in practice and hindrances from my own self as well as from people around me. Some force behind me guided me to remain determined. That same force was my inner voice forcing me, "Come what may, continue". So there was some kind of divine force and it is still persisting and protecting me and making me continue with my daily yogic discipline.

Luckily, you are all in a better position by birth than me because you have been guided in the right path from the start of yoga. Probably, the circumstances are more favourable to you than they were for me when I took to yoga. Despite those unfavourable circumstances I could continue, then why not you too? How fortunate we are when we have been given a good chance in life to practise yoga! This is how you have to see and go ahead with what you have learnt. Do not expect the result without efforts. Even do not hanker for maximum benefit with minimum effort. But they come on their own. It came to me because I persevered persistently even with repeated failures and agony. If you put in maximum effort, it may result in some achievement. As you get fruit from the tree when you pay total attention, you get the fruit of yoga if you practise with devoted dedication. As you have a good background to practise yoga, you minimise the effort by discarding unwanted or wasteful efforts. No doubt, in the beginning a lot of donkey-work is required, only then can you discard that which is not needed. For example, I can do *Uttānāsana* without any strain but can you do it in the same way? I can be in *Śīrṣāsana* without any strain. Can you? I get the maximum effect because my effort is effortless as that effort educates me throughout. In the beginning the benefit was less but the effort was more. It is the same for every beginner to struggle to stand on his head. Will he learn without struggling? All these have to be understood first. As a practitioner I will not bloat with words for the pupils who are learners, because in the early stages I knew that I had to put in a lot of efforts myself. Gradually, the efforts became natural; in that naturalness, the power or strength that I exerted began reducing. For me, it was not a collapse, but a release both inside out and outside in. Now extension of my body is there, as well as a tensionless alert mind. My practice for you seems that I am stretching my muscles and tendons. For me it is a soft process from the core of my being. It means that bodily, mentally and intellectually, the efforts are less, but the maximum expansion of my self is there. This you have to learn as you progress in your *sādhanā*. Patañjali has said, *tīvra saṁvegānām āsannaḥ*,[1] meaning that the effect will come faster to him whose intense efforts are no more felt as intense. Those practitioners are very swift in uniting the cellular body with the organic body and the organic body with the mental and spiritual bodies.

---

[1] The goal is near for those who are supremely vigourous and intense in their yogic practice (*Y.S.*, I.21).

If this "uniting" is difficult, then one has to struggle. That is why I say that if you are a mild practitioner, the benefit is mild. If you are average, the benefit is average. If you are casual in efforts, you're also casual in effects. If you are intense, then the effect is intense. This is very logical. But we have to experience this. That's why Patañjali uses the word *tapas*.

The word *tapas*[1] has been used for us to understand that there should be no darkness in any part of the body. The inner body remains in darkness if the mind does not reach there. Perhaps, you may understand with this analogy. If the president of your country is driving down the street along with his cavalcade, a red signal doesn't affect him. He is allowed to cross through them. Can you go like that? If you go like the president, you are caught and you have to pay a fine. Does he pay the fine? The diseases, the obstacles, the darkness, are like a red light for us to think and act. We have to take care of them, otherwise we pay a big fine. In yogic practice, we make the Self to travel in our body without hindrances anywhere and everywhere it likes. There is no red light for the Self at all. No disease, no obstacles, no red light, no penalties at all. We practise yoga so that we do not pay any fine! We practise so that the *ātman* travels within and without with no hindrances at all.

The problem is not one of "how long". The problem is with our patience. Do we have the patience and tolerance to wait and get the genuine experiences?

Q.- You said the *ātman* was travelling outside also. How?

The soul within is an embodied soul or an empirical soul. But the soul inside and the soul outside are not different. The whole world, the cosmos is in that Universal Soul. The *Bṛhadāraṇyaka Upaniṣad* expresses the *Brahman* as *Otaprota*, meaning, *Brahman* is interwoven cross-wise and length-wise. The universe is soaked in that Universal Soul.

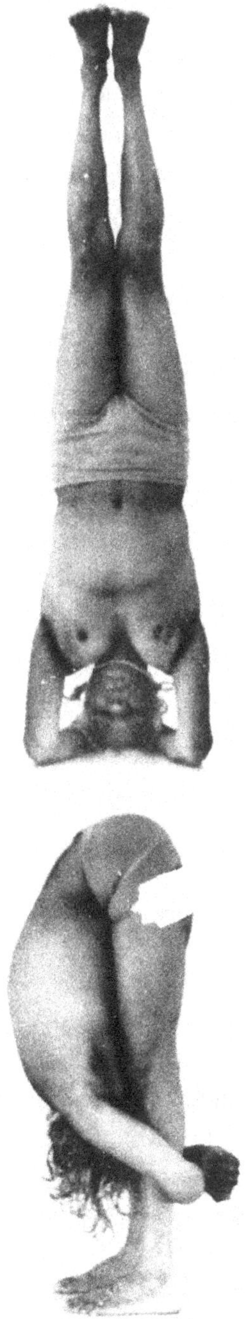

Plate n. 8 – *Sālamba Śīrṣāsana* and *Uttānāsana*

[1] *Kāya indriya siddhiḥ aśuddhikṣayāt tapasaḥ* (*Y.S.*, II.43). *Tapas* (self-discipline) burns away impurities and helps in kindling the sparks of illumination.

Now, how to experience this? Patañjali says: *Viśeṣadarśinaḥ ātmabhāva bhāvanānivṛttiḥ.*[1] *Viśeṣadarśinaḥ* means the one who sees distinctly. The one who sees distinctly is the "real seer", because he sees the *ātman*. He sees the very seer separate from the seen. He realises that the seen is not the seer. The consciousness is not the seer. Due to the want of knowledge *(avidyā)* the *sādhaka* identifies himself with consciousness. But when the knowledge comes, this identification ends. He realises the distinction between *citta* and *ātman*, consciousness and soul. And the search of the Self comes to an end.

With the practice of yoga, the organs of action, senses of perception, body and mind are purified; as pure as the Self and transformed to the level of the Self. Therefore I say, see the Self everywhere while practising *āsana*. To those who experience this state, Patañjali says, *viśeṣadarṣinaḥ*. Lord Krishna calls them *samadarṣina*. *Sama* means equal, so the one who sees with equality. This state comes only when the *sādhaka*, the practitioner, gets clarity and purity of *jñāna*, without having even a tinge of *ajñāna* or ignorance. Such a *sādhaka* becomes a seer. First he is a seeker. After seeking he finds and realises the truth that he is no longer a seeker but a seer. Such a seer looks at everyone with the vision of equality. Lord Krishna says that such a seer who is *viśeṣadarṣin* or *samadarṣin* (*B. G.*, V.18) sees with equanimity even those who are not equal; whether one is a *brahmin* or a cow, an elephant, a dog or a dog eater. A common man may love or hate according to his tastes or likings. His feelings depend on his likings and dislikings. But a *samadarṣin* sees and respects all with the feeling of equality, because he sees that the soul within himself and the soul in them are the same.

- How about us? -

I said that the practice has to be such that you have to learn to see the soul spreading everywhere. It is not just the stretch of the body. The stretch and extension of the body is one thing, but experiencing the extension of the soul everywhere, and realising the freedom of movement within is a different thing. The stretch, correction, adjustments and so on are the instruments to experience the freedom of the Self. This inner freedom brings outer freedom also. How I see the outside, I begin to see inside also. This is what you have to develop through yoga. This comes with your religiousness in practice. If *Brahman* is *Otaprota* - occupied in and out and remaining beyond -, in the same way your practice also has to be complete in and out and out and in. Nothing should be covered by unintelligence. Each *āsana* should culture in order to change the attitude of the mind. One has to learn to make use of this mind that goes on culturing. As the milk is taken from the udders of the cow, one has to learn to take that

[1] *Y.S.*, IV.25. When the difference between consciousness and the projector of consciousness is recognised by the seeker, the search of Self-realisation ends.

nutritive nectar from practice and filter it to get the best out of it, or the *sattva* out of it. From this shines the pure illuminative consciousness, which is equal to the soul. Finally, the soul shines and the darkness is eradicated.

Q.- If we stay just with our practice of *āsana* and *prāṇāyāma*, do we progress in *yama* and *niyama?*

This is the same question that you asked about *abhyāsa* and *vairāgya*. The question is coming from the brain and not from the heart. It is possible only if there is a total involvement and such involvement comes from the heart. The brain doubts, the heart does not. What is *yama, niyama?* The ethical disciplines, are they not?

- Yes. -

Āsana and *prāṇāyāma* help to control the motor nerves and sensory nerves. When we say that *āsana* and *prāṇāyāma* have to be done judiciously, it implies the ethical discipline to bring harmonious function in the motor and sensory nerves. While you are doing an *āsana* and *prāṇāyāma,* if your mind goes on wandering, can you do justice to your body, your mind, your intelligence? Did I not question you, when you stretched in *Setu Bandha Sarvāṅgāsana,*[7] what happened to your mind? You said that your mind goes inside. What is that? Is it not a discipline? This way you learn to study, adjust, observe and reflect. When you observe, you have to put it into practice; after putting into practice you have to re-reflect on that practice, between what you did and what you are doing. After reflecting, you observe again. Then the wheel of mind with the spokes of the body moves on in your presentation. When you reach precision, the spokes and the wheel stop moving, but in the process of moving, these spokes like facets of the mind move. Suppose in *Sarvāṅgāsana* your right leg is alert while the left leg is not, then do you call it an ethical practice or a non-ethical practice? It's easy to say that you have a defect on this side or on that side. This is pure escapism from facts. As the pride in you doesn't accept the faulty approach, you bring some reasons to save your self-respect. This does not come under honest approach. You have to give it a thought and honestly find out what you do and at the same time see whether your intellect is attentive or not. In this attention, penetration takes place and you feel how the cells, the fibres, the ligaments, and which part of the joints work. Then you study which part doesn't work. Which part of the ligament does not work, which tendons do not stretch. In this way of observation, you have to have a multifaceted or multi-channelled mind to

[1] See plate n. 7.

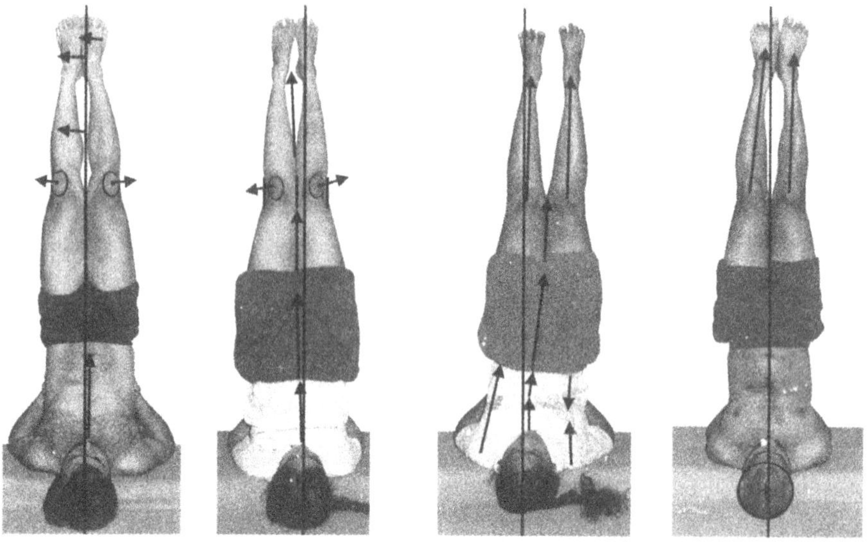

A central perpendicular line has been drawn from the eyebrows.
The arrows show the direction of distortion from that centre.

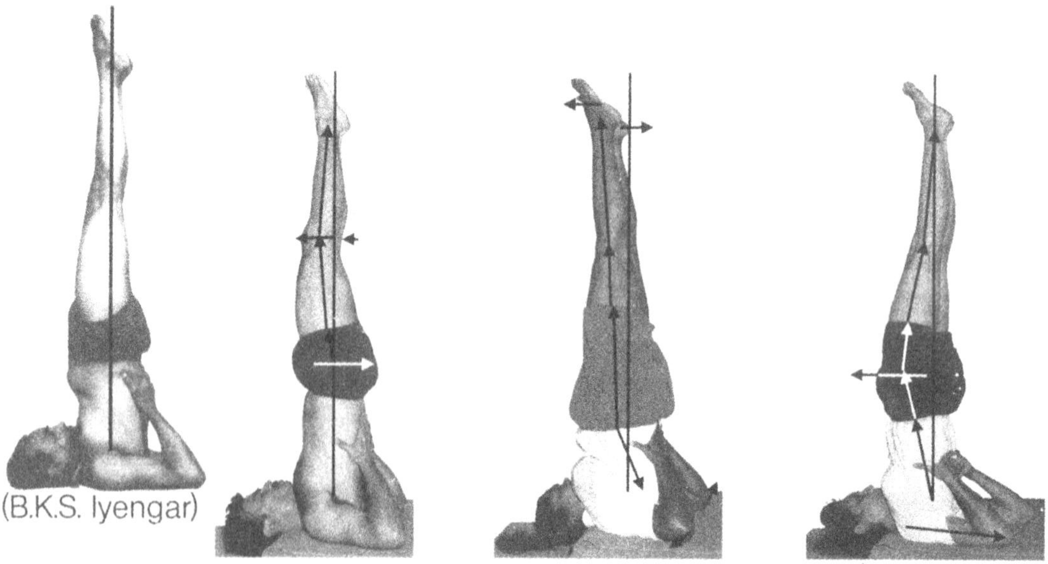

The perpendicular line is traced from the centre of the armpit.
The arrows show the direction of distortion away from that line.

Plate n. 9 – *Sālamba Sarvāṅgāsana* showing defects

see everything in a fraction of a second. Patañjali says that the yogi with exalted knowledge grasps clearly, instantly and wholly on all objects without thinking of time.[1] And then you bring unity in these multifaceted minds and in your actions. When you bring these multifaceted actions into a single action, what happens? Then what is that state called? Tell me.

– Purity and sensitivity! –

Correct. So the sensitivity and purity gets set in your mind. Now what is ethics? The meaning of ethics is to be pure. You can see that all those principles of *yama* and *niyama* are meant to bring purity in *citta*.

Q.- But in our practices, when we are doing, how do we understand *ahiṁsā?*

If your right leg is stretching and your left leg is not, you believe that the left leg is in *ahiṁsā* and the right leg in *hiṁsā;* you are doing *hiṁsā* to your right leg and *ahiṁsā* to the left. The one that you do not stretch is in a non-aggressive state, while the other, which you are stretching, is in an aggressive state. You think that the stretching is *himsā* and non-stretching is *ahiṁsā*. In both cases, you are creating *hiṁsā*. If one is a deliberate aggression, the other is a non-deliberate one. The moment when both legs are equally stretched or equally relaxed, there is neither violence nor non-violence. This is how you have to study the ethics in *āsana*.

Q.- How to follow the principle of *satya* in *āsana?*

You know, we have sensory nerves and motor nerves. The motor nerves act very fast and receive messages also fast through the sensory nerves. These nerves spread all over the body like a net. Sensory nerves follow motor nerves, and motor nerves follow sensory nerves. Sensory nerves are known in yogic terminology as *jñānanāḍī* and the motor nerves as *karmanāḍī*. They run parallel to each other. In order to understand these hidden sensory perceptions in your practices, I say to bring your attention to observe the felt feelings. This observation makes the motor nerves to react accurately. Through the *jñānanāḍī* you develop perception and through *karmanāḍī* you act and adjust. When I say, "Lock the knees" or "Tuck in the top of the patella", what does it convey?

---

1 *Tārakaṁ sarvaviṣayaṁ sarvathāviṣayaṁ akramaṁ ca iti vivekajam jñānam* (*Y.S.*, III.55).

It conveys the message to the motor nerves to act and not on the sensory nerves. But if I say, "Find out whether both the knees are locked equally, or the top of the patella is tucked in equally", then, in order to feel the equalness in locking or tucking, you have to apply your sensory nerves. You need to check truthfully the feel of evenness. This awareness is the quality of *satya*. Communicating with the motor and sensory nerves and bringing communion through action is *satya*. We are keen to see the truth in the outside world, since we cannot tolerate injustice being done, but how far do we truthfully do justice in our own practice? Why do we slip from the truth in our practice? Seeing these escapes, I stuck to *yama* and *niyama* all the time, to see how far one can follow those principles within one's individual efforts. That is why I ask while doing the *āsana* whether we are responding to *jñānanāḍī* or not. Do our *karmanāḍī* react or not? This observation and right adjustment between these two nervous systems is for me *satya*. The popular meaning of *satya* is, "Be truthful. Be honest". We try to be honest in society as much as possible; but when it comes to the *sādhanā* of yoga, I find the real depth of truthfulness lying within. When this surfaces, you follow *satya* on your own.

Q.- Can you tell us a little more about the other principles of *yama* and *niyama*?

I think I have explained it so many times in the classes while teaching and on several occasions while lecturing, and you are asking me again.

Now let me speak on *asteya*. *Asteya* means non-stealing. Now men like us will not go to steal. We are not thieves. We can preach ethics to a thief, not to steal. So what about us? How do the principles of *yama* and *niyama* apply to us? We need to study the psychology behind "stealing". It is mental greediness more than the actual need. A needy person may beg but he won't necessarily steal. A thief has a mental attitude to steal. His mind as well as the *karmendriya* cause him to do so. In our case, we may be greedy; temptations may come though we don't actually go to steal. But *tapas* demands tremendous discipline, which controls the greed and temptations. Know that *tapas* is religiousness in *abhyāsa*. *Tapas* is a methodology to apply for our progress. Similarly *santoṣa*, satisfaction. Is satisfaction physical or mental?

- Mental. -

That's it. Here the *jñānanāḍī* should be sensitive. Do you know how one becomes physically affected if one is mentally dissatisfied? One can suffer from dissatisfaction like acidity or heart trouble, hysteria or schizophrenia. I have come across such cases on account of dissatisfaction. The unhappiness *(asantoṣa)* is a slow sapper of the nervous energy, which later

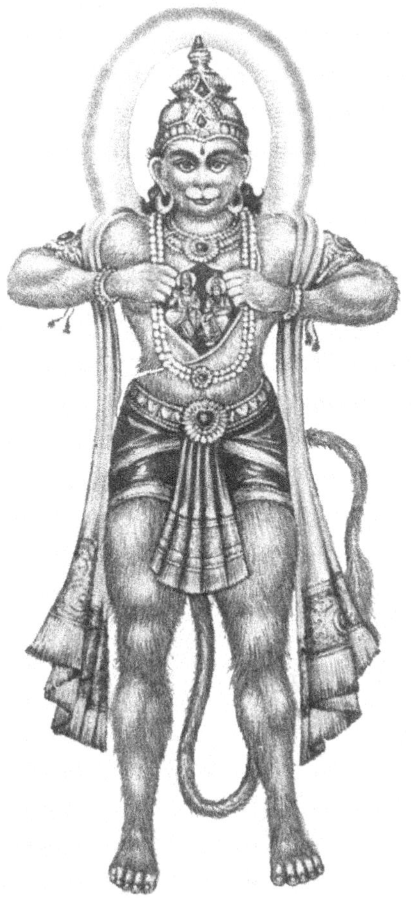

Plate n. 10 – Lord Hanumān

affects the mind. When the brain and nerves are affected, the *karmanāḍī* and *jñānanāḍī* get deranged.

Hence, it is important for us to take care of the *karmanāḍī* and *jñānanāḍī* so that they do not get affected by disorders. This is *nāḍīśuddhi* or cleansing of the nerves. This cleansing is possible only with the depth practice of *āsana* and *prāṇāyāma*.

Śauca means cleanliness. Purity of word, thought and deed is cleanliness . It is external as well as internal, physical as well as mental. The physical cleanliness is known to all, but do we know about the internal cleanliness? Here come *jñānanāḍī, karmanāḍī,* mind, intelligence and conscience. If these are polluted, non-cleanliness sets in.

Regarding *brahmacarya*; *Brahma* means the Ultimate Truth, Supreme Soul, the God; *cara* means to move. The one who always moves towards or in *Brahma* is a *brahmacārī*. It also means celibacy, which covers physical and mental strength, vigour and valour. Patañjali mentions the effect of *brahmacarya* that knowledge, vigour, valour and energy flow in abundantly[1].

According to the Indian heritage, students are called *brahmacārī* since they are made to study. Study is *svādhyāya*. *Sva* means self, and *adhyāya* means study. To understand *Brahma* and to know the Self that resides within is *brahmacarya*. This is the period of study of sacred books, so that he uses this knowledge practically in later life.

Each cell has to move with God. Each cell has to vibrate with Self and God. There is a story in the *Rāmāyaṇa* where Lord Hanumān tears open his chest and shows Rāma (his God) existing in his heart. It is a very symbolic story. The God is within and we have to be in God. God is here, God is there, God is everywhere.

---

1 *Brahmacaryapratiṣṭhāyāṁ vīryalābhaḥ* (*Y.S.*, II.38). When the *sādhaka* is firmly established in continence, knowledge, vigour, valour and energy flow to him.

Aparigraha is to learn to be non-possessive. We want to possess of what we like. We love so many things and like to own them and this makes us to remain attached to things. It is also possible for *aparigraha* to build up good *saṁskāra* (latent impressions). *Aparigraha* may uplift the *sādhaka* or cause downfall. Attachments change often with our varying tastes. But attachment to God is something unique. One can have attachment to chocolates, as well as coffee. If one gets intoxicated with either of the two, then one develops toxins, which lead to disturbance in health. Intoxication with God does not bring diseases. It brings elixir only. So *aparigraha* leads one towards *Īśvara praṇidhāna*.

Now about *āsana*. The *sthiratā* or stability in *āsana* is not possible without non-violence and *abhyāsa*. *Sukhatā* or steadiness of intelligence in *āsana* is not for the sake of pleasure but to develop desirelessness through *vairāgya*. *Prayatnaśaithilya* is effortlessness that comes only with *aparigraha*. Attachment to the body, love towards the body and undue protection, does not transform effortfulness into effortlessness. Effortlessness leads to *ananta samāpatti*. *Ananta samāpatti* means reaching the infinite and this is nothing but *Īśvara praṇidhāna*. When one attains the state of *ananta samāpatti*, there comes the freedom from the shackles of dualities or *dvandva* (*Y.S.*, II.46-48).[1]

Yoga is an evolutionary subject that makes an incomplete man complete. It teaches one how to become eclectic; it guides how to economise energy so that nothing is wasted but allowed to flow towards the Supreme. This is the economy of the progress of the body and skilfulness of the mind in thinking and in action and saves one from worldly indulgence.

Q.- During classes, you often refer to the five elements. How does one feel their action in the body?

I talked about it at Panchgani and later in France.[2] I think you have to read that article. What is the quality of the element 'earth'? It is the heaviness. If your foot is lightly placed on the floor in *Utthita Trikoṇāsana*, can you perform the *āsana?* When you do *Utthita Trikoṇāsana* you move one hand up and one down. When you move your hand upwards, this movement is with the element of air. The one that is down acts as the element of earth. The right hand is used differently than the left. Adjustments, forward or backward movements, firmness and heaviness

---

[1] *sthira sukham āsanam* (*Y.S.*, II.46). *Āsana* is perfect firmness of body, steadiness of intelligence and benevolence of spirit.
Prayatna śaithilya ananta samāpattibhyām (*Y.S.*, II.47). Perfection in an *āsana* is achieved when the effort to perform it becomes effortless and the infinite being within is reached.
Tataḥ dvandvāḥ anabhighātaḥ (*Y.S.*, II.48). From then on, the *sādhaka* is undisturbed by dualities.

[2] See also *Aṣṭadaḷa Yogamālā*, vol. 2, pp. 210, 234, 257-259, and vol. 3, pp. 51-52, 118-119.

of the hands differ. It is the same with the legs. In *Śīrṣāsana*, the forearms become the element of earth and the legs become the element of air. In this way you have to understand in each *āsana*, how the elements change the frame of the body and the attitude of mind. In fact, one has to understand the way of using the elements of the body to bring firmness, softness, lightness, heaviness, heat and cold with the elemental adjustments. In *Pascimottānāsana*, don't you feel the coolness of the head and the warmth (element of fire) in the abdomen?

In *Sarvāṅgāsana*, the base of the neck, shoulders and upper arms are firm like the element of earth. You push your hand to open the chest, that is the element of fire. The more you involve the mind, the fire element increases. You have to see whether you feel that same warmth everywhere. Fluidity is the quality of water. If one leg is active and the other leg is

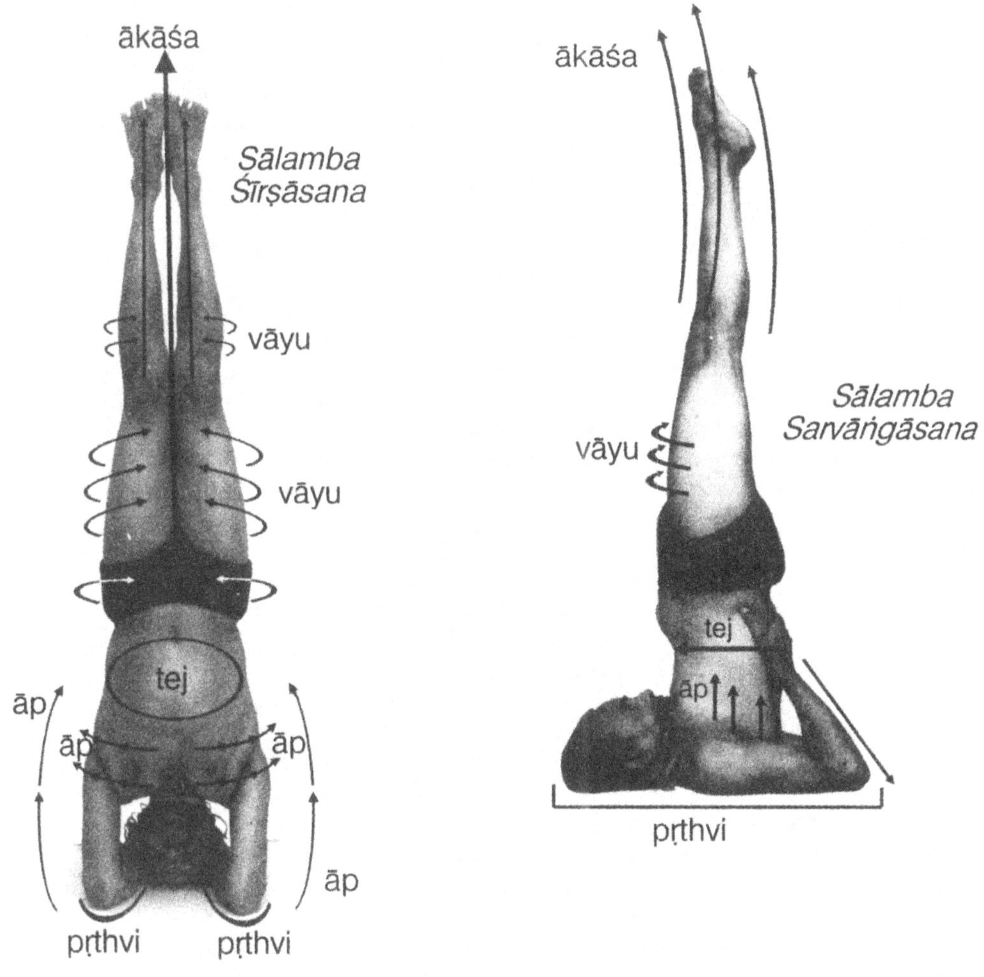

Plate n. 11(a) – Elemental attributes in *āsana*

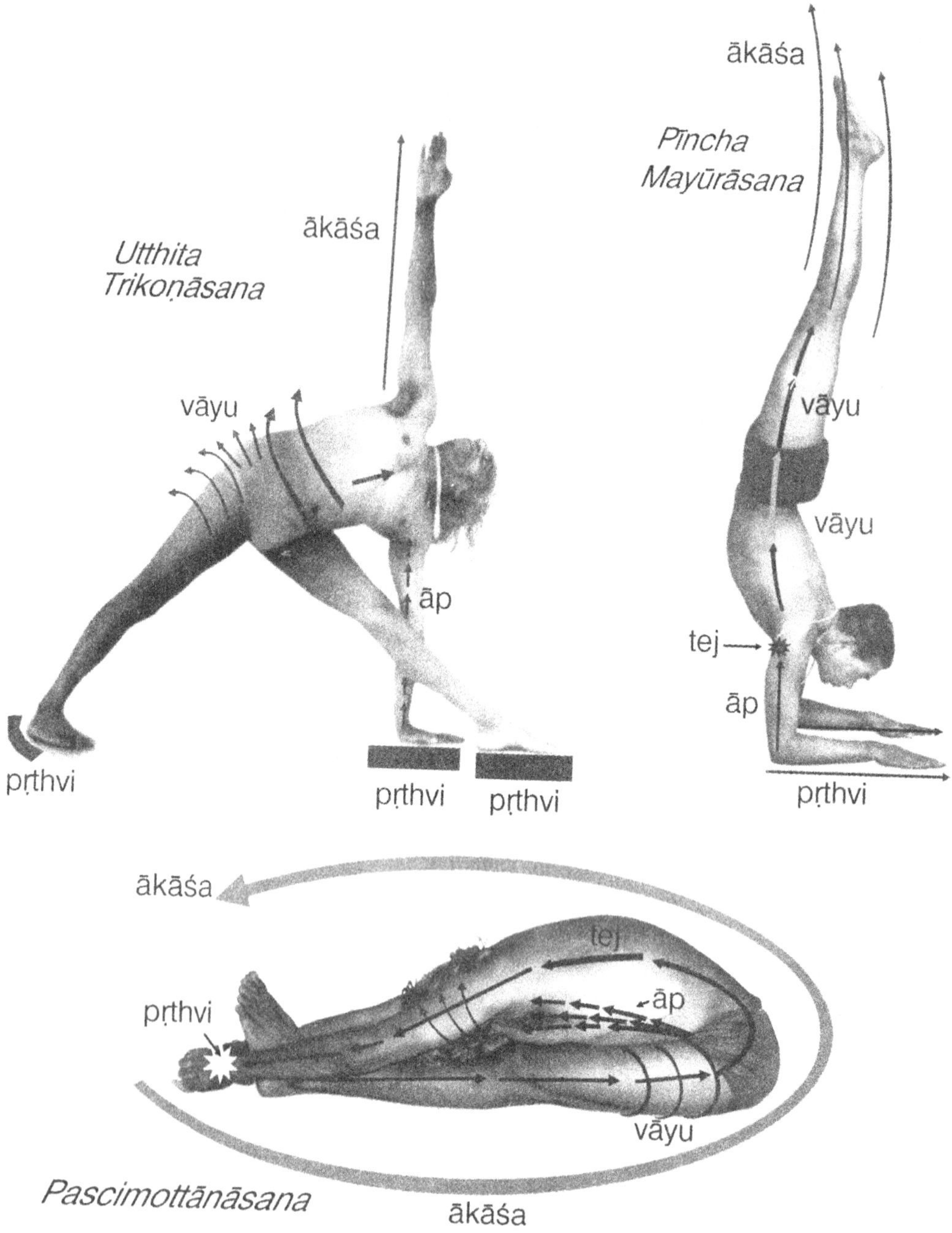

Plate n. 11(b) – Elemental attributes in *āsana*

inactive, will there be a proper supply of blood? Does water flow, if it does not find its level? Similarly the blood is liquid and can't flow if the legs are inactive. Even the energy that is like fire spreads in the body. The heaviness is of earth, flow is of water, warmth is of fire, the sensation of touch is air, and the expansion or contraction is space, which is ether. As all these elements are inter-woven, one has to observe their interactions.

When one is doing the *āsana* one has to constantly observe all these movements of matter. Sometimes one takes the elbows inside and contracts in space in *Sarvāṅgāsana* or in *Pīncha Mayūrāsana*. When one opens the chest, one expands in space. Similarly with the legs. This way one has to observe the character of the elements in each *āsana*. It is a subject to understand through the experiential ways by balancing them evenly and clearly.

Have you read the *Light on the Yoga Sūtras of Patañjali?*[1] There I have given the qualities of the five elements. Read and memorise so that it remains firm and useful in the *sādhanā*. Observe the rhythmic adjustment of the elements and the changes occurring within yourself.

Q.- I think you may have already answered the next question. What are the priorities of observation while performing an *āsana?* What are the signs that indicate that the work in an *āsana* is achieved in the most desirable way?

The element of air is the element of intelligence. The element of fire is the mind. The skeletal body is the element of earth. The fluidity in the body is the element of water. Warmth is the element of fire. Contact is the element of air and contraction or extension is the element of ether.

You have to study and understand that the firmness in the *āsana* is the element of earth. The flow of energy in the system is the element of water. The element of fire is in the presentation. The element of air is the right feel of the *āsana* and the expansion or contraction is of the ether. This is how you have to study.

Out of the five elements, the first three, earth, water and fire, are gross elements. The subtle elements are air and ether. When we begin to learn yoga, we use our skeletal body, the element of earth. After some time, we create room in our body so that the element of water (blood) may feed the body. Then we allow energy, or the element of fire, to feel the warmth. This makes us feel the inner contact. This inner contact alerts the intelligence, which belongs to the element of air and through the element of air, we penetrate the space within. This is the element of ether. These subtle experiences come only at later stages. In the beginning, there is a maximum effort resulting into minimum effect, since we have to cross through the first three gross elements – earth, water and fire. This journey takes its own time. Then we have to build up from the gross

[1] See *Light on the Yoga Sūtras of Patanjāli*, by BKS Iyengar. pp. 226 – 227, Harper Collins, London.

towards the subtle elements, namely air and ether. When the practice is at the level of air and ether, your practices are close to the self.

Q.- In class you say that there is good pain and bad pain. How can we recognise when the pain is caused by incorrect practice?

Any beginner will have pain as they have not used their muscles. But when the pain persists even after practice, it means one has unknowingly made some wrong movements. If the pain comes at the time of practice, but you do not feel it afterwards, then that is not a bad pain. Sometimes when you are stretching you get a pain that is very soothing. This is a healthy pain. Sometimes the pain is excruciating and continuous. That pain is a wrong pain. Something may be going wrong to cause this unhealthy, excruciating, unbearable pain. This type of pain is a bad pain. Sometimes you say that it is a good pain and you want to stay in that pain. This is a healthy pain.

Pain that hinders the regular movements and causes disturbance and imbalance is a wrong pain. The pain that does not obstruct movement cannot be called pain. Yesterday you saw the man with atrophy from U.S.A. You know about the atrophy of the muscles. But do you know about the atrophy of the mind? Who knows about the atrophy of the mind? You don't use such words. By looking at the patients you say that the atrophy is of the muscles. But what about the mind? The mind doesn't travel there and hence the muscles and nerves get atrophied. So, yoga teaches the art of making the mind to move in the body to understand how muscles that are atrophied can be corrected. The mind does not work on that area and therefore the muscle gets atrophied and loses control. Here the body does not have any pain but hardness and shortness. Yoga works to remove shortness and hardness by using the mind with discernment.

We ask the affected person to bring the mind there and activise that area so that he gets some action, vibration and pain in stretch. The unactivised area is penetrated by the mind and activised, so that he stands with even weight and moves his limbs with equal pressure. Such movements bring pain, and one has to accept that, because that pain brings elixir to the area.

Even in healthy people, the untouched areas may remain non-painful and the moment it is activised it becomes painful. The area that is in a sleepy, dormant state gets awakened. Such kinds of pain are healthy. The unactivised area may not be atrophied but may have no sensation and no feeling; when such areas are activised, they become painful. Yet this is a healthy pain. So one has to analyse the right and wrong pain by adjustment and study.

- Does this man from the U.S.A. have a virus? -

Yes, he had a virus infection also, but it could be on account of a disease like fever. It may be viral or genetic, or may be congenital. A healthy person may also get such problems due to wrong behavioural patterns of walking, standing, sitting, and wrong usage of certain muscles. These things do happen. But here I am using a particular example that you have seen. The reason why we practise *āsana* is to see that no atrophy takes place in our brain, mind and cells or in the tendons. The one you saw is a known atrophy of the muscles. But what about the unknown atrophied muscles? There is no name for such untouched and unactivised areas where such atrophies occur. Even while teaching, don't we tell you to know the black holes in your body? We don't know the depth of the body because the intelligence does not penetrate. You need a lot of torchlight to go into the dark areas or dark caves. Similarly the torch of intelligence has to be used in the body for penetration, to see and break the darkness inside. And that is to search the atrophy from within. This understanding comes with practice.

Q.- You have said that one of the weaknesses of Westerners is want of emotional tolerance. How do we deal with this problem through yogic practices?

Are the attachment and aversion the emotional or intellectual problems?

- They are certainly emotional. -

That is why I say that yoga is not only an intellectual subject, but also an emotional subject. Rather it deals with emotions and organises them. Patañjali speaks of five afflictions. Among them *avidyā* and *asmitā* are intellectual defects, *rāga* and *dveṣa* are purely emotional and *abhiniveśa* is instinctive.[1]

Abhiniveśa means fear of death. In other words, it is an attachment to life. If *rāga* (attachment) and *dveṣa* (aversion), are objective emotional feelings, *abhiniveśa* (fear of death) is a subjective emotion. From the subjective inborn emotions, objective emotions sprout out in the form of attachment towards happiness and aversion towards sorrows.

---

[1] *Avidyā asmitā rāga dveṣa abhiniveśaḥ kleśāḥ (Y.S.,* II.3). The five afflictions which disturb the equilibrium of *citta* are namely, spiritual ignorance *(avidyā),* the sense of 'I' *(asmitā),* attachment *(rāga),* aversion *(dveṣa),* clinging to worldly life *(abhiniveśa).*

Abhiniveśa is a very subtle, sensitive, interior hidden emotion. If this is understood properly, I would say that it is a stepping stone for Self-realisation; because birth and death are in the unknown region but the life in between is in the known. It is this known region that has to be known first, then the unknown too becomes known. If one begins to analyse the emotions affecting you from outside, then you can reason out the inner subjective emotions and come out of them also.

Actually, yoga is the only science that is learnt with emotional involvement. It deals with emotions and corrects the emotional defects and also shows the way for an emotional tolerance and equipoise. Patañjali is the only person who has said that the afflictions are the cause of emotions. The emotions are symptoms of afflictions. The emotional defects and intellectual defects are conquered when you attend to the physical body and mental states. Fear of death is the root cause of all emotions. Once stability is built up in body and mind, you will not be so much afraid of death. The conquest of the fear of death is possible through the intelligence of the heart. As a river takes birth and flows to meet the sea, we too move from birth to death like a river. This has to be realised not by logical dogmatism but by the intelligence of heart and emotional maturity.

– *I have the feeling that in the West, we suffer from different forms of emotional distress.* –

I do not think that emotion is a question of the West. It may be true that the fear complex is more in the West than in the East. For example, in the West if a woman marries, begets children and becomes fat, then she worries because she thinks that as she has become fat her husband may divorce her. Right?

– *Yes.* –

Similarly, with menopause the fear is that husband may leave the family and go after someone. Right?

– *Yes.* –

Such things are possible in western countries because the importance is given to external appearances. That is the way of living in the West. In the East, it has not reached to that extent. This is why it is called emotional disease and not an intellectual one. The hidden fear bothers everyone. Clinging to life is clinging to worldly pleasures and the hidden fear is that one may lose that pleasure.

When a woman becomes fat, there is a fear of divorce, which becomes a big question mark for women. "Oh! What have I to do, how am I to face, how am I to remain young and beautiful?" These unfortunate things lead to stress factors. If a man becomes fat he does not bother himself. He only charges the woman, as if he is perfect. These problems are created by society. No one sees the beauty of the heart. They love only the external appearances and not the inner beauty. Emotions like fear of divorce, fear of losing the family, are common in the West. Lack of emotional intelligence is the main reason for these. Horizontal development of intelligence is emotional intelligence. Technology and science cannot develop this. Manufacturing nuclear bombs is an intellectual development. Man has walked on the moon. It is an intellectual achievement. But has he come closer to his wife or wife to her husband? Do they come closer to each other? When they come closer and understand each other, it is horizontal intelligence or emotional broadness. The intellectual western growth is vertical. The eastern intellectual growth is horizontal. Asians are emotionally happy, but Westerners are not.

- *Sure, sure!* -

If the intellectual intelligence is from the head, the emotional intelligence is from the heart. The language of the heart is compassion, hatred, anguish, friendliness or love, and so on.

Studying academically to get a Ph.D. is a vertical intelligence of the head and living and communicating with men and matters is horizontal intelligence of the heart. Yoga helps us to blend both together. When a *yoga-sādhaka* blends the intelligence of the heart and head harmoniously, he is called a matured person. He is called a *prajñāni* – a divine being.[1]

In yogic texts we come across the word *vāsanā*. It means desire. Desires existed since eternity. Each action and each thought of ours leaves its impression and memory, which have their own tendencies and potentialities, and express themselves as *vāsanā* or desire. These impressions may be favourable or unfavourable. The unfavourable impressions such as anger, greed, lust, pride, envy, infatuation, anguish, are the ones that bring defects in us. These can be called as emotional distress. Similarly, there are healthy, favourable impressions and emotions, which bring a spirit of joy in us. If unfavourable ones make one desperate, favourable ones, inspire. Patañjali explains the favourable emotions in the first chapter, like friendliness, compassion, joy and indifference. These need to be cultivated so that one gets the emotional maturity. The unfavourable ones may grow like weeds or moss in water. They have to be controlled and got rid of. Patañjali uses the word *bhāvanā*. *Bhāvanā* means feeling. This feeling is very sensitive. The feeling comes with deep understanding and reflection.

[1] See *Aṣṭadala Yogamālā*, vol 1, pp. 169, and vol 2, pp.185

When the mother sees her baby, the milk flows from her breast though she does not think about it; it just happens. Does it not? This is *bhāvanā*. Patañjali wants this quality of emotion, which is pure. Similarly he wants the healthy emotions to follow *yama* and *niyama*. Do you think that these principles haven't got an emotional base? Can you be non-violent without love, without emotion, without compassion? Can there be contentment *(santoṣa)* without emotional satisfaction? Even *Īśvara praṇidhāna* is based on emotion. If we develop a tolerant mind and accept both favourable and unfavourable upheavals in life, real satisfaction is felt. This is *ahiṁsā* of mind.

- People have the belief that their existence is based on what they feel, or think they know. When you talk about the intelligence of the heart, this is something that they cannot rely on, as they believe their existence is linked to their knowledge or thinking brain. They live in an intellectual world and not an emotional world -

You are right. The intelligence undoubtedly exists in the head. The ego too exists close by. The intelligence of the head gets tainted with the ego. If it is a ripe intelligence then it brings humbleness. This real ripe intelligence is guided by the conscience. When the intelligence is guarded by the conscience, that person truly becomes a wise person. This is the intelligence of the heart, which is free from ego or I-consciousness.

Egoism - *asmitā* - is a defect, it is an affliction. It is partly an intellectual defect and partly an emotional defect. *Asmi* means "am", "I am". This is *asmitā* - full faith in one's existence. *Saṁprajñāta samādhi* explains four types of awareness. The first awareness comes through thinking *(vitarka)*, the second by reasoning *(vicāra)*, the third with bliss *(ānanda)*, and the last is of knowing the pure state of being *(asmitā)*. This *asmitā rūpa samprajñāta samādhi* is the auspicious state of *asmitā*. This ego which is very near to the core of the being is made pure and *sāttvic* through yogic discipline to witness its core. As long as *asmitā* is not purified or has not become auspicious, it is an affliction. When we get attached to the continuity of life and small self, it converts into pride or ego. This is the subtle psychology of the ego. When we fail in our attempts, watch the state of pride, which is negative. When we achieve or acquire something, observe the pride that leaves a permanent mark on us. We get attached to what we have. We become involved in it and like to preserve it, cherish it. This pride is *svarasavāhī* - the current of love of life. This pride attaches us to our life. Even wise men are not free from it. This pride or *ahaṁkāra* or ego is the impure *asmitā*.

Ahaṁ means I, and *ākāra* means shape. *Ahaṁkāra* is that in which the "I" expresses itself or identifies itself as that which belongs to it, or is near to it. The English language has no word for *ahaṁkāra*. When we say, "This is ours", we identify the "I" with what belongs to us. The belonging cannot be 'I'. This is mistaken identity. Even a learned person will have this misidentification. Therefore he, with all his knowledge cannot be free from ego or *ahaṁkāra*. He forgets that his intelligence is not "himself". He forgets that his intelligence is separate and different from his "Self", and therefore, at this stage, though he is near to "Self", he remains far away from "Self". For learned and wise people the Self-realisation can never get actualised or factualised, until they drop this subtle ego which misidentifies itself with the Self.

The moment one gets illumined by removing the veil of erroneous knowledge, the intelligence of the heart shines. The saints are free from ego because they remain one with the intelligence of the heart. The philosopher only philosophises, that is why he remains closer to the intelligence of the head. The intelligence of the head flourishes with ego, whereas the intelligence of heart flourishes with the feeling of friendliness and compassion. That is where the saint has his mind in his heart, whereas the philosophers, thinkers and intellectuals have the mind in their heads.

So the problem is not only with people like you, but also with all. Society can produce scientists but not saints. That is why I said that the vertical intelligence is growing because of advancement in science. But horizontal intelligence is fading because of want of humane feelings.

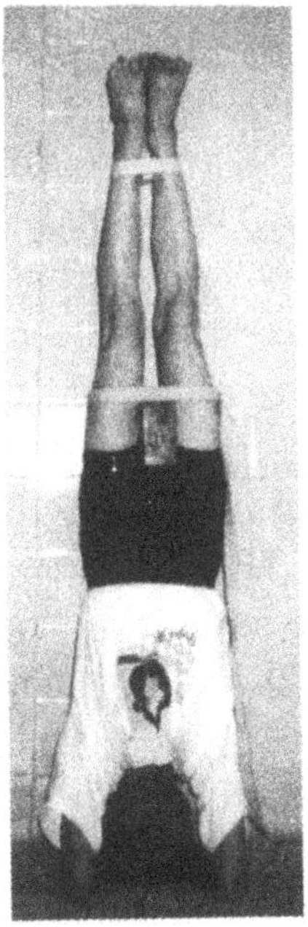

Plate n. 12 – *Sālamba Śīrṣāsana* using a brick between the legs

Q.- Yes, it is clear but very complicated and hard to accept, since we don't have the experience of intelligence of heart. But when you taught us *Vīrabhadrāsana* II, yesterday, you were talking about the auspicious feeling and I think that we have had a glimpse of it.

Good, that you felt it. Yes, that is correct. Well, even others had that experience. Didn't you feel that quiet auspicious moments yesterday in *Śīrṣāsana?* I kept a brick between the legs and the tailbone went in. At that time wasn't your ego auspicious? When the brick was not there you disturbed the tailbone with your egoistic intelligence. This is how you have to understand the functioning of the ego, which expresses through your action, through your posture and gesture as well. Someone may question how the brick controls. It happens because of accurate and precise adjustment, which changes mental attitude also. This way you develop sensitivity and from sensitivity you go towards purity. When Patañjali says, *sthira sukham āsanam*, one should know it is not just the stability of the body, but also the mind and ego. This brings the auspicious feeling.

– *Thank you, Gurujī. It is enlightening and at the same time exhausting. Should I switch over to some light question?* –

Yes.

Q.- Should the general practice of women differ to that of men?

The practice does not differ, but the approach might differ. If the needs differ, the purposes differ. Positioning the body accurately with the disposition of mind is to see that there is no difference between the outer body and the inner body. Basically there is no difference between the inner and outer body. But we create the difference. Men want to do yoga as an exercise and women to keep the nerves calm. If women want to do jumping during menstruation, will it make the mind quiet? When one is suffering from abnormalities, one has to stay in the *āsana*, and not do them as an exercise. The circulation has to supply, and the body has to be supplied with energy. Hence, staying with delicate adjustment is needed. These delicate adjustments are the qualities of yoga, as yoga means to bring the state of equanimity in body, mind and sou

During menstruation one cannot do the *āsana* such as *Ūrdhva Prasārita Pādāsana, Nāvāsana, Jaṭhara Parivartanāsana, Śīrṣāsana, Sarvāṅgāsana, Halāsana*, or hand balancing such as *Adho Mukha Vṛkṣāsana, Pīncha Mayūrāsana* and *Bakāsana* and so forth. If you raise the legs up and down in *Ūrdhva Prasārita Pādāsana*, then excessive bleeding takes place, during menstruation. The period may even prolong due to pressure on the abdomen. With this understanding, one has to do yoga without disturbing the natural cycles of the body. Many women do balancing exercises such as *Bakāsana*. When they do so, they strain the abdominal organs, as their arms are not strong enough to lift. This incorrect movement may rupture the organic body or the blood vessels. Men have strong arms, hence they use arms. Women need to learn to lift from the back of the arms and not strain their vital organs. So women should avoid such wrong practices.

Women have a double responsibility of working in the office as well as taking care of the house and family. Naturally the stress and strain on the nerves is more on women than on men. Men think that they are intellectuals, and think that they can solve all the problems with

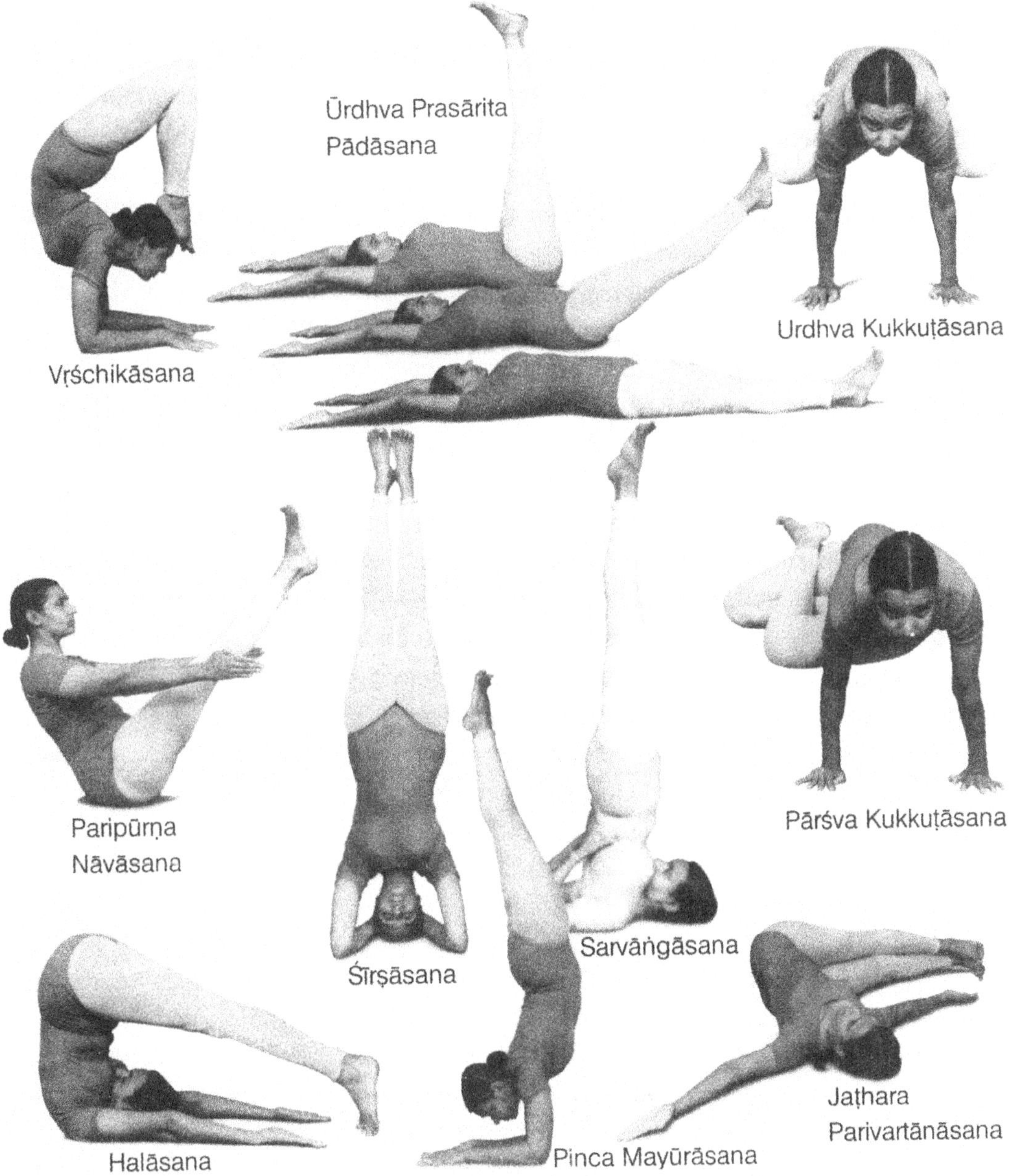
Ūrdhva Prasārita
Pādāsana
Vṛśchikāsana
Urdhva Kukkuṭāsana
Paripūrṇa
Nāvāsana
Pārśva Kukkuṭāsana
Sarvāṅgāsana
Śīrṣāsana
Jaṭhara
Parivartānāsana
Halāsana
Pinca Mayūrāsana

Plate n. 13 - Women's practice of inversions, balancings and abdominal *āsana* (not during menstruation)

their heads. They don't realise that the ego also is growing side by side with the intellect. They think that the emotions cannot touch them. But can friendliness be cultivated by the intellect? Can compassion come from the intellect? Does sexual joy come from the intellectual head? It is emotion, it is from the heart. Women have more access to the emotions. Men always think on an intellectual level and not on an emotional level. Women always speak on an emotional level. When marriages take place the intellect of the heart and the intellect of the head are brought together. It is the marriage between emotion and intellect. But often, as in your countries, these two entities are at loggerheads. In our country these two entities form a good combination. Here, we are taught both, the value of emotion and feeling, and the intellect. If emotion is *bhakti*, intellect is *jñāna*. If somebody suddenly comes to visit at your house, the man will say, "Let's go out for a meal", but the woman naturally feels, "No! They have come specially to visit us" and says, "I shall cook for them". This is how frictions or differences arise. Women see compassionately, "Let me prepare the food myself", but the man sees intellectually, "Why not go to a hotel and enjoy food there". In India, whatever people may say, a husband respects the wife and the wife respects the husband. You may not be knowing these things. Often in India a husband will never stand and argue with his wife. If he sees that his wife is losing her temper, he remains quiet. Or, if the husband loses his temper, the wife remains quiet and harmony is maintained. Indian culture allows room for one another. And that is how relationships are maintained. In your country, both argue and argue for nothing. Here, we know that if we keep on arguing, tempers flare up in the house. Either the man may go out for a while, or the woman goes to the kitchen to do cooking. You can see these things happening in the Indian home. You can see that though there are differences, oneness is maintained.

So, when you practise yoga, find out the *āsana* to cultivate your emotional life, which feed the heart more than the head. Sublimation of the ego is the key of yoga as the head is the seat of the ego.

- What do you mean by sublimation of the head? -

Sublimation of the head means making the brain an object. It should be transformed into a reflective process. Then the brain loses the power of pride and yogic practices help one to transform the seat of the brain – a storehouse of pride – into a state of compassion.

As the woman has the load of responsibility in running the house and family, she gets exhausted quicker than man. Keeping this in mind, we help them in removing their exhaustion and rejuvenating their system so that they are able to withstand the pressure with ease in all the household affairs. As man thinks that he is strong, our teaching will be in a way to test his power and to realise that he is not. This way we humble his ego and bring him closer to the heart. Thus we make a man or a woman understand the value of yoga according to their needs.

Q.- *Gurujī,* since you spoke about the difference in approach while teaching yoga according to the situation or the demand, I would like to know, what are the limits of therapeutic yoga?

First of all, the therapy is the side product of yoga. It is just a branch of the tree of yoga and not the main part of yoga. And there are no limitations in therapeutic yoga. The moment you say that there is a limit, then, it cannot be called a science. You have to explore. Treatment is nothing but exploration. The moment you start exploring, you come closer to the right type of treatment. If you cannot explore, you are not sure of the treatment, then you limit the science of yoga as you are limited in its knowledge. Therapy is just like the twigs of the tree. Therapy is like branches and twigs of a tree. Every twig is made to act for a right treatment. You may chop off a twig, yet it grows. In yoga too, each aspect, each movement is a twig and each twig of movement is an exploration. So, you should know full well how to explore yoga to accurately and promptly benefit the entire human system.

The practice of *yogāsana* makes one to learn and know the minutest part of each cartilage, the minutest part of each tendon, ligament and muscle. The mass is made to dissolve into minutest parts such as molecules into atoms.

For example, when you do *Vīrāsana*, what do you do to your ankles? It is like a mass, which you have to adjust and readjust and break the mass into atoms for the blood particles and life force to reach there. Here, when I use the word break, it means to dissect consciously each area of the ankles. Unless one learns and know all possible movements of the ankles, it won't be possible to bring life into the ankles. Similarly, one has to know all the possible movements of the body to endure or eradicate the diseases by applying various facets and directions in several *āsana* that work on the afflicted part. These various facets and movements of the body are the twigs of the yoga tree. As the twigs grow in different directions, one has to search and research the twigs of the *yogāsana* and *prāṇāyāma* tree for the benefit of the suffering people. Each *āsana* has several varieties. For instance, in *Vīrāsana*, there are several ways of keeping the feet, knees, ankles. You have to find out what happens if you turn the ankles one way, or if you stretch the ankles backwards or outwards or inwards. Feet move like twigs. The joints of the feet have that power to move in any direction, provided you know how to move them. If you don't know, then it cracks or breaks. As you trim the tree, you have to know how to trim the joints. Then the treatment has no limit. Then you know how to treat particular areas.

Similarly, how do you treat arthritis of the metacarpals? Unless and until you know the various movements and the range of movements of the wrists and palms, each and every knuckle in which direction they move, you cannot treat. Each joint and its movement has to become familiar to you. You have to see where the calcification is, in which position it can be dissolved and eradicated through blood current and energy flow. You have to search ways of movements with various adjustments. This needs a deep sensitivity in the teacher. In this way, you can enhance your knowledge and understanding for yogic presentation. It is same with *prāṇāyāma* too. So why limit it? Even to treat the mind, you need to know the other aspects of yoga as they are meant not only to stay within the limits of the body and mind, but to cross beyond them. As medical science progresses continuously, so also yoga is a continuous process. Only what we need is the application in practice and devotion.

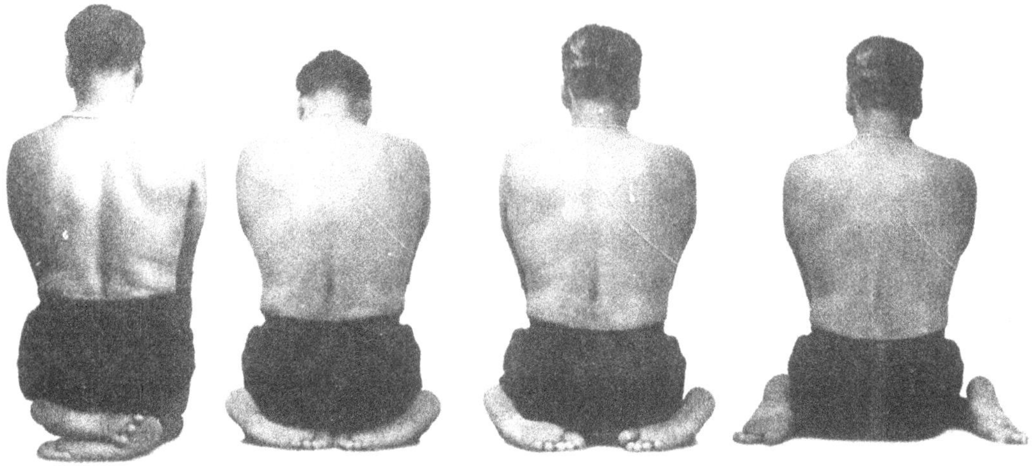

Plate n. 14 – Movements of the ankles in *Vīrāsana*

- Thank you very much, Gurujī! -

Thank you. I hope you have gathered some knowledge and understanding by throwing the light on yoga through these questions.

- Yes. -

God bless you!

A PATH OF EVOLUTION AND INVOLUTION*

Shirley: Ten years ago, I had the privilege of interviewing you accompanied by two Australians. This time, it's two Canadians and one Australian!

It is a good international exchange, I think!

Shirley: We have a lot in common – our countries are large, the population is small and spread out, and culturally we share a common heritage.

***Guruji*, it is ten years since the book *Iyengar: His Life and Work*[1] was published. I wonder if you would comment on the direction your life and work have taken since that book was published.**

Life moves dynamically, and changes do take place in each individual's way of living, practices, contacts, and so on and so forth; but I do not wish to add anything about me here, as the world knows me well. Instances in life are such that if we speak the truth it hurts a lot of people: that is why an autobiography is a very difficult thing to write. To be straightforward and honest means embarrassing many people. And that's why I don't want to complicate anything about anyone through an autobiography.

My pupils and people who have seen me, who have known me, who have watched the progress and who are well acquainted with the new thoughts taking place in me – they can certainly do more justice than I. So, it is for all of you to think of the coming generation to know that it is not just a book written for one time but putting the new thoughts and ways of my present approach to the subject which may be added with consultation and conversation with your peers. Many of you have seen how evolution in the field of yoga has taken me and you all

---

* Interview realised on 16th October 1995 at the Library of the Ramāmaṇi Iyengar Memorial Yoga Institute, Pune. The interviewers were Shirley Daventry French of Victoria, Marlene Mawhinney from Toronto and Kay Parry of Sydney, Australia. Published in *Victoria Yoga Centre Newsletter*, July/August 1997.

[1] Timeless Books, U.S.A., 1987

to higher dimensions, across different frontiers. So it is good, if someone like you could purposefully work for the future development of yoga. One should not write emotionally, but with facts.

Shirley: Perhaps this is something we could think about for your eightieth birthday.

Yes, whether it is the eightieth or ninetieth birthday God alone knows, but I have heard that *Iyengar: His Life and Work* may not be published again, and if it is not published, with the evolution you and I have made, naturally it is going to be a loss. Today, of course, most of my senior pupils have a copy of this book, but after fifteen or twenty years, the juniors who are interested would like to know something of me and my work after its publication in 1987. I think the Iyengar Yoga Associations all over the world can come together and bring out the new edition to date by comparing the notes, discussions and consultations.

Shirley: That book is such an inspiration! When young people read it – well not just young people – people who have only known you since you have been successful, when they see how you struggled in your early days it encourages them to keep going.

As my work in yoga goes on spreading, naturally people would like to know more and more about the founder. For example, I never thought *Iyengar: His life and Work* would be reproduced in India. The very first publication itself was a great achievement, because *Light on Yoga, Light on Prāṇāyāma, Tree of Yoga, Light on the Yoga Sūtras of Patañjali* have been published outside India. However, *Iyengar: His Life and Work* published by an Indian publisher was amazing to me because it is not a technical book – it is nothing except the life of an average man who did *sādhanā* starting from a rudimentary level to reach the present height.

- The life and work of one man! -

For me, it was something amazing as Indian publishers never thought of my classical books that are published outside India, but published *Iyengar: His Life and Work*, which is something astonishing. May be the coming generation will be inspired or interested to know more and more about my life. Hence, I feel that it would be a good thing if the Iyengar Associations and representatives compiled what they have collected up to date, my sayings and ways of conducting, my way of advice in the classes, the guidance that I gave would act as pillars of encouragement for the new generation to pursue the art.

- There is so much more now. -

Well I would be happy if others could bring out in case the present publishers do not bring out.

Kay Parry: That's a task for us!

With due respect to those who do work to compile with new and additional thoughts, I would be very happy to go through the compilation and give my suggestions if somebody wants to publish it.

Shirley: Sir, Geeta talked to us yesterday in the question and answer period about our responsibility as your students to make sure it is known that your work is spiritual yoga...

It is true. Probably God did choose me to go deep into the study of the spiritual ground and aspects of *āsana* and *prāṇāyāma* and prove the divineness in them, but it is taking time for people to realise the spiritual value. Even today I explained the higher values of *āsana* by the authoritative words of the *Yoga Sūtra* alone. How much attention he has paid to each and every part of human growth from body to the soul is amazing. He has not left even the minutest points out. If you ask me I say, "All aspects of yoga are yoga" to experience the divinity in us. First, we have to learn not to demarcate art. Can you tell me when music is physical and when it is spiritual? When painting, what is physical and when does it become spiritual? People are creating barriers, frontiers, and we succumb to them. We have to break that frontier!

In *The Art of Yoga* I have clearly written that for the sake of convenience, the body has been divided into three parts: the gross body, the subtle body, the causal body. And it has got five sheaths: the anatomical, physiological, mental, intellectual and spiritual bodies. This is for the common people to understand of humanity as a whole by knowing its various parts.

Man the Unknown, is a famous book written by a Nobel Prize winner.[1] How many of us know the body? "Man the Unknown" means that the body, which is a part of man, is also

[1] Alexis Carrel, who won the 1912 Nobel Prize for Medicine & Physiology.

unknown. Yogis, knowing very well that many things of man remain unknown, presented the knowledge from the known to the unknown bringing to the surface layer after layer, by removing the veil of the sheaths which were covering the soul.

I have not read anywhere in the treatise that so and so is physical yoga, so and so mental yoga, so and so spiritual yoga and so forth. This is the verbal gymnastics of the intellectuals who started demarcating to show their intellectual superiority. I say there is no division at all in the subject of yoga. Patañjali speaks on the elemental body up to the non-elemental soul. Hence, it is possible that one can start from the periphery towards the core or from the core towards the periphery.

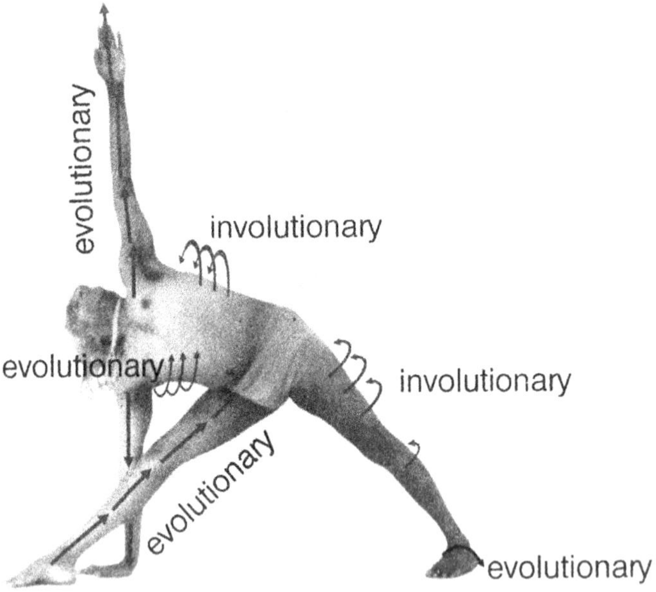

Plate n. 15 – Evolutionary and involutionary aspects of *Utthita Trikoṇāsana*

Now when one speaks of *jñāna* or the path of knowledge, can the path of knowledge improve without *karma*, without action? The more one purifies one's action with an honest approach and pure intention, naturally the better the knowledge flows. The more one cleanses the inner body, the more one understands and comes closer to the soul. Otherwise, how does one understand the soul? Tell me? Subjective experiences are quite different from objective words. How do we put the expressive, objective words to subjective experience? One has to work layer after layer to express the hidden knowledge. Today when you did *Utthita Trikoṇāsana* on the right side, I said energy and intelligence move out or evolve, whereas in the left leg they move inwards or involve. Similarly, the right hand has to follow the involutory process and the left hand the evolutory process. The right side of the trunk evolutes and left involutes. In an evolutory process, the expressive intelligence surfaces in the exterior. In an involutory process the flow of intelligence reverses. One has to find out where the evolution and involution meet. You can call the evolution as the active phase and involution the passive phase, since evolution expresses its progressive action and involution expresses the resolution of action to become quiet and passive. In that situation, when there is the evolutory process, the awareness –the light of the Self surfaces on all the frontiers of the body. At the same time one experiences the sensitive contact of the energy with the intelligence as well. In *āsana* practice, the *prāṇa* and *prajñā* have to reach every nook and corner of the body. In the involutory process, the same awareness gets folded towards the core. The *prāṇa* and *prajñā* reverse their flow from the frontiers of the body to the Self.

Body is the frame. We are not working on the actual frame, but we are working for the contents that are hidden within the frame so that the Self occupies and expresses that the content and the container are not divided. That's why one cannot divide yoga into various facets as physical, mental or spiritual. The content is unknown. The content is nothing but energy and intelligence, *prāṇa* and *prajñā*. Unless one is not in contact with the Self, the other contents or vessels are not felt, recognised or understood. There needs to be this contact *(saṁyama)* with the core of the Being. Otherwise the content in the container does not evolve. The medium between energy – *prāṇa* – and Self – *ātman* – is *prajñā* or awareness of intelligence. *Prajñā* connects the consciousness *(citta)* with the other contents of the body so that everything becomes absolute without any division, that's why it is called absolute consciousness or a state of aloneness. Here there is no division between body, mind, soul or the three sheaths of the body namely, gross, subtle, causal. Yoga teaches us to experience this oneness. As I said several times: we are expressing our inner hidden force through the expression of the body: Can a soul express without a body? Tell me. This much explanation is enough to understand the spiritual value of *āsana* and *prāṇāyāma* to guide the future yogic enthusiasts.

– Well, not in this world. No. –

If there is no cross in a church, would you call it a church? The cross is there; the outer frame is also there, which is known as the building. There is a cross inside which is known as the soul, and there is a building around it which is known as the body. These two have to be inter-linked to experience the unalloyed bliss. Divisions have to be shaved off, layer after layer, as you peel the skin of a fruit and eat the inner part – the content. Similarly you have to peel yourself from the skin to move deep within. What we are doing is exactly this – to come in contact with the content. We are peeling the skin so that we get the real taste of the fruit. That real taste is dynamic health, dynamic movement of life force. And that is what yoga teaches! As Geeta said to you: we have to announce what we have experienced to remove that misunderstanding, and these misunderstandings have to be rectified by all of us.

- We were talking about this yesterday, and we all feel we have to do what we can in order to stop this criticism springing out from total misunderstanding. -

Yes! When the *sādhanā* touches the heart, know well that there is an element of spirituality, otherwise we do not feel that inner presence. In the nineteen thirties, yoga was relatively unknown. My *guru*, Krishnamacharya, did not have many pupils, but he had a few who could take this subject, to reach the people. If we had not done that basic work of our *Gurujī's* teachings, *Gurujī* would have remained unknown to the world. In the nineteen thirties, we could count the *yogi* in India on our fingertips, but today it is impossible, because the zeal is there, but as the zeal is there unscrupulous people are taking advantage. Because average people have taken the burden of popularising yoga, some intellectuals might have been afraid that they may not be recognised; so they attack which is known as the best form of defence. Unfortunately, we have been forced on to the defensive. But the truth is different. So let us explain the truth.

At the end of the *Yoga Sūtra,* Patañjali says that through the practice of yoga, actions will be free from afflictions.[1] What a great thinker he is! He has spoken of the spiritual life, but he has said that when the afflictions are washed off, then there is an automatic cleanliness in the intelligence, purity in the consciousness and clarity in conscience, hence, there is illumination. That means all actions or *karma* are done not through dependence on books, words or mere logical inferences, but directly from the soul, which has not got even a tinge of taint.

It is very interesting to see what Patañjali says in the first and last chapters - *Samādhi* and *Kaivalya Pāda.*[2] When the practitioner refines his intelligence, his intelligence develops a special faculty of insight, or a truth bearing wisdom, or a highest state of matured wisdom that is called as *ṛtaṁbharā prajñā.* This wisdom cannot be gained or gleaned from books, testimony or inference. It is a self-evolved knowledge. This knowledge or *prajñā* is not tinged by any

---

[1] *Tataḥ kleśa karma nivṛttiḥ* (*Y.S.,* IV.30). Then comes the end of afflictions and of *karma.*

[2] *Ṛtaṁbharā tatra prajñā* (*Y.S.,* I.48). When consciousness dwells in wisdom, a truth-bearing state of direct spiritual perception dawns.

Śruta anumāna prajñābhyām anyaviṣayā viśeṣārthatvāt (*Y.S.,* I.49). This truth-bearing knowledge and wisdom is distinct from and beyond the knowledge gleaned from books, testimony or inference.

Tajjaḥ saṁskāraḥ anyasaṁskāra pratibandhī (*Y.S.,* I.50). A new life begins with this truth-bearing light. Previous impressions are left behind and new impressions are prevented.

Kṣaṇa pratiyogī pariṇāma aparānta nirgrāhyaḥ kramaḥ (*Y.S.,* IV.33). As the mutations of the *guṇa* cease to function, the uninterrupted movement of moments, stops. This deconstruction of the flow of time is comprehensible only at this final stage of emancipation.

emotion, prejudice, desire, will power or ego. It is totally devoid of impurities. Even the *guṇa (sattva, rajas* and *tamas)* cannot influence this *prajñā*. This highest *prajñā* remains entirely with the *ātman* all the time. This *ṛtaṁbharā prajñā* has no chance of fluctuation or modification. It is constant, ever fresh, ever shining. There remains no fissure in the consciousness that can pollute this *ṛtaṁbharā prajñā*. Time does not affect it. Our knowledge changes as the new findings eradicate the wrong knowledge, which is conceived by ignorance or perverted intelligence. But the knowledge that comes through *ṛtaṁbharā prajñā* does not get affected or changed. It is totally refined, filtered, nurtured and matured. A yogi whose intelligence is essentially filled with such *prajñā* has fulfilled his aim since nothing remains to be achieved. He is beyond time. We need the time factor if we want to achieve something or lose something. Here the yogi goes beyond it. So his living (life) moment to moment is clean, clear, pure and divine.

Patañjali defines: *yogaḥ cittavṛtti nirodhaḥ*, yoga is the cessation of movement in consciousness (*Y.S.*, I.2). Everybody quotes this *sūtra* and begins to talk of what yoga is, but what are the ways? Does anybody think about it? He begins the text with *ānuśāsanam* - code of conduct - and explains in detail in the second chapter what *anuṣṭhāna* is. *Anuṣṭhāna* is devoted practice. These two words, *ānuśāsana* and *anuṣṭhāna*, are very important as they show the way. What is the code of conduct in yoga? He says that the code of conduct in yoga is *yama, niyama, āsana, prāṇāyāma, pratyāhāra, dhāraṇā, dhyāna* and *samādhi*. So the *ānuśāsana* is explained much, much later, though mentioned at the beginning.

The problem is that in ancient times, the authors were explaining from just the beginning alone the final approach of knowledge before elaborating the subject matter further.

In olden days, this was the adopted formula. The authors used to give the conclusive values and then proceed to explain what the subject is, where it leads to, what the goal is and the way in which the subject is related to reach the goal. Within three lines they were giving a synopsis of their entire work, and later they were elaborating the subject. Accordingly, Patañjali concludes yoga in three aphorisms. First he says yoga is a codified discipline. He defines yoga as cessation of consciousness and in such a situation, the seer abides in his own grandeur. In other words, one lives in the abode of one's own Self when the waves of the consciousness are restrained. Do you mean to say that you can live in the abode of the Self at once by reading the first three lines? If that were so, then the whole book would have ended in three lines. They knew the aim and the way to reach the aim in order to have the vision of the Self. They could teach the means to touch the goal. From this, you have to imagine the intellectual standards then. Today's standard is not that high. So what we do is to go step by step from the perceivable things and then hop towards the goal. We need to see the means, which have been explained in depth. We do not go into the depth of the means. We do not think of what we have to learn. It is our responsibility to pay attention and follow thoroughly the means, the method, the way, the code of conduct given to us as *ānuśāsana* (discipline) and *anuṣṭhāna* (devoted practice).

In India we had to make people get interested in the field of yoga as very few were showing interest. In the earlier days I had to think of ways and work to make this subject educative and attractive. The question arose yesterday about *aṣṭāṅga yoga*. Myself and Pattabhi Jois both learnt under the same master, Sri T. Krishnamacharya. You have seen my film of 1938. It was my first film in which my *guru* also presented his practice. If you see the film again, you will know the method that was practised then as a mobile form of yoga. My practice in the 30's and today's Patabhi's teachings are not different. In those days my *Gurujī* was teaching youngsters in *vinyāsa krama* (sequential jumping), we were following the same. For adults he was giving static *āsana* and for youngsters, with *vinyāsa krama* to reach the *āsana* and then to come out of the *āsana* in the same form but in a reverse way. Why I left that method was due to the complaints of aches of fatigue on the body and mind. God guided me by sending me to Pune so early to face the challenges of elderly people then. Elders were not interested as they were exhausted in those fast movements. People of Pune were exercise-conscious and exercise-lovers. Pune was famous for wrestlers and martial fighters. Here you find more wrestling arenas than anywhere in India. Obviously, they were doing what you call push-ups. My jumping was more like push-ups for them, and they wondered why would they do yoga when they were already acquainted with such movements.[1] This opened my eyes and made me think of how to interpret yoga to fit into their way of life. If they had not raised their problems, I would have been teaching *āsanas* with *vinyāsa* like my colleagues. Though I do once in a while take sequential jumpings for the final *āsana*, yet I evolved the subject to suit various age groups and disabled people. Many of my *guru's* pupils, of my time never called on him after they began teaching. Perhaps I was the only one from the earlier group who kept contact with my *guru* until his last breath. So please know that my *guru* on the other hand appreciated my finer adjustments of the *āsana*. Not only was he appreciative of my finding the subtleties of each *āsana* but I was touched when he honoured me with a gold medal inscribed *Yogāṅga Shikshaka Chakravarti* in 1961. Regarding my colleagues they lost the touch of a creative mind and stuck to a routine that was taught in the 1930's. Pune opened my eyes because the people never accepted *vinyāsa*. They said, we are doing two thousand to three thousand *Sūrya namaskar* a day and we do not need this. That changed me. I respected their thoughts and I began to think of finding means not for muscle power but for sharpening the mind.

---

[1] See *Aṣṭadaḷa Yogamālā*, vol. 2, "*Vinyāsa Yoga*", pp. 245-253.

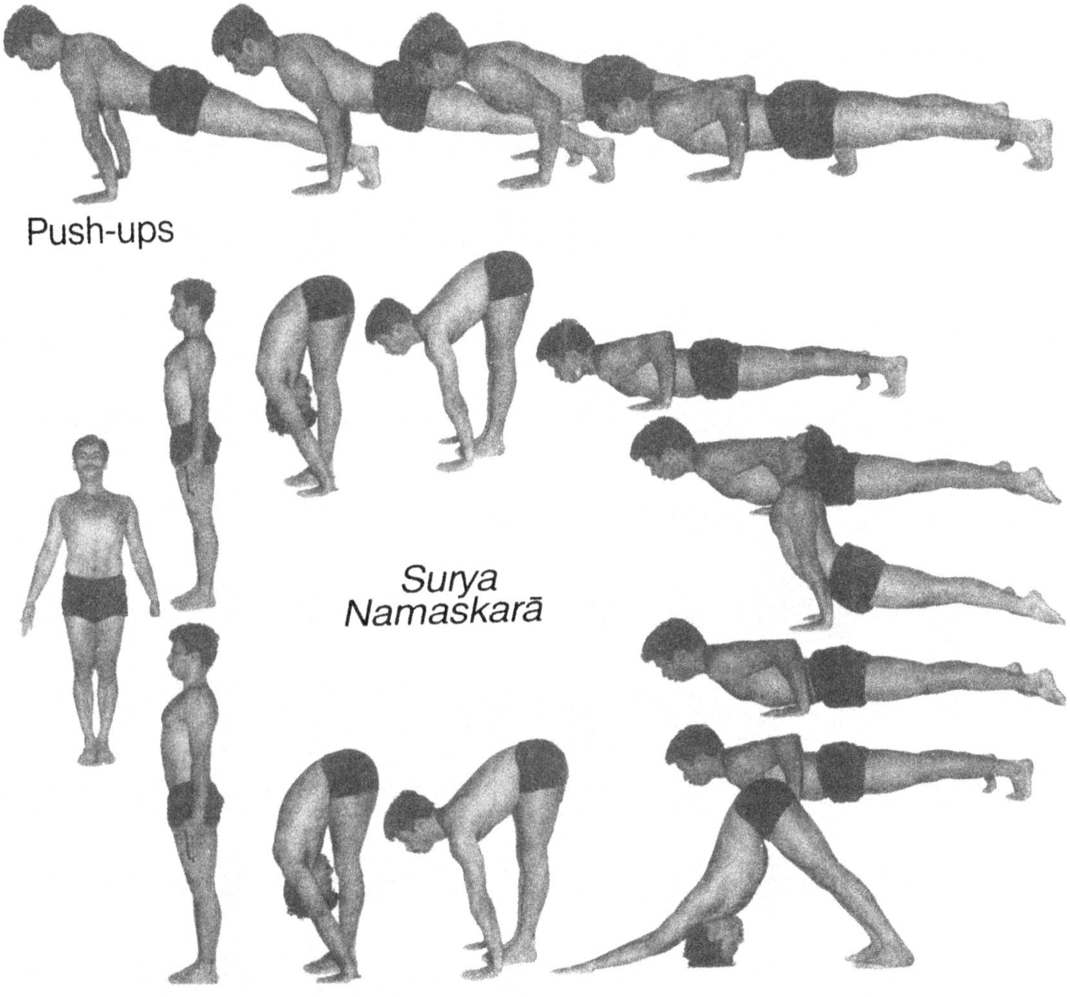

Plate n. 16 – Push-ups & *Sūrya Namaskar*

This brought skill in me to refine the art and you all have it now, which you have to stabilise and establish. Even if you cannot add, at least you can maintain it. If creation is difficult, can you not maintain at least what is given with a subtle touch? Think that way and work on it to establish that it is not just physical but has many things beyond it.

Shirley: Sir, the other day when we were here, in the library, you talked about students who practise very hard and they can't understand why they are still suffering and have pain. You said that their practice is vibrant, not illuminative. Could you speak about the difference between vibrancy and illumination?

It is said that man has the qualities of *bala* (power) and *ati-bala* (extreme power). Philosophically the *bala* stands for *tāmasic* and *rājasic* qualities, *ati-bala* for *sattvic* qualities. Yes, I did say that their practice is vibrant. It is the *rājasic* quality of nature. It is an expression of pride *(bala)* in one's self whereas illumination is a *sattvic* quality *(ati-bala)* which helps one to sublimate the pride.

I have already told you long, long ago, and even in the classes, that practice with discretion slows your movement. In *vinyāsa,* your body moves faster than your intelligence. Does your intelligence move so fast when you are jumping?

- No. -

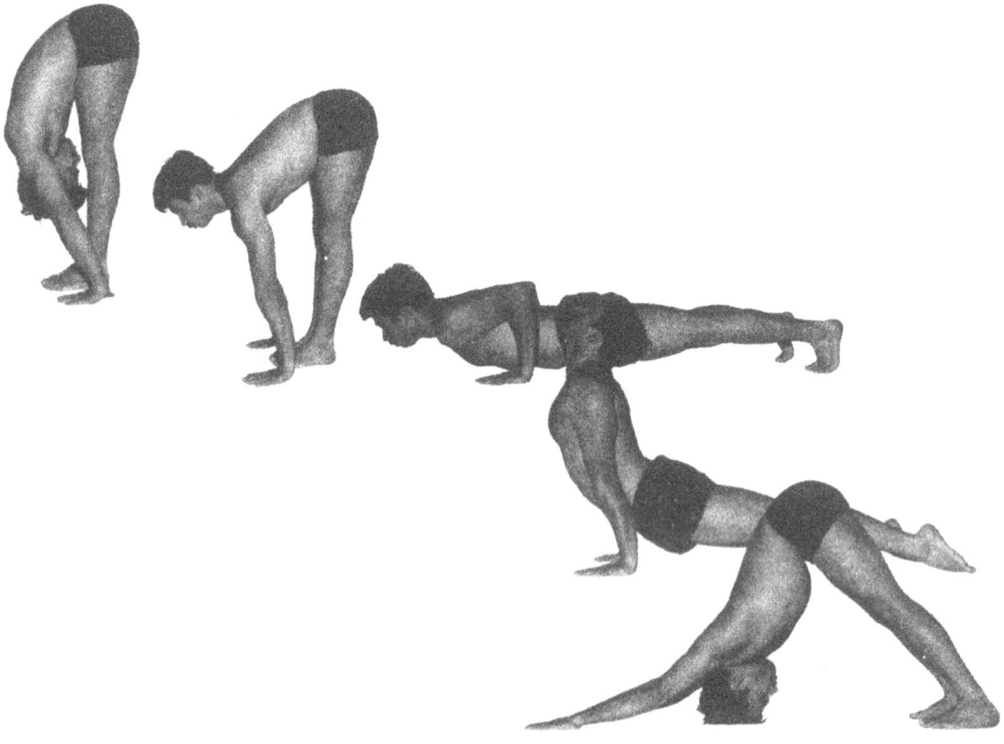

Plate n. 17 – *Uttānāsana, Chaturaṅga Daṇḍāsana, Ūrdhva Mukha Śvānāsana* and *Adho Mukha Śvānāsana*

If I ask you to do *Uttānāsana, Chaturaṅga Daṇḍāsana, Ūrdhva Mukha Śvānāsana and Adho Mukha Śvānāsana* fast, you just follow, isn't it? But can you inner-penetrate and build up the inner body?

- No. -

This is exactly what happens in *vinyāsa*. One sweats physically and gets excited. This makes one arrogant as if he has physical power but it does not illumine the practitioner. It is just a workout process. They don't allow the intelligence to sweat to penetrate inside. There is no looking in, in the *vinyāsa* process. In *vinyāsa krama*, does one know how the energy moves in the body? It is easy to get carried away with motion and not in the in-depth action.

Do you watch how the energy moves in the body? Do you watch the state of intelligence whether it is reaching the unknown parts of the body?

- *Occasionally!* -

Occasionally! It means 'yes' or 'no' for me. Now stretch your hands. Both hands like *Utthita Hasta Pādāsana*. See how the energy moves in your hands. Did you feel it when you were stretching or afterwards?

- *Afterwards.* -

Now slowly extend the hands without jerk or force and feel how and where the energy moves.

- *It flows deep inside.* -

This is how one has to notice the reflective action. These subtle movements of energy and intelligence will not be reflected in *vinyāsa krama*.

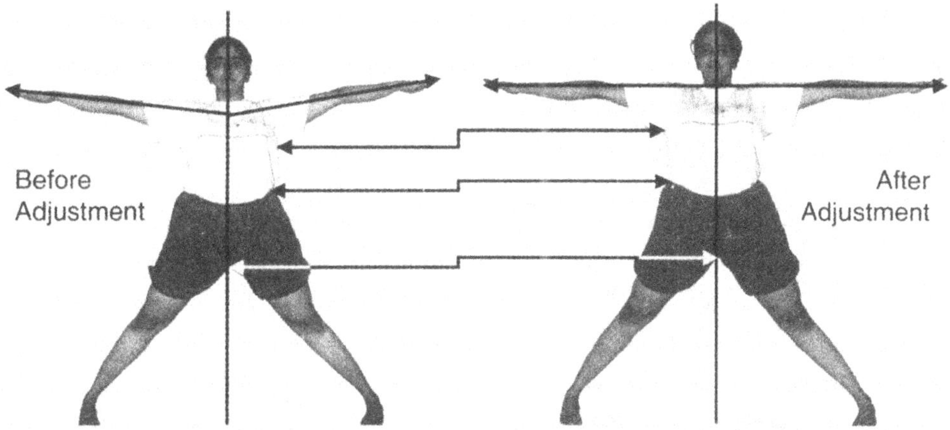

Plate n. 18 – *Utthita Hasta Padāsana*, with adjustment to bring changes in intelligence

You felt deep inside the stretch and flow of energy and intelligence. This is the lesson one has to follow in the practice. Without observation, practice is not a *sādhanā* at all. Bend your elbows slightly. What happened to the energy?

- It goes forwards. -

Now, like a filter paper, stretch up your arms slowly. See how much time the intelligence takes to feel the flow of energy. When you just stretch the body, the intelligence gets introverted. The body expresses itself with outward flow and the intelligence expresses with inward flow. It is neither physical adjustment, nor intellectual adjustment. And when discrimination and discretion are not there, is it yoga?

As you have done it, is the intelligence flowing evenly around the right and left hand? Understand how much time it takes for you to know that. You do not think, and so you do not feel. When I question, you become aware of it. Until then you don't. People want to show that they are working hard, and that is exhibitionism. Haven't you seen me? Find out each and every time when you practise, what mistakes you commit and what good things you bring in. Your intellectual sheath has to be like a mirror reflecting all these. The object has to be the in-depth study of the subject. In *sādhanā*, there has to be an interaction between you, your intelligence and your *āsana*. The doer, the instrument that does, and the *āsana* done have to be one. *Āsana* is the object and you are the subject. You have to structure the rightness of the *āsana* through your intelligence and receive the *āsana*. The body does the *āsana* but the doer is you. The intelligence being the connecting instrument between the doer and the body, the doer has to notice through his intelligence as a witness in the *āsana*. The doer has to sensitise the body. By doing fast movements, many things are left unnoticed.

Imagine that I take you on a round the world trip and from an aeroplane show you all the countries. Then would you say that you have visited and saw all the countries of the world? The aerial view does not take you to the heart of the city. You see the landscape. That is vibrancy; but when you see the land after landing, then you see clearly. This is the illuminative approach.

Earlier, my teaching was such that I made the newcomers to have this aerial view. I wanted them to know how the body can be utilised in the practice of yoga. Now, I ask them not only to utilise the body but to direct it so that it is under their command. The earlier process of my *Gurujī*'s teachings of *vinyāsa krama* is a demanding process and what you see in my teaching is a commanding process. When the students have not understood their own body, mind and intelligence, the teacher needs to ignite them. Mental discipline of the teacher is needed, so that the students learn to govern themselves. This process is the seed of evolution.

The first instrument, the body that is dull, slow, stupid, *tāmasic*, inert and insensitive is ignited by doing the *āsana* fast and quick, through *rājasic kriyā vinyāsa*. Once the body is ignited, then the process is reversed. We learn to connect the body to the mind, the mind to the intelligence and the intelligence to the seer. The intelligence enters and lights the unknown corners of the body in order to gradually reveal itself to the seer. This is the involution process. My practice and teaching are nothing but an illuminative *sāttvic* practice. For instance, while I give public demonstrations my attention is more on the external body, attracting people towards the presentation and not on how the inner body is touched. This type of presentation is an evolutionary subject, but when I practise, it is totally an involutionary subject. People can see only the evolution. They cannot see the involution.

– Right, it's an outward form when you are performing. –

We use the outer form, to inspire people and draw them towards the art. While practising at home, it is not exhibitionism but inhibitionism. This, one has to learn. In the class you are not exhibiting. You work on yourself for yourself by yourself. Today in the class, I choose the best body and the worst body in *Trikoṇāsana* to educate you all. The worst body presented better than the best toned body. That is known as right observation. With discretion we have to work, to learn. Today we are doing yoga not for the health of the body, but for the intelligence to understand the body. That is why I said to read the book *Man the Unknown*. Let me take you a little deeper. Do you know your cells? Do you know your circulation? Do you know your breathing processes? Fifteen breaths will have fifteen different movements. Are you doing fifteen breaths per minute the same way, or different ways? Do we know even that? Do the majority of people know that? Which part does each breath touch, which part inhales and which part exhales? It is not at all the same each time in each breath. The time differs, the place differs, the touch differs, the length, velocity and density differ. The yogis studied all this, and that's why they brought the science of *prāṇāyāma* for us to practise. They wanted us to study and observe the various sensitivities of our inhalation-exhalation for one minute or two minutes: where does it touch and what is its quality of touch? Where did it touch the first time? Where did it touch the second time? Where did it touch the third time, the fourth time? Put all the various cycles of breath together, and study. I presume that the yogis were studying and accumulating, and then they found the ways of connecting all these various movements of breath together and called it *prāṇāyāma*.

Similarly in the *āsana*, when you do it from one end to the other end, it is like a string. For example, in *Utthita Trikoṇāsana*[1] I watch from the left end of the foot to the right end of the

[1] See plate n. 3.

foot and connect them into a single string and stretch. This way I watch each part of the body, each limb, each organ and each cell. If you practise like this, then I say the real practice has set in, in you. Ripeness in intelligence has to set in. Otherwise it is just a manual effort. I am not denying manual effort. It is needed. You can't just sit and say, I am going to do *Vṛschikāsana*. To do *Vṛschikāsana* you have to know how you should create space within this body and the thirty-three spinal vertebrae. I showed you yesterday one *swāmiji's* photograph of *Vṛschikāsana* and people say, wonderful! But did you not see the compression of the spine and the collapse of the shoulders? Instead of compression, expansion and creating space demands discrimination.

See, this is *Vṛschikāsana:* compare this *Vṛschikāsana* to my *Vṛschikāsana.*[1] I am heavier than him. His ribs are predominant, sunk-in. See, where is my head, how my energy moves. See in the other, compression and flop, whereas my body flies in the air. That yogi may say, "I am perfect". Then which one is perfect? Tell me? Please do not think that I am being vain about myself. I am presenting the science of yoga and not myself.

- Of course, your āsana *is showing the maturity. -*

This way, learn to watch. Then you too may develop the quality of bringing the best in *āsana*. Again compare *Vṛschikāsana*. See how the energy is ascending, and how the calf muscles, the knees and the trunk express in these two similar presentations. Compare this flow here with my own earlier *Vṛschikāsana*. See this one, taken when I was 20. There is a definate evolution. Now you can see an elegance, there is a balanced geometric icon. This is the meaning of Patañjalis *sūtra; rūpa lāvanya bala vajra saṁhananatvāni kāyasaṁpat* (III.47).

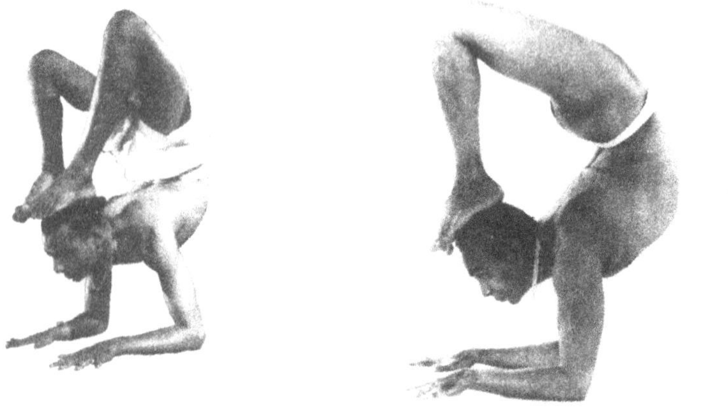

Plate n. 19 – *Vṛschikāsana* – earlier and later

[1]They were looking at the *āsana* in a yoga magazine

Does anybody observe such differences? Because one is done by a *swāmi*, it is considered spiritual, me being a householder, my presentation is seen as physical. This type of prejudice by so-called yogis and journalists is what I do not understand. People get carried away with the outer appearances. Fortunately, I do not wear saffron robes but I try to see whether I can progress further than where I am now.

Sometimes I allow the intelligence to be soft; sometimes I make the intelligence dynamically hard. Similarly, when the intelligence is hard, I make the *prāṇa* to be soft. When the *prāṇa* is hard, I make the intelligence *(prajñā)* soft. And I try both. I make both hard and observe what type of movement comes? I will never waste the energy of the body. The energy has to resist my intelligence to move and vice-versa. Is this not an inner awareness to remain in contact with the core? My intelligence is all the time on *prāṇa* and awareness as with the core of the being.

See my *Ardha Matsyendrāsana*. Can you see the vastness I create? Can you see how I am creating room for the muscles to remain in their places without distortion or contortion? See how *prāṇa* (energy) covers the frame. This is how I study and practise. When intelligence interpenetrates, what happens to energy? Does it outer penetrate? Then I try both ways. With outer penetrating intelligence, what happens to the energy of the body? I strike a balance. One cannot strike a balance till one studies and understands this outer and inner-penetration of intelligence and energy. Your intelligence may be aggressive; your energy may be regressive, or your energy may be aggressive but your intelligence may be regressive. Doing from the brain and repeating over and over again not knowing where the energy is, it appears as if one is struggling very hard. One cannot keep on struggling forever. It happens only in the earlier phases. Later one has to see that the intelligence and energy are balanced and moved in concord.

Kay: *Gurujī*, mostly people are introduced to *cakra* by intellectual means, but in Rishikesh this year you gave practical experience of the *cakra* through *āsana*.

Yes. I spoke. Have I spoken about those things again?

– A little bit. Not much. –

When?

– You talked about movement of energy but not calling it cakra. –

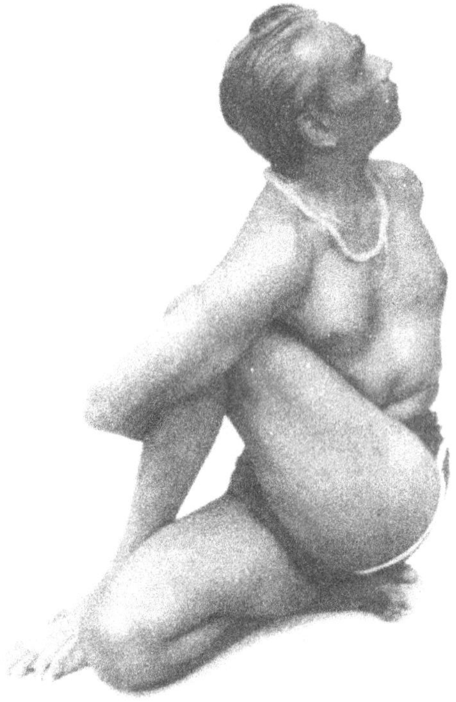

Plate n. 20 – *Ardha Matsyendrāsana*

In Rishikesh I had to speak about the *cakra* because the *sannyāsi* and *swāmijī* at Rishikesh said that I do not know what *cakra* and *kuṇḍalinī* is but was teaching only physical yoga. The moment I spoke on *cakra*, what did they say: "We never knew. We have never heard this". And I proved to them, that I also know about all those things. But I am not the one who uses such knowledge as saleable goods.

Kay: Of course, we understand the depth of your knowledge and we know that you teach from the sole to the soul... (Laughter) –

Yes, but I will not take it as a base every time to explain. In Rishikesh, I just spoke of how *cakra* can be worked. And I always say, *cakra* are within the spine, and plexuses are outside the spine. Only one cannot give a comparative study because they are subtler and closer to each other. On the other hand I say, 'as the body is the temple of the soul, the plexuses are the temples of the divine *cakra*.' As the body is the outer sheath of the soul, the plexuses are the outer sheath of the *cakra*.

Shirley: You made a very nice analogy the other day about a river – when the water is flowing in the river with twists and turns the water touches unevenly both banks unless there is damming or diversion, and then you talked about how we have to adjust the energy and consciousness to touch evenly on either side of the body as well as the front and back in twists, backbends, forward bends and inverted āsanas so that all should be like the balance of the scales of justice.

Even Patañjali indicates that you have to be like a farmer who builds dykes for making water to seep in before he breaks the dyke for the water to flow through to the other fields. You tame the river by building reservoirs. Here you tame your energy. *(Gurujī shows a book with photographs of his Guru Krishnamacharya performing yoga-āsana)*

When you speak of evolution, even from my *Gurujī's* presentation of *āsana* I can show you how I built from where he left off. See the *Utthita Trikoṇāsana* of my *guru*, do I do the same way or have I evolved from his presentation? See there is *Utthita Pārśvakoṇāsana*, ...*Bakāsana*, *Nāvāsana*. Do I do them like this or have I evolved those *āsana* further? At least you get an idea because you don't have a book of my *Guru*.

– Oh, yes! There is a vast difference. We see a perfect balance and evenness. –

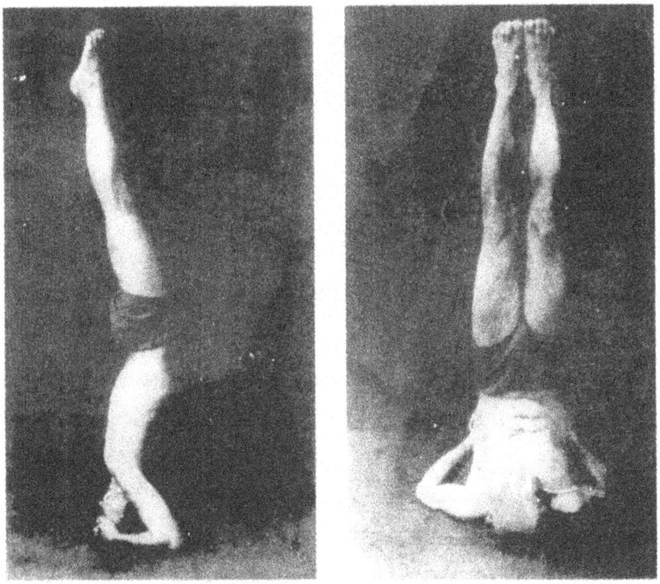

Plate n. 21 – Shri T. Krishnamacharya performing *yoga-āsana*

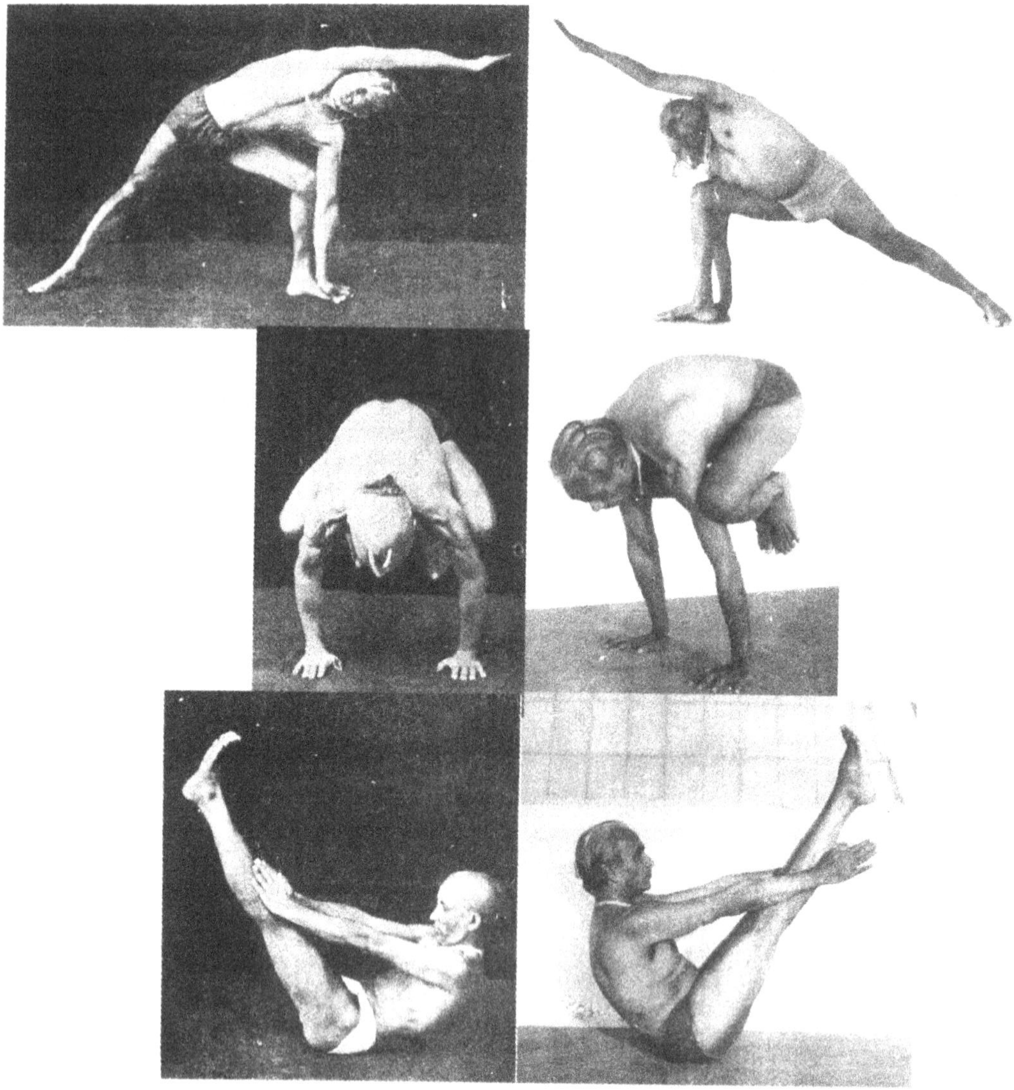

Plate n. 22 – *Utthita Pārśvakoṇāsana, Bakāsana, Nāvāsana* of Yogācārya B.K.S. Iyengar and Shri. T. Krishnamacharya

The base for my growth is my *guru.* In those days he was a top class practitioner. According to the time, he was the master. We had seen so many people but not one could present like him. Then I asked myself, is that the end or is there something further? I took his presentation as a starting point and proceeded further. Here is my *Jānu Śirṣāsana* and here is the other's *Jānu Śirṣāsana.* See the *Halāsana, Paschimottānāsana.* But method is not different. We can't say we are different. We follow his line only. Do you do *Pārśvottānāsana* like this? If I do like this, what will you say now?

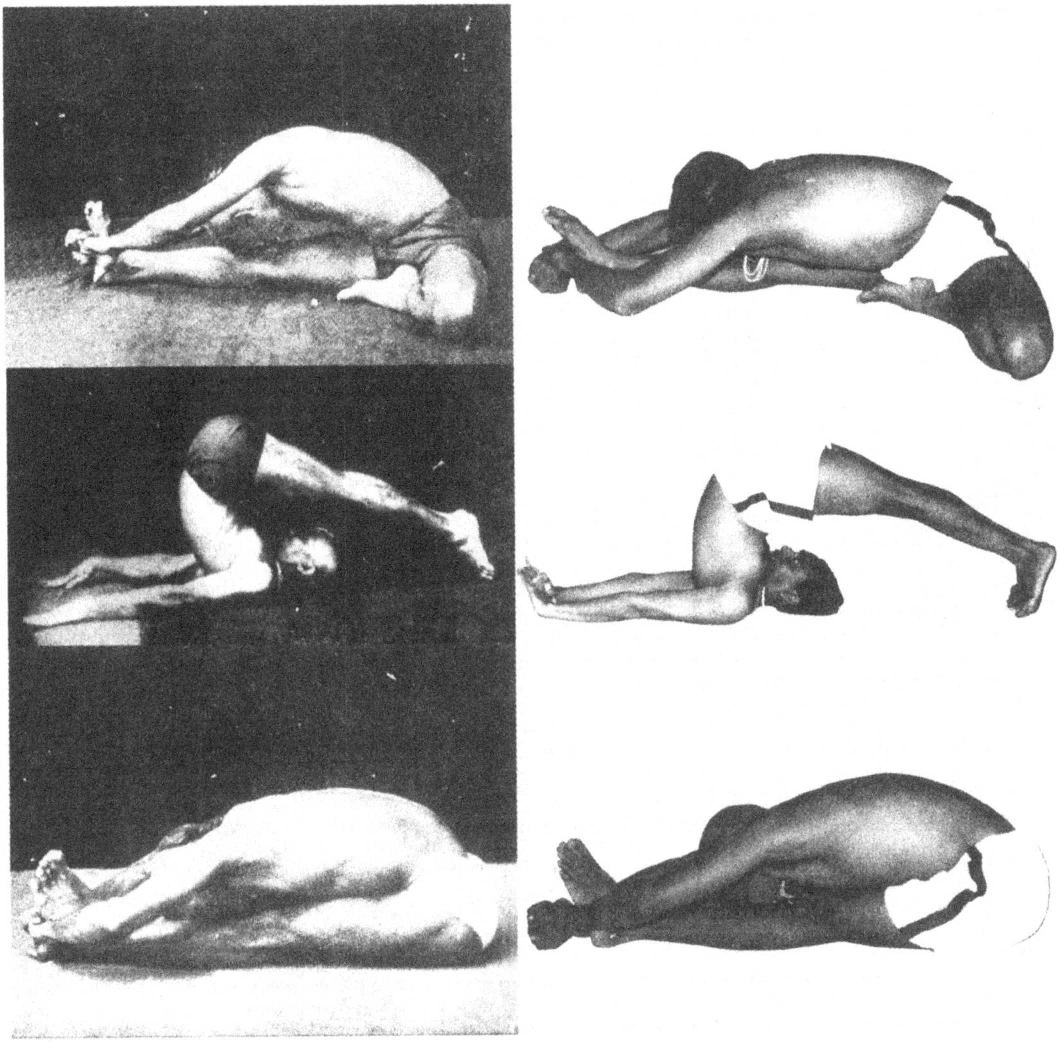

Plate n. 23 – *Jānu Śirṣāsana, Halāsana, Paschimottānāsana* of Yogācārya B.K.S. Iyengar and Shri. T. Krishnamacharya

Marlene Mawhinney: We know what you would say if we did like this!

Try to understand this evolution. I worked and trained to observe myself what is right and what is wrong. Where is the balance? Ah! Scale of justice. This is how I worked on balancing that scale of justice in *āsana*. This way I evolved. I involuted in order to evolve the subject. Now you see *Śirṣāsana* and compare. Do I do *Śirṣāsana* like this? Many of you do like this, even now.

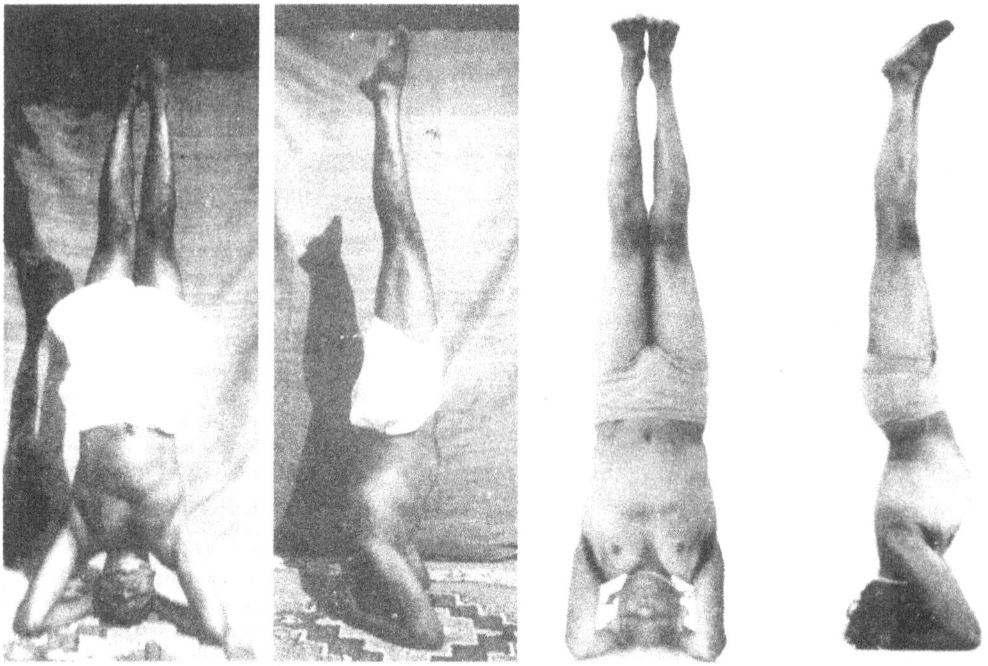

Plate n. 24 – Early and later *Śirṣāsana*

Thank God my *Gurujī* showed us the way. I thank God for having learnt from him. I have shown you someone else's *Vṛschikāsana* and my *Vṛschikāsana*. I have shown you my *Gurujī's āsana* practice and my *āsana* practice. This is the way to progress from where you are stuck. And if I had not come to Pune probably I would have practised and followed as I was taught in 1934-1936. So I am grateful to the people of Pune who demanded new things from yoga. Thanks to their criticism of yoga as exercise, I could take their criticism into an advantage to improve my practice artistically. I took their criticism as advice and worked to study the inner-body rather than for going towards muscle building. I developed for nerve endurance and intellectual growth and changed from physical building to nerve endurance, mental tolerance and trained the body to tolerate the timings by staying in each *āsana*.

Shirley: And this is what we see when we see in your practice now. –

Even today at the age of seventy-eight, I do one and a half hours of *Sālamba Śīrṣāsana* and *Sālamba Sarvāṅgāsana*. Even yogis say that one should not do more than three minutes I am doing this daily with no ill effects.

– A lot has happened! (Laughter.) –

Yes, a lot has happened in my way of practice. No more does my mind see whether I sweat or exhaust. I enjoy the juice *(amṛta)* that comes out of my practice.

Now have you understood how one has to work for one's evolution? With very little guidance of my *Gurujī* in *āsana*, I proceeded further. I did not stagnate his subject. But I dynamised it. So I ask you not to stagnate but to maintain the quality.

In *The Bhagavad Gītā* Lord Krishna has said to do well what you know, and not to worry about the criticism of others. Let me show you in the *Bhagavad Gītā* what I wanted you to read. *(Gurujī gives a copy of the Gītā to Shirley and asks her to read out loud.)*

Shirley: *"In this path no effort is ever lost and no obstacle prevails. Even a little of this righteousness, dharma, saves from great fear, no step is lost, every moment is a gain, every effort in the struggle will be counted as a merit." (Bhagavad Gītā, II.40)*

Is it not enough for you to get confidence in what you are doing? What more proof do you want, when the scriptural authority says so? Is it not an *āgama pramāṇa?* Now remember that even if you are doing *āsana*, do not bother about others' criticism. Are they better than Lord Krishna? The others are *yogī*, whereas Lord Krishna is a *yogeśvara*. You may be knowing the difference between *yogī* and *yogeśvara*. We are all *yoga sādhaka* but Lord Krishna is the *Yogeśvara* – the Lord of Yoga. So, whose word has more weight? Ours or His?

– *Of course, His.* –

Shirley: Sir, with your Indian students, do you find the same mind-body split as in the West?

Fear swallows the East, pride and power swallow the West. There is only one difference between the East and the West. The intelligence of the Indians is mostly emotional, not intellectual. And the Western mind is less of emotion, more of intellectualism. And that's the difference.

Shirley: How does this affect their practices?

The East doesn't use their head, and the West doesn't use their heart. *(Laughter.)* You use your head, they use their heart. If the heart of the East and the head of the West join together, then probably the practice of all will be quite different. The Asians do with feelings whereas the

Westerners calculate and don't reflect. The Asians will not be thinking of what words they should use; intellectually they remain silent but consciously they are open. Yet without intellectualism one cannot bring attention. In Asians awareness will be there, but attention will not be there. In Westerners attention will be there and not the awareness. This is not a scale of justice. A scale of justice awareness and attention should be equal everywhere.

Shirley: That's one of the things we learn from coming to Pune to study and seeing the difference in India... –

Indians work from the back brain and Westerners work from the front brain. Indians look from the back brain, and don't use the front brain at once, whereas Westerners work from the front brain and don't use the back brain to feel what comes from action. This is the difference.

Shirley: Well that explains another statement that was in the *Haṭhayoga Pradīpikā* that Westerners want to make sense of everything, but Asians accept mystery as a fact. Would you say that is true?

The question of mystery does not arise. You have to understand in which situation they spoke and in what frame. We accept the spiritual life as a fact; for you, it may take time to understand and undertake the mode of the spiritual life. We do not think there is an agent between the spiritual and the mental body, what you call "psychic force" or "psyche". We don't use the word psyche; we say it is a direct path to contact the Self. You say there is a medium and we don't accept that.

It appears that the spiritual life is a mystic life, but it has a practical way. As it is difficult to explain one terms it as mystic, but it is not. One can speak about Self; one can explain about the Self, but one cannot explain the experiencing state of the Self. One can explain pain, one can explain pleasure – but the actual experience of pain, experience of pleasure is not the same as you express it. Even the word happiness is a mystery for many. Therefore, one can understand why the word Self or Soul remains a mystery.

Kay: Most of the students only hear from you through newsletters. Is there anything you would like to say to our communities?

My friend – everybody asks the same question. There is nothing for me to say for the community. Just now I quoted from the *Gītā*: the more you do the better the understanding comes; but correct practice comes with right approach and correct discrimination, then the light will come on its own. Now I am soon planning to present the depth of my experiences to all of you in the *Aṣṭadaḷa Yogamālā* volumes to know more of yoga.

Shirley: It's wonderful how the network in yoga has grown in fifteen years or so since Newsletters started on yoga and how we are sharing it. –

Yes, newsletters and network on yoga give a chance to have a comparative study which is important to develop both intellectually and practically. If you strike two stones there is light. Exchange is growth and so we have to think constructively, but not to oppose each other for criticism's sake. As I said in the class, this high-tech of mine sparks the pride in many. So my advice is that all of you should cultivate a humane quality to get a healing touch. Technique with a healing touch is the quality we all need to learn to be true in our yogic practices.

Marlene: Those of us who have felt it know... –

Yes, you have felt, that I know: but the world will not know. I am not speaking for others, but for my own students. When I have got the healing touch through yoga, do you mean to say you cannot get that healing touch in your own presentations? That's what Patañjali said, that techniques with friendliness, compassion, gladness, and when required by the *sādhaka*, indifference[1]. Now do *Marīchyāsana* III[2]. Remain like that and move the thoracic dorsal spine to touch your sternum and feel your armpit. What happened?

– *It comes alive.* –

So this is healing. See whether there is a nourishing feeling in the healing touch. What you are doing; did it nourish you? This comes back to your earlier question: many practise vibrantly and do so repeatedly, but is there a nourishing feeling of the healing touch in such practices, is the question mark. As one says, "know thyself", we know the world, but do we know

[1] See *Yoga Sūtra*, I.33.
[2] See the author's *Light on Yoga*, Harper Collins, London, for a description of this *āsana*.

ourselves? So learn to get this nourishing feeling, exhilarating feeling, then you begin to know yourselves and learn how to exactly heal a person. This is what I want my pupils to learn, and not to depend upon techniques only.

In the early days I too was showing off. I think I have given hundreds and hundreds of demonstrations. I do not know if others have given so many publicly. My *guru* made me demonstrate publicly two or more times a day. Then I had to learn to do solo: one man on the platform like a concert artist. Who can do that today? It came with me, and it may go with me. I don't blame myself for that, but today you can give performances in groups but singularly you cannot. You cannot give three hours' performance non-stop. But I have kept people spellbound for three hours. You have seen my performances. I did this because I needed to attract more and more people towards yoga. And I did it, and am happy.

– It worked! –

It worked. So I say to you people: once in a while for your own students, your own group and association, call senior students for a demonstration, and let the juniors see. Let the juniors do one day, and let the seniors observe. Inter-exchange. Then you see, when you did it, what did you miss. When they did it, what was new. If you catch that, it becomes education. There is plenty of room for education. At my time there was no room for education, or for exchanging views. I went ahead and my colleagues remained static. So I could not accept them, they could not accept me. I built up cell by cell, what is right, what is wrong. This is how God blessed me to do the *anuṣṭhāna* of yoga and I am sure that God will bless you all if you work the way I did so that you feel its good effects and act as messengers of yoga.

Shirley: Thank you Sir!

YOGA PRACTICE NEEDS WILL POWER AND DISCRIMINATIVE POWER*

In August 1996, Yogachārya Shri B.K.S. Iyengar, Gurujī, *was talking to some senior pupils at the Ramāmaṇi Iyengar Memorial Yoga Institute, in Pune, India. Questions were raised by the pupils to which* Gurujī *responded.*

Some of Gurujī*'s senior pupils from the U.K. approached him and interviewed asking for clarity.* Gurujī *replied with patience and cleared the doubts.*

Gurujī *and Shri Pattabhi Jois, both learned yoga under the guidance of the late* Yogachārya *T. Krishnamacharya.* Gurujī*'s teaching is recognised by his pupils as* "Iyengar yoga." *The method of Shri Pattabhi Jois is recognized as* "aṣṭāṅga vinyāsa yoga."

Q.- Though you and Pattabhi Jois learned from the same *guru*, why is there a difference in your methods?

It is a fact that we both learned from the same *guru,* and therefore I do not think there are differences. He stuck to *vinyāsa krama* and I to the alignment of the intelligence in the *āsana.* I never wanted my pupils to call my method "*Iyengar yoga*". Yet they continue to do so. For me, yoga is yoga. In yoga, individuality has no accountability. Only the subject of yoga should be held in high esteem. Yoga is universal. Even Patañjali, who codified the 'yoga' that had been practised and taught by the sages of yore, does not call himself its originator. Maybe Patañjali's followers might have "named" him so, as it was compiled by him.

My *guru,* Shri T. Krishnamacharya, made us do a lot of jumpings, known as *vinyāsa.* One may ask, what are "jumpings?" Let me explain. As in *prāṇāyāma, dhāraṇā, dhyāna* or *samādhi* there is *sabīja* (with support) and *nirbīja* (without support) forms, so also in the practice of *āsana,* there is the *savinyāsa* and *avinyāsa* systems. *Savinyāsa krama* is a sequential movement to go into a final *āsana.* For example, take *Paschimottānāsana.* The *savinyāsa krama* is like this: it begins with *Tāḍāsana* or *Samasthiti,* then comes *Uttānāsana, Chaturaṅga*

---

* This interview was taken at the Library of the R.I.M.Y.I., Pune, by senior pupils, on August 1996.

Daṇḍāsana, *Ūrdhva Mukha Śvānāsana*, *Adho Mukha Śvānāsana*, *Lolāsana* and the main *āsana*, *Paschimottānāsana*. Then to reverse back to *Tāḍāsana* from *Paschimottānāsana*, one is made to go back to *Lolāsana*, *Chaturaṅga Daṇḍāsana*, *Ūrdhva Mukha Śvānāsana*, *Adho Mukha Śvānāsana*, *Uttānāsana* and *Tāḍāsana*[1]. This is *savinyāsa krama*. This *vinyāsa krama* is smoothly connected to the main *āsana*. Sometimes my *guru* would sequence the standing *āsana* and link them with jumpings. He would link forward extensions with backward extensions and so on. Sometimes he was demanding any *āsana* any time with or without *vinyāsa*. Sequences of programmes as methods were not given regularly, however they were there. Demanding any *āsana* in an unsequential way is *avinyāsa krama*.

As long as I was under his guidance, he never mixed the *āsana* practice with the *prāṇāyāma* practice. He always kept the practice of *prāṇāyāma* separate from the practice of *āsana*. He did not teach anyone *prāṇāyāma* before they mastered *āsana*. Only in special therapeutic cases he used to combine the techniques of *prāṇāyāma*, including *Nauli*, *Uḍḍiyāṇa*, *Trāṭaka* (gazing) and *Bhastrikā* in specific *āsana*, but not in all the *āsana* and never all the time. He used to introduce these things when required as per the condition of the patients, and never for healthy people. All these were his facets and ways of practice. As *Gurujī* worked, I also worked on the *āsana* along with *Nauli*, etc., which many of you have seen in the 1938 film[2] with my *Gurujī* and my sister.

I won't say that the difference in methods is to show individuality. I progressed in my own way to reach the core of the being as well as the core of the subject.

Q.- But is this the right way of doing the *āsana*? Can one introduce *Uḍḍiyāṇa* and *Nauli* in between the *āsana*?

I am not a judge to give a judgement. It was in the experimental stage and my *guru* might have been working to get a feedback by introducing these. One should know that in those days yoga was not as popular as it is today. The students/practitioners were few, so chances were taken to study the consequences. Methods were dropped when found not congenial. *Gurujī* too dropped this method at a later stage. These days people go in for some excitement in yoga and *Nauli* is one that creates excitement. Actually, the *Haṭhayoga Pradīpikā* explains that *Nauli*, *Dhauti*, *Basti*, *Neti*, *Trāṭaka* and *Kapālabhāti* are not part of yoga but are known as *ṣatkarma;*

---

[1] See *Aṣṭadaḷa Yogamālā*, vol. 2, pages 249-253 for illustrations. The only difference that you may find between this *vinyāsa krama* and the ones described in volume 2 is that in volume 2 *Ūrdhva Hastāsana* is included after *Tāḍāsana*.

[2] It is now available on videotape.

cures for certain abnormal diseases. So it is yoga therapy and not a yogic discipline[1]. Only *Uḍḍīyāna* is introduced as *bandha* in *prāṇāyāma*.

But one should know what perfect health is and then learn the proper way of doing *Uḍḍīyāna* and *Nauli*. Not many people have the patience to wait and build up inner strength in order to learn these complicated things. People want everything instantly like an instant coffee. My advice is to first build up strength in the body, have a control of the breath and develop stamina in the nerves through the practice of *āsana*. Thereafter learn certain simple but vital *prāṇāyāma* such as *Ujjāyī*, *Viloma*, before learning *Nauli* and *Uḍḍīyāna*.

– *What you say is true, because some women did such things like* Utthita Trikoṇāsana *and then* Uḍḍīyāna, *then the next standing* āsana *and again* Uḍḍīyāna. *Then they developed problems like leucorrhoea, heavy bleeding and other gynaecological problems.* –

I do not know how this type of practice came into existence. I have not seen my *guru* teaching like this. So I do not know how it is in vogue. In my experience I feel that *Uḍḍīyāna bandha* is not harmful compared to *Nauli* provided they do not tense their throat and shrink the chest while doing *Uḍḍīyāna*.

It is better to practise *Uḍḍīyāna bandha* separately. If one's mind is halfway in *Trikoṇāsana* and halfway on *Uḍḍīyāna*, how can one do justice to both? When a beginner has not scratched the subject, does he/she know ever the correct *Utthita Trikoṇāsana* or correct *Uḍḍīyāna bandha?* What benefit will come if incorrect practice is done? Do they have sensitivity to know exactly where and how the grip on the abdomen should be? Have they studied what is the connection between the standing *āsana* and *Uḍḍīyāna?* There should be a real cause for doing such practice; otherwise it becomes 'mad' practice. Let them refer to *Haṭhayoga Pradīpikā* again.

I feel that many practise *Uḍḍīyāna* and *Nauli* thinking that their *kuṇḍalinī* will be awakened. On the contrary, they suffer from wet dreams, looseness in the abdominal organs and prolapse of the uterus. By such practices, women develop menstrual problems, like a heavy flow or irregular periods with spotting. When my *Gurujī* was teaching, very very few women were doing yoga. As far as I know, he never asked these women to do such things.

---

[1] *Medahśleṣmānivṛtyarthaṁ ṣaṭkarmāṇi samācaret /*
anyathā nācarettāni doṣāṇaṁ samatāyataḥ //

(*Haṭhayoga Pradīpikā*, II.21)

When fat or mucus is excessive, *ṣaṭkarma;* the six cleansing techniques should be practised before *prāṇāyāma*. Others, in whom the *doṣas*, i.e. phlegm, wind and bile, are balanced, should not do them.

Dhautīrbastī tathā netī trāṭakaṁ naulikaṁ tathā /
kapālabhātīścaitāni ṣaṭkarmāṇi pravakṣyate //

(*Haṭhayoga Pradīpikā*, II.22)

Dhauti, basti, neti, trāṭaka, nauli and *kapālabhāti;* these are known as *satkarma* or the six cleansng processes.

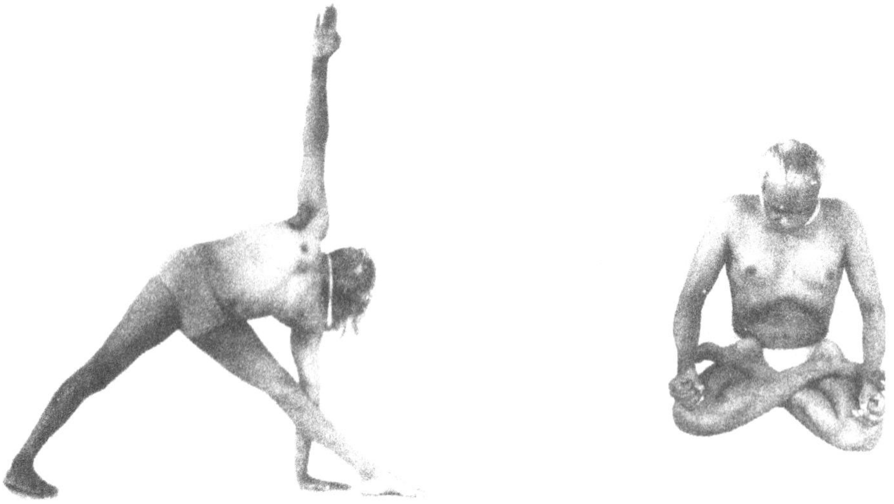

Plate n. 25 - *Utthita Trikoṇāsana* and *Uḍḍīyāna Bandha*

For *Uḍḍīyāna* one needs to establish inner contact with the abdomen. The grips should not go wrong. Tension on the cells of the brain should not be felt and the chest box should not be narrowed. In order to do this well, attention and caution have to go together. Do we not demand attention in standing *āsana?* Do we not ask to keep even flow of attention everywhere? It takes time to learn and adjust. That is why we ask you to stay in *āsana,* to feel the body, interaction of body-mind, interaction with breath and mind, breath and nerves, involvement of intelligence and awareness as well as your presence of consciousness everywhere as a witness in each *āsana.* When you do one *āsana* and one *Uḍḍīyāna* and *Nauli,* what is the connection between that *āsana* and *Uḍḍīyāna* or *Nauli?* How can these co-ordinate in harmony?

- They keep on doing... -

I feel it is dangerous to play with the nerves like this. Know that it is not from my *guru,* hence no comments from me are necessary.

Regarding jumpings, *Gurujī* himself never did them but made us do them. Youth needs fast, vigorous, dynamic, powerful movements and strength. Hence, it is all right for them but not for elderly people.

Actually, one has to see whether one is practising just for movement or to organically penetrate. One has to watch whether the vital energy is reaching everywhere. Those who do not know the depth of penetration, they do as keep-fit workouts. Doing for keep-fit purposes is only pride. It is like "all smoke and no fire."

- Yes, it does not ignite any intelligence. On the contrary one invites problems. -

Yes, it is the ignorance of the practitioners. They do not know what problems are waiting for them. Yogic practices need discrimination. They are to be practised to eradicate the impurities for the right knowledge to dawn[1]. One has to help those who are suffering, guide them in the right direction.

Q.- Did you change the method?

How can I change the method? If I change the method, then I cannot call my *guru* as my *guru*. He gave the foundation and asked us to evolve. That progression is not the change of method. How can I change the method? If I say that, then it is my stupidity and pride. I have said that our *guru* taught us one method, jumpings. He taught another method without them. The base for my practice is what my *guru* taught me. From that base, I evolved to get the alignment of the body; extending the intelligence in par with the stretch of the body evenly and then making the consciousness not only to reach the remotest areas of the body but spreading it evenly in all the complicated *āsana*.

If one continues to do the fast movements, the power of the body fades after some time and intelligence too loses its awareness. One does not realise which way the energy is sucked and how exhaustion sets in. One has to question oneself whether yoga is meant for rejuvenation or exhaustion.

Recently, medical science has come out with the name "chronic fatigue syndrome". Those who combine things as I stated earlier, suffer from this type of fatigue. Therefore, it is for them to discern and not me. How can I help such fanciful people in yoga who complain and keep repeating the mistakes?

Yoga is certainly an ancient subject, but it is not a stale subject. Life is not stale. As one squeezes the fruit to get the juice, one has to draw the juice from one's practice. Know that yoga cannot be done without tasting the flavour that is generated by the practice. As one practises, one goes on improving. I too did fast, dynamic movements, but I began observing what I was missing in such a practice. I found the missing points and linked them, when I thought of alignment. I learned action, observation, absorption and through absorption, readjustment of action for re-absorption. That is how I learned right alignment, precision and rejuvenation.

---

[1] *Yogāṅgānuṣṭhānāt aśuddhikṣaye jñānadīptiḥ āvivekakhyāteḥ* (*Y.S.*, II.28). By dedicated practice of the various aspects of yoga impurities are destroyed: the crown of wisdom radiates in glory.

Āsana is not an exercise, but if it is done with the combination of jumpings, then it is purely on the physical level. Please know that there is a lot of difference between *āsana* and other exercises. *Āsana* acts mostly on the organic body, and not on the skeletal body. *Āsana* develops organic or physiological body, psychological aspects of the mind and hence they are not to be called exercises, but positionings.

People these days have become health-conscious, but only work on the keep-fit basis. They enjoy heavy breathing, perspiration and exhaustion. They do not want to work the body with a conscious mind. When I use the word "conscious", I am indicating that we have to learn to feel and look how the *āsana* reaches from the external layer towards the inner and innermost layers of the body. In the practice of *āsana,* the physical development that occurs is natural; but this is not the end. One has to think and question whether or not the intellectual development is also interplaying and interweaving. No doubt with any sort of exercise, the toxins of the body will be thrown away, and the purification will be happening to that extent. This is known as *aśuddhikṣaya* – diminishing the bodily impurities. But where is *jñānadīpti* – shining lamp of wisdom? The eight aspects of yoga have to yield both[1]. One may decide to do the *āsana* quickly, but one has to question whether such speedy movements flashed the knowledge or understanding to the intelligence. Does one reflect on the movement and motion in fast changing positions? Does one see whether the inner body is charged? Does one treat both the sides equally? Does one develop the sensitivity within to find concord? I am asking not only to observe the expansion and extension, but also the density or firmness, and how the area is filled with energy and awareness, both within and without. If energy acts as attention, total expansion of consciousness acts as awareness.

Further, does one grasp the quality of *āsana* when there is no pause or space to see and reflect on the feedback from the nerves? Can one discern what is right and what is wrong? Then how will one know the subtle points? Patañjali said that the practice of *aṣṭāṅga* yoga is meant for diminishing impurities and to kindle the light of wisdom. Isn't it our duty to see and assess whether we are achieving that or not? With quick, fast movements we certainly benefit on the surface level. We feel the health and lightness *(aṅgalāghavam)* in the body. This comes because *vāta,* which remains in an arrested and immobile state, is made free and mobile through the practice of the *āsana* in the *vinyāsa* method. Therefore, the body experiences lightness.

You know the word *bala* (power or strength) and *ati-bala* (more powerful). *Bala* stands for *rajasic* and *tamasic* qualities and *ati-bala* for *sattvic* qualities. Actually, the quick and fast performance makes the *tāmasic* body light and the dull brain active. But still the question remains to be faced, where will you allow the now activised brain to flow? How will you utilise

---

1 *Yoga Sūtra* II.28.

or apply the intelligence of the awakened brain? This is known as *viniyoga.* Patañjali says, *tasya bhūmiṣu viniyogaḥ*[1]. Thus, which way will the newly generated energy be engaged or directed?

The people who do jumpings do not know the subtle points of adjustments that are necessary for culturing the body and the mind as well as the intelligence. There is very little chance in the jumping system for correct understanding and corrections. This conative action in *āsana* certainly leads to a dynamic and active life. Only this is a positive gain. When you do *vinyāsa* way, it is hard to find out how or in which position the lungs work in *Chaturaṅga Daṇḍāsana, Ūrdhva Mukha Śvānāsana* or *Adho Mukha Śvānāsana* and how the positioning of the legs changes in these *āsana.* For this one needs *vicāra* – reflection, absorption, synthesis, and this calls for time. When cognitive reflection takes place, analysis and synthesis play their role further. Due to cognitive reflection and re-action, one's consciousness is brought to get woven and entwined with the practice, which becomes a spiritual way of practice. The former one is a blind process, the later one is an alert, watchful and discriminative process.

As you all have experienced many subtle points, why don't you take these felt points to the pupils who come to you to get the taste of yoga?

- Our trained teachers who haven't had much contact with you are mixing up the method to attract more people. -

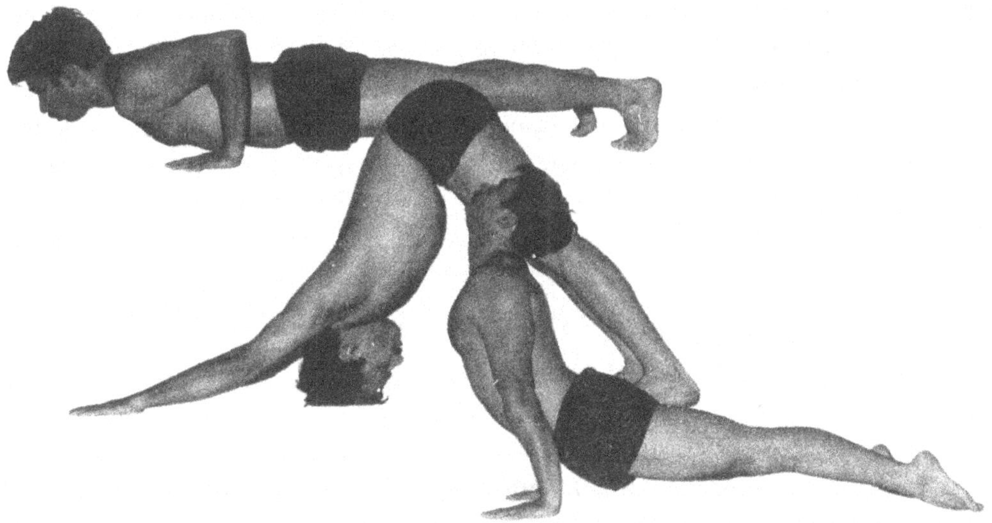

Plate n. 26 – *Chaturaṅga Daṇḍāsana, Ūrdhva Mukha Śvānāsana* and *Adho Mukha Śvānāsana*

[1] *Saṁyama* may be applied in various spheres to derive its usefulness. *Y.S.,* III.6.

You are asking me to address those teachers who are in touch with you all but not have come in contact with me. Is it not your duty to guide them as they are in contact with you all? My experiential knowledge in the method is a gold mine for teaching. If you allow those who were trained by you to use my name, then who has to be blamed? You should speak to them about the ethics of yoga. If they do not heed your guidelines, mix up and teach, then for me, it is hocus pocus yoga or yoga salad. This is most unethical in the philosophy of yoga.

Q.- Some newcomers and fresh pupils like fast, quick and dynamic movements. These pupils walk out of these classes when they get injured.

This is a personal question. It means that you do not want to lose students and hence teach according to their tastes. Knowing that they get injured, is it ethical on your part to continue teaching like this? Is it not your fear that makes you do what is not right by your own conscience? For a true teacher, it is not what students demand that has to be given, but what is needed to uplift the students towards the evolution of the mind and intellect. This is the *dharma* of a teacher. See yourself what you have in your mind. Is it not just greed in you that makes you teach what your students demand? As a teacher, you have to think whether your students get the poison or the nectar. Take it as their misfortune if they walk out when their indiscriminate demand is not met, and not yours in losing them. Don't you know honesty pays at the end? So stick to your conscience and teach with your honest approach. If they leave the class, it is their loss, not yours. As your conscience is clear, you are closer to the spiritual discipline. Mixing up various styles is against the moral principles until those styles are qualitatively superior to the one you know. Do not have any selfish interest. Treat yoga as a divine subject and not as a money making subject.

Going to several teachers and gathering knowledge is not love for yoga but building up a trade for business. It is better to practise diligently and conscientiously and gain a solid foundation with confidence. Use yoga to gain knowledge, equilibrium and contentment. Teach to live gracefully, but not for amassing wealth and fame.

Q.- Being arthritic, I am very much concerned by all this because of my own concerns about healthy practice for all, to allow all to benefit by your views. But after discussing with other teachers and seeing the requests of some of my students, still some doubts remain which don't allow me to be very firm in my position.

I am really sorry for your doubts and at the same time the fear of losing your position and status. The expression of your physical condition is a weakness combined with fear. Imparting deep knowledge is important. In *āsana-sādhanā*, the *vinyāsa* is an intermediate stage of an *āsana*. Jumping from position to position was maintained by my *guru* from 1932 up to 1942, or so. I have seen my *Gurujī* demonstrating with us but he never did jumpings. He made us to do them during demonstrations in order to attract people towards this art.

Have the guts to announce your arthritic problems and show what you can do with that stiffness and how much better they can do without them.

From 1937 to 1940 I was teaching *āsana* in the *vinyāsa* way in the schools and colleges, because they were young. As they grew in age, they began feeling the exhaustion and wanted yoga free from fatigue. This request of theirs ignited me to search new avenues in yoga.

Pune was a Mecca of physical activities like *mall-khāmb*[1] and wrestling. Having done *mall-khamb,* they were unhappy to do yoga on the conative level. It was a challenge for me to work on myself and search, penetrating the inner body to go closer to the mental and spiritual bodies.

People with diabetes, high or low blood pressure, arthritis, backache, restlessness and nervous breakdown, were getting flashes and hotness in their eyes and ears through *vinyāsa krama*. I thought that *yoga* might not flourish with the introduction of *vinyāsa*, I changed the method towards the interpenetration of breath and mind.

Even in performances worldwide, I did *vinyāsa* to show external expressions and dynamism. It does attract people but that does not allow them to get the depth of the *sādhanā*. When I began working to reach the inner body, it gave me a great deal of understanding of the real aspects of yoga. It helped me explain the action, and made my pupils experience it. They loved these in depth feelings and began to show interest, as the mind, intelligence and consciousness began percolating throughout their bodies. This brought respect to this art.

My view is that *vinyāsa krama* ends only on the physical level. It is not bad practice to start with, but as the outer body is toned and tuned, one has to penetrate the space in one's own body as the mind gets immersed in the inner alignment; from the body towards the mind and soul. For me, alignment is enlightenment. This enlightenment brought in me the light of wisdom to impart to others and helped me in synchronising action with knowledge and live close to the core.

First of all, be clear that *vinyāsa* is *yama* to *samādhi*. It is a process for reaching the Ultimate in the *sādhanā*. If one has to experience and deliver the *āsana*, one has to know how

---

[1] *Mall-khāmb* is doing *āsana* postures on a polished wood pole fixed to the floor and twisting, rotating and back-bending around it.

to go with the motion, action, stability of each area and each cell that carries us to the final position of the *āsana* and to advertently come out from the *āsana*. *Vinyāsa* means *viśeṣa nyāsa* – specific placement.

Coming to your individual problem such as arthritis, how can you expect to do *vinyāsa* with jumps? Yet undoubtedly you do *vinyāsa*. When your knee, ankle or fingers are going crooked, getting swollen, there are certain sequences of *āsana*, which you follow to work on specific affected areas, intelligently applying your mind. If you neglect this sequence and do fast inattentive movements, *you* invite more problems. Then it is neither *bhoga-yoga* nor *yoga-yoga* (neither *preyas* nor *śreyas*) but *roga-yoga* or sickening yoga. Yoga has to be done by igniting discrimination – *viveka* – in every step of *sādhanā*. Yoga cannot be done in a competitive spirit. If one tries to do that way, one loses judgement of the *sādhanā*.

In classical Indian music, several styles of expression are practised and evolved by original teachers. Such styles are called *gharāṇā*. Similarly, yoga is the music of the mind and soul. First learn from one method. Digest it and let it mature before you think of changing your style of practice.

IYENGAR YOGA, THE FOUNTAIN OF LIFE*

While teaching and practising yoga, Iyengar doesn't present himself to the world as a guru, or a master but a humble disciple. Having dedicated his whole life to yoga, Iyengar shares his knowledge with others to help reach this inner-peace, which will bring us health and happiness.

During his tour of Europe, Mr. Iyengar visited our country to inaugurate various yoga centres in the principal cities. At 78 years of age, although he doesn't admit it, he is one of the important authorities in the world of yoga. B.K.S. Iyengar has his main school in Pune, India. Thanks to his books, Westerners have access for the first time to the material necessary to initiate themselves in the practice of yoga that, above all, has brought balance to many men and women of our society.

Q.- You were sick as a child, and were recommended the practice of yoga as a last resort...

Yes. I was a sickly child. My brother-in-law suggested that I do a few *āsana*. As my joints were rigid, my body was like a log of wood and weak. On account of this I say I was in a disastrous condition. Thanks to those few *āsana*, after five years of practice I began to feel better. As years went on, I was able to understand what it meant to be healthy. Once I gained health, interest in yoga set in.

Q.- What is yoga to you?

Years of illness created distance between my body and my mind. The sick body made my mind negative with no interest in life. I developed pessimism and became a non-receiver. I gained

---

* Interview by Montse Batlle in September 1996. Published by the Spanish magazine CuerpoMente in April 1997.

health through *āsana* as well as receptivity. From this point of view I mean and feel that yoga refines and unites the body and mind to work together to experience the "fountain of life". For me, this is yoga.

Q.- What was the motivation behind acquiring such an exact understanding of the human body?

Since I had very little education there was no possibility to find a job. The only thing I knew was *āsana* to practise and teach to make a living. I began with public demonstrations to attract possible practitioners. Yet at the same time my primary motive was subsistence.

Though I continued practising for subsistence, my heart was telling me not to block my mind with the idea of making a living but to keep my mind open to see what yoga could really offer. With this motivation, I began to concentrate on understanding how each *āsana* was directing my mind to feel the most remote corners of my body to experience the life force, strength and vitality existing in those areas. This led me in understanding the living force of the human body.

Q.- Is the Iyengar system the only one that uses ropes and supports for the *āsana*?

If we read Indian mythology, we see that yogis historically practised this method hanging upside-down from trees.

I began to construct the ropes to resemble the branches of trees, and practise as if attached to a strong and straight tree. I started working with rings and hooks to substitute the trunks of the trees and to see in what ways they could be used. Now one can do with zeal and enthusiasm almost all *āsana* with supports. Thanks to these innovations many classic *āsana* from my book, which appear very difficult, have become easier for students to do.

There are many people who have physical problems or handicaps: for this I thought of access for them to practise yoga to gain maximum benefit.

Yet, props alone do not signify the Iyengar system. If one thinks that the Iyengar system means props, one is misdirected. At the same time it is wrong to brand my practice as the Iyengar system, I only systematised to some extent the approach, which my students recognise as the Iyengar system of yoga.

Q.- What are the *sūtras?*

Sūtra means a thread. As one weaves the flowers to form a garland or the pearls to make a necklace, so are the *sūtra* woven together like "pearls of wisdom".

Patañjali codifies his experiences of yoga not only with the philosophical approach but also gives a methodology to make the aspirant reach the core of the being. His work is recognised as *Yoga Sūtra*, which is a treatise on yoga. The whole subject, which is vast, has been reduced to 196 aphorisms. Each word has a great potency conveying its depth. He aptly explains everything in the form of *sūtra* without leaving room for any loose ends. His exposition in the form of *sūtra* are what yoga is.

Q.- Do you believe that there is a direct relation between our attitudes and our bodies?

Of course! There is total relationship between the attitudes of body and mind. Outwardly our bodies, represented by bones, muscles and organs, are identical; each individual differs as far as the mental attitude is concerned, which itself is known as the science of psychology. But yogic science penetrates deeper than modern psychology.

Yoga teaches how to develop and deliberate right mental attitudes in a sound body to have the purity, sanctity and divinity of our existence.

Yoga practice consists of integrating the disintegrated body, senses, mind, nerves, intelligence and consciousness. We strive to unite all these constituents of the body for purification to come close to the purity of the soul so that both appear as one unit.

Q.- Can one prevent physical and mental disorders through yoga?

Yoga has gained popularity in recent years for its preventive and curative value. It was known to our ancestors as a remedial science from time immemorial. Patañjali wrote three treatises – one on grammar, one on medicine and one on yoga. He presented through all these three treatises the way to prevent and cure the physical and mental disorders.

Coming to your question, let there not be any doubt about yoga as a therapy, an oriental method of healing. In order to get health, Patañjali speaks from the holistic and wholistic point of view on body, mind and intelligence. His message is to prevent the disease on the physical, moral, mental and spiritual levels and to maintain that health. Since diseases affect all these phases of the human being, his eight aspects of yoga are based on this theme of health, as man is susceptible to physical, mental, moral and intellectual diseases, as well as those of consciousness.

Practice of *āsana* and *prāṇāyāma* works on improving the immune system, as they work on the cellular and organic body making all the systems function together healthily and harmoniously. They work directly on the nervous system and brain, which stand as the threshold between the body and mind. The glandular system, nervous system and mental apparatus get balanced in the practitioner. This is how prevention becomes possible.

According to Patañjali, the root cause of physical and mental disorders is deeply rooted in the mind. There are five types of afflictions. Want of knowledge, ego or pride, attachment, hatred and fear of life or death are the causes of diseases. Basically, want of knowledge, lack of understanding, misunderstanding, misinterpretation, negligence, forgetfulness, lack of sensitivity, cause afflictions. They express themselves in four states. These could be dormant or latent, slender or attenuated, alternately interrupted with ups and downs, or remain fully expressive. Yoga heals them on all these four stages.

When the illness is very serious, work must begin from the periphery, as in the psychosomatic sciences, using body and mind to confront the illness. If the illness is hidden or dormant, then the practice of yoga brings such diseases to the surface. As the hidden diseases come to the surface, they are recognised for treatment with yogic discipline. The future awaiting diseases can be prevented. Some of the diseases may not be serious but may bother off and on, which can be combated. But the diseases, which are fully active and take one to the door of death will be reduced and endured. That is the beauty of yoga.

Patañjali asks the yoga practitioner to reduce the intensity of affliction gradually with the practice of yoga. In order to prevent the diseases, one has to practise the eight aspects of yoga first to diminish and then to finally eradicate them from the body, mind, intelligence and consciousness.

Q.- What would you say for you is an ethical life?

It is something very difficult for me to explain since the ethical or moral path is very subtle. It is *sūkśma dharma* - subtle religious path. On the mundane level it builds the character of an individual. Our character is completely tied to our physique, our nerves, our blood, our skin and our neurons. If we abuse the ethics of the cells, the fibres, the respiratory or energy systems, they deteriorate. Ethics raises a person and allows evolution in life. That which destroys the growth of a person is by no means ethical. To cultivate one's character against wrong tendencies is the base of ethics. One needs to peep inward into one's conscience in order to eradicate bad tendencies and build up good tendencies. Patañjali says that purity of body brings purity of mind. This is the work of the *āsana*. Those who practise *āsana* for indulging or appeasing their appetite for food and sex are for me immoral. Ethics is the foundation of all religions, and are meant to uplift human beings from a subhuman plane to the human plane and above.

Q.- What do you think is the root of the actual violence in the world?

If there is competition, there is jealousy. Some years ago, I went to see a bullfight. It is pure violence; it is not worth watching. In the Olympic games, which were celebrated recently, we have seen athletes who were like living rocks; not one was a natural athlete, all of them were artificial. When we practise yoga our endurance is natural because we are not trying to compete with anybody. The only healthy competition is in measuring our development, the growth of our intelligence.

Nowadays, a person believes that his possibilities are limitless, and from there he begins to experience physical stress, mental stress and nervous tension. When competition ends, violence ends. There is competition on all levels. Even war takes place because of it. Competition leads one towards dissatisfaction. If the capacity and endurance of each person were appreciated, then there would be no competition, no jealousy, no dissatisfaction. Rather, each would strive to do their very best. "Live and let live" should be the attitude.

Q.- Do you believe that in order to obtain happiness we should reduce our necessities and belongings to the minimum, just the opposite of what our current society implies?

No. What we must do is to understand our true needs. However, it is very difficult to determine where needs end and where desire begins. The answer ought to be in one's level of contentment, but people are discontented even though they have more than they could possibly need. This is the reason why there are so many misgivings between human beings. I am not saying that we should live precariously; our needs should be in accord with the times we are living in.

If I were to live in the Himalayas, my necessities would be minimal, but if I must move among this society, I must adjust my needs so as to not be a parasite on the rest of society. If things come of their own, all is well, but I will not waste my energy trying to force it. Every individual must analyse and comprehend where necessity ends and desire begins.

Q.- Why are there such problems between religions if each one is looking for something similar?

There are two types of religions, religion created by God and religion created by man. There are only problems in this second category, not in the first. Man, for power and position, divided religion creating problems. There are similarities in all the religions of the world: Buddhism, Jainism, Sikhism, Islam, Hinduism, Christianity... In all, the base is exactly the same. Yoga too expresses religiousness as its core. There are some who, acting as impostors of religion, create differences between man and man. If I wear a red line on my forehead, some will say that I am from a different sect, someone else who wears a cross forms another sect. Why fight about these outer marks when all these symbols mean the same to God. We should begin to look at the points where the religions coincide; then we will be able to reach mutual understanding.

Q.- Why do you present yoga as a science of religions rather than as a religion in its own right?

Because yoga is for all humankind. Patañjali said that what one experiences doesn't just stop at him. It belongs to all humankind. Hence it is universal cultivation of good experiences; it is not individual but universal. Hence yoga acts as science to build one to be righteous and that righteousness is true religion.

Yoga works for this, to cultivate, educate, embellish and purify the body, mind, intelligence, and the I-ness so that the journey is made towards the Self. Yoga acts as a science to build up auspiciousness in oneself, which is nothing but an asset of all religions.

Q.- Are there not many paths for one to take toward the Self?

Yes. There are many ways to climb a mountain: zigzagging, round and round, straight up... In the mountain one can enjoy the aroma of the flowers, the trees, the rock formations. Similarly, one can climb the tree using any branch. However, the mountain or tree has the ground as its base. Therefore, the path may differ but the ground is the same.

Each person has distinct tastes. Paths too are distinctive and in accord with the thoughts of each individual's taste. Through knowledge one can begin to live better, through right action to develop one's inner source of knowledge. Both knowledge and action lead us to live a harmonious life.

Q.- What is the difference between *rāja yoga* and *haṭha yoga?*

The word *rāja* means a king. As the mind is the king of the senses, intelligence is the king of the mind and Self is the king of all. To reach the king – Self, one has to be near the Self, and to feel that is *rāja yoga*.

Haṭha has the two syllables *ha* and *ṭha* signifying sun and moon. *Ha* means sun, and *ṭha* means moon. Actually the psychological and spiritual aspect of this word is forgotten, and its physiological aspect is emphasised, saying that *haṭha yoga* is physical yoga.

In reality, the moon represents the consciousness *(citta)*, which is similar to the moon, has varying cycles of fluctuations. The sun however shines constantly without fail, like the Self.

Haṭha yoga is the science that reveals and upraises the fluctuating mind to the level of the Self. Hence, I do not see the difference between *haṭha yoga* and *rāja yoga*. If *haṭha yoga* is the strength of the will, *rāja yoga* is the method of restraining the consciousness. If *haṭha yoga* is the process of practice, *rāja yoga* is the result. With the practice of *haṭha yoga* one purifies the body, senses, mind, intelligence, I-consciousness, and conscience; and finally the pure *citta* reaches the Self as *rāja yoga*.

Q.- Can the soul be described?

The soul cannot be described, but it can be experienced. For example, watching a sunset, we cannot observe our mind because it gets dissolved in the sunset. When we concentrate on the beauty of the panorama we forget ourselves. In yoga when there is purity of consciousness, we experience the soul. But if we begin to describe it, it can only be words and not actual experience. It is like two sides of a coin: if the mind appears, soul disappears, if soul appears, mind disappears. Soul is mute and mind is talkative. It speaks within itself. Here I use the word 'mind' for the whole mental apparatus that is intelligence, I-consciousness and *citta*.

Description, expression, apprehension and comprehension come from the mental faculty. If I express through this faculty, then I am giving a form to the soul. Soul is formless, eternal, self-luminous, non-perishing, non-diminishing, free, ever pure, mute, dumb, deaf and immutable. The science of yoga refers to soul as *ātman*, *draṣṭā* – seer, *puruṣa* – one who dwells in the body, the dweller of the body, *jñātā* – knower. But this description is beyond a common man's intelligence.

The practice of yoga sublimates the power of the mind so that the hidden soul shines with luminosity. This Self-luminosity is what one commonly calls "intuitive understanding".

Q.- What does it mean to be a *guru*?

Guru is he who eliminates the darkness and brings light. *Gu* means darkness or heaviness and *ru* means light, weightlessness, and illumination. The *guru* eliminates the heaviness of the body, the darkness of the mind and illuminates the intelligence of the disciple.

These days, the teacher is considered to be a *guru*. The word *guru* has become cheap. I think some clarity is required here. *Guru* is strictly one who directly shows a practical path to reach the soul, by eradicating the wrong and perverted knowledge as well as ignorance and arrogance, uplifting the disciple from the ocean of desires and wrong tainted imprints, which stick stubbornly in the pupils. *Guru* takes the disciple from the bank of the physical towards the bank of the spiritual, crossing all mental hurdles. As you asked me whether the soul can be described, *guru* does not describe the soul but takes the disciple towards that journey in order to experience the soul.

Q.- What is for you a disciple?

I am only a *guru* when I teach what I know; when I practise I am a disciple. In each *guru*, the discipleship has to exist as a base, which seems missing these days. A *guru* needs to have the potential discipleship in him.

When I practise each of the *āsana*, I enquire of the *āsana* to guide me as to what I must do, and not do. Here, I am a student of yoga. I still remain a disciple of yoga, with the exception of when I am teaching others.

The innocent students are like hard soil with confused mental ground, even sometimes they appear like impenetrable rocks. In order to sow the seeds in the soil, one has to loosen the soil to make it useful. Similarly, the field of consciousness of the student needs to be nurtured. The *guru* sees that the field of consciousness is qualitatively improved with right imprints. The field is burnt to remove the weeds. The seeds of knowledge are sown in that field. The watering of compassion and discipline is done, with the expectation of a harvest of knowledge of the Self in disciple.

Q.- Are there currently more people in the world who are reaching a higher level of spirituality than formerly?

I cannot say, as it is beyond my comprehension. But I feel that there is more interest than before. There is an increase in enthusiasm and curiosity. *Jijñāsā* is the first step of self-realisation in which one begins to make self-inquiry. People have started having this *jijñāsā*[1]. For me a disciple is he who receives the guidance and instructions with open mindedness, having no tinge of doubt (hard soil with non-productive weeds); flourishes with the knowledge which is received in the seed form and continues the *sādhanā* in order to protect and preserve the experience without allowing the consciousness to divert from its goal.

The farmer reforms the field for a new crop. Similarly, the *sādhanā* has to be continued to remain close to the soul. A disciple is he who continues with discipline. The life of a disciple is discipline.

As I said, curiosity and enthusiasm is there in the new generation, actually masters are few and difficult to find.

It is not so easy to become a *guru* or find a *guru*. It is not the clothes that distinguishes one, but inner purity. There is a big difference between a *guru* and a preacher: a *guru* preaches what he practises; a preacher guides you, but doesn't practise himself. For this reason there are few true *guru*. The people however have a genuine desire to experience the "elixir of life" or the truth of existence. We must build up step by step and grow on the spiritual path, so that new generations are able to find wise teachers.

Q.- Don't you think that to marry and have children is a hindrance along the path toward total union with God?

I am a married man with children and grand-children. If I had not known the suffering involved in the upheavals of an ordinary human being, I would not have evolved in life in a true sense.

Married life does not create a barrier. In fact, the married life, which is known as *gṛhasthāśrama*, teaches the *sādhaka* to develop qualities such as tolerance, endurance, patience, forbearance, and to face adverse circumstances. It teaches the value of love and affection. If the husband and wife do not love each other how can they learn to love hundreds of people in society? For me marriage is the starting point to experience the divine marriage between body and mind, mind and soul, soul and God – the Supreme Being.

---

[1] There are seven steps of incitement or instigation. 1.*Prepsā* – wish to gain, interest in self-realisation. 2.*Jihāsā* – Aversion towards those desires which come in the way of self-realisation. 3.*Jijñāsā* – enthusiasm to know newly about the subject of self-realisation. 4.*Cikīrṣā* – to have direct action, dynamic participation. 5.*Śoka* – To have sorrow for past activities going against the process of self-realisation. 6.*Bhaya* – To have the fear that a new problem may arise in the process of self-realisation. 7.*Atṛpti* – discontentment and dissatisfaction, inclining towards self-realisation.

My *guru* was a married man, and his *guru* was also a married man. The highest authorities in the history of yoga have also been married persons. Vaśiṣṭha, Viśvāmitra, Ātreya – all these *ṛṣi* were married. Vaśiṣṭha had one hundred children, but his mind all the time dwelt in the soul. He was great *ātmajñānin* who showed the light and enlightened to follow his precepts.

Married life teaches us how to grow despite the difficulties. The life of a renunciate, on the other hand, does not represent these ups and downs and sufferings of life.

Q.- When one reaches inner peace, is it a permanent state?

Yes. However, one mustn't stop and experience only that. One must develop and have compassion towards the rest of the world and guide and help others to find and share that permanent peace which one experiences. Being in contact with others, our own peace increases. Peace is not something that should stay only inside oneself. It is for sharing with people. In fact, the inner peace becomes the field for the expansion of freedom to establish peace in the world.

Q.- You are considered an authority. What do you believe has been your greatest contribution to yoga?

I do not think that I am an authority. I know what I know, but that which is unknown about yoga is much greater than what I know. People say that I am an authority, but I don't pay attention to this kind of praise. The only authority in yoga is the great master, Patañjali. We are but followers after understanding his detailed explanation of yoga. We are under his shadow of knowledge. He is the protector of our aspiration. A person such as I, who was unhealthy, to have arrived where I am today, cannot consider myself as an authority when the credit and merit belong to Patañjali, with whose blessings I live in yoga.

Whatever I have contributed, it is by the will and grace of Patañjali and not my own. I have been crafted to be as an instrument.

Just as people buy various colourful scintillating dresses and wear them to beautify themselves, I try to beautify the inner Self with the garland of shining imprints (*saṁskāra*) of yoga. Just as many people use cosmetics to appear more beautiful, I use the yogic cosmic light to beautify and adorn the consciousness. My practice of *āsana* and *prāṇāyāma* is to bring the beauty of the soul to the surface.

Q.- What is your message?

Without doubt, the wealth of a nation lies in its health. The nation flourishes with physical, moral, mental and spiritual health. If the health improves then the economy improves. Such comprehensive health can develop well through the science of yoga that cultivates body, mind, intelligence and soul. There is no greater nation than our own body and our own inner-Self. Through yoga one can achieve a better life and greater happiness.

SIMPLE MAN – SIMPLE ANSWERS*

The premises appeared more like a temple than an institute – calm and peaceful, with the chirping of the birds breaking the silence. The evening breeze was cool and fragrant. Hurriedly I and Rumu (my friend), walked towards the office. We were led to the office by Mrs. Sunita, Gurujī's daughter who was friendly and gentle. I was a little tense, for we were late, keeping my fingers crossed I cursed the traffic jam, and whispered to Rumu that perhaps the great man I was to interview would be annoyed. But to my surprise, I saw Gurujī walking briskly into the office with a radiant face and a big smile. Gracefully he occupied his chair and reciprocated our greetings warmly, he was the world famous Yogachārya *Shri B.K. Sundararaja Iyengar.*

Born on 14th of December, 1918, Shri B.K.S. Iyengar is a man of principles. The life and work of Gurujī (as he is respectfully called by one and all), are of epic proportions. Yogachārya B.K.S. *Iyengar has pursued the yogic art with great devotion, without compromising its purity and divinity. Through this art and science he has brought to the troubled mankind a new hope of health and tranquillity.*

He is a legend in his own time, a teacher without peer. He has faith and confidence in himself, which he instils in his pupils. Throughout his life, from days of grinding poverty to days of affluence, he has preserved his faith and equanimity. Words are too scarce to narrate his achievements.

Q.- What motivated you to start this Institute?

It was not a motivation, but a tragic juncture in my life that led me to begin this institute. In 1973 I had purchased a small piece of land for the construction of a house. But unfortunately, my wife Smt. Ramamani Iyengar suddenly passed away. Relatives, friends and well wishers suggested that since there was a need of a yoga institute it would be appropriate to build the institute in her memory. Thus began this Institute.

The Institute is presented to me by my pupils.

* Interview published by *Pune Today*, 15th September 1996.

Q.- What is the mission of the Institute?

The mission is to create universal health awareness. Health is wealth, of every human being. Yoga cultures the mind, and purifies the body. These days life is full of tensions; no one is tension-free. Pollution plays its own role in disturbing the atmosphere. All this has become a part of our lives. Under such circumstances, the only way to purify our body and have contended mind is the system of yoga.

By the practice of yoga, the body and mind gets transformed to the level of the soul. For example, a drunkard leaves drink, an ill-tempered person becomes gentle and humble.

The zealous practice of yoga, whether he be young or old, infirm or diseased or those who are enfeebled, unfailingly leads them towards health and fulfilment. Health is the true foundation for securing the aims of life – righteousness to salvation. Yoga helps one to achieve peace of mind and happiness both externally as well as internally.

Q.- Tell us about the history of yoga.

Narayana, the *Hiraṇyagarbha* (the golden womb) is the creator of yoga, there is no one beyond him. Yoga is a part of the ancient Indian culture and spiritual approach to life. The *ṛṣi*, *muni* and later Patañjali, author of the *Yoga Sūtra*, codified the relevant points of yoga from the ancient scriptures such as; *Veda*, *Upaniṣad*, *Saṁhitā*, *Araṇyaka* into *Yoga Sūtra*.

Yoga means communion. It means discipline of all the powers of the body, mind, intellect, emotions and will, bringing poise on the soul, enabling one to look at all aspects of life in a calm, unruffled manner. Yoga is like music, for the rhythm of the body, the melody of the mind and the harmony of the soul creating the symphony of life. Yoga draws out the best in a person and provides the finest system of education.

Q.- How and when did you start practising yoga?

I was born into a large and poor family, I suffered from malnutrition and a number of diseases. All this made me very weak and underdeveloped. In 1934, at the age of 16, I went to my sister's house in Mysore. Keeping my health in view, my brother-in-law, Prof. Krishnamacharya, initiated me into yoga. In a very short time I learnt the practical side of yoga.

Q.- When did you start teaching yoga?

In 1935 I used to teach yoga in the *yogaśālā* of Mysore. Then went to Hubli, Dharwar and Belgaum to demonstrate and teach if asked. I was invited to Pune in 1937 by the Deccan Gymkhana Club and joined as a yoga instructor. Initially, I faced many problems. It was very difficult to make both ends meet. 1940-1947 was a crucial time in my life. In 1947, the members of the Rotary Club of Pune invited me to teach yoga. Slowly people started recognising my talent.

The seed of yoga planted by me nearly sixty years ago germinated and sprouted into a huge fertile tree with many branches. The seed remains in Pune and the institute here is the Mother Institute to many institutes, propagating this universal culture. Now, I have more than 180 institutes all over the world and a number of institutes in India, with millions of students. Also there are Iyengar National Associations in each country, where propagation of this system of yoga takes place.

Q.- Since, various *āsana* are taught in the Institute, how do you adapt these *āsana*?

There are as many *āsana* as living species in this world. *Āsana* are innumerable. They have been there from the beginning of time but were forgotten. I learnt and changed certain techniques to suit people in these modern times according to their limitations of will and as per their ailments are concerned. I had to alter and make the *āsana* suitable for easy practice. A few *āsana* I changed as a challenge from within. For the sake of progress and evolution, I had to create some *āsana*. I have evolved a unique system of teaching yoga through my assiduous personal practice, and the study of the needs and problems of people around me.

To distinguish my system from the other systems, my pupils call it 'Iyengar yoga' and describe themselves by this name. The system is entirely based on Patañjali's *Yoga Sūtra*. The emphasis is on *āsana* and *prāṇāyāma* and instruction is given in both by incorporating the principles of *yama* and *niyama* as yoga cannot be divorced from discipline and morality. The higher aspects of yoga such as *dhāraṇā*, *dhyāna* and *samādhi* are taught only to those who have gained a measure of proficiency in *āsana* and *prāṇāyāma*. Any attempt at bypassing these vital steps, which render the body, mind and intelligence to remain fit and pure so that complications may not occur in their higher practices. Therefore, my emphasis is on the practice of *āsana* and *prāṇāyāma* to remain stable in work, speech and mind.

Q.- Through yoga can any ailment be cured?

Yes, there is a huge scope and tremendous possibility for curing various ailments and diseases through yoga. Sincere practice of yoga under the guidance of a competent *guru* can always work wonders. We conduct special classes three times a week to help persons suffering from severe problems. Some mentally challenged children also come to us.

Q.- Any do's and don'ts while practising yoga?

Neither freedom nor beatitude is possible without discipline. Yoga being the most subtle science and supreme art, calls for different qualities of the head and heart. Discipline is the foundation for the practice of any art. Yoga demands the highest discipline. Regularity and punctuality are essential parts of discipline. Yoga demands cleanliness and purity. A pupil should wash hands and feet before entering the classroom. The body is sustained and influenced by the food we eat. Hence the food should be ideally vegetarian. Courtesy in speech and conduct to all involved in the instruction of yoga is expected.

Teachers occupy a unique position in the yoga system. Faith and respect for the teachers is a must.

Q.- How do you feel with all these life-time achievements?

I am fully a contented man; I have felt the worst and the best in my *sādhanā* as well as seen the worst and best in life. Now the only thing I pray God is to die with the thought of yoga.

STRESS BUSTERS!*

They live life king-size. Speeding in the fast lane and thriving on the blaze are some of Pune's celebs, who after years are still fired up and raring to go. Their secret? Finally it's out!

He has a star in the Northern hemisphere named after him. His disciples range from J. Krishnamurthi to Jayaprakash Narayan, from Achyutrao Patwardhan to Yehudi Menuhin. He practises yoga for four hours daily at least (incidentally he is over seventy-five years old!). He has cured ailments, which had no cure in the medical annals. All this he has achieved during his "bonus life". At the age of thirteen, when he contracted tuberculosis of the lungs, the doctors gave him only two years to live, resigning him to fate. But yoga multiplied it by thirty and B.K.S. Iyengar is the living proof.

– *Physical well being equals success...* –

Health is wealth and is essential for success in life. Yoga is a psycho-physiological subject which aims at arresting psychosomatic fallouts, such as stress-related problems and cardiac arrests. Yoga enlivens every cell in the body, bringing the presence of mind in every cell. Common people like you and I cannot disconnect from the impediments of our body, only people like Ramakrishna Paramhamsa could do that. Physical well being brings mental well being, which in turn cultivates harmony leading towards peace.

– *I tackle stress by...* –

...Stressing on practice of yoga.

In fact, I don't suffer from any stress. For me life is dynamically positive. There could be stress due to environmental fluctuations, but because of yoga I can relax in the midst of it.

---

* Interview published by *The Citadel* in October 1996.

– Burnout according to me is... –

...Because of bad actions, wrong decisions and over-ambition make one's life desolate, and yoga burns out these impurities. Otherwise they burn out the person.

All stress problems are basically due to guilty conscience, which plagues most people today. Most of us are guilty of having cheated friends, subordinates as well as near and dear ones to achieve our goal. Having played such tricky games, we are scared that the same may boomerang on us some day, hence this increase in burnouts. As one sows so one reaps.

– My diet consists of... –

...Simple, homely, clean food.

I do not advocate a special diet, because of my background where I couldn't even afford a one-time meal. I eat whatever other normal people eat.

If one's salivary glands are not functioning, then even the best food becomes poisonous. One should not make a fad out of this diet theory.

I do not prescribe food. I emphasise the practice of yoga, which consequently changes one's food habits.

– Yoga according to me is... –

...*Kāyā kalpa.*

Kāyā is the body and *kalpa* means an elixir to keep oneself healthy. Yoga helps in maintaining sound health with awareness from within. It is a preventive measure to avoid illness and nurtures the thought to acquire clarity.

– I exercise to avoid... –

...Not the fatty tissues but the "tissues" of faulty actions.

– Yoga versus modern exercise technique is... –

...Wisdom versus showmanship.

Yoga has its age-old beliefs in the cellular system, which scientists today talk about. Modern day keep-fit programmes, gyms, callisthenics merely burn you out, without inducing any positive energy. Yoga builds up positive energy eradicating negative stress. Yoga helps in changing unhealthy people towards health and at the same time keeps the healthy people healthy in all aspects – physical, moral, mental and spiritual.

– I keep fit by... –

...Practising yoga.

– I think allopathy is... –

...A good remedy.

But health has to be earned, not bought. Yoga is not an alternative cure. It has a major role to play like modern medicine. If you balance the five elements in the body, you will be healthy. Imbalance in them will lead to disease.

– The best way to live life is... –

...To be content in spite of having a persistent and patient perseverance of one's goal.

When you have done your job well, satisfaction will come automatically.

– My personal recipe for a healthy life is... –

...Love, labour and laugh!

"LIKE A SEA DIVER, YOU DISCOVER NEW DEPTHS"*

At the young age of twelve a doctor told him that he was suffering from an advanced stage of TB, and that he would live for three years or so, today he turns 78. He is none other than the world-renowned yoga exponent Yogachārya B.K.S. Iyengar.

On the occasion of his 78th birthday, the man who is Gurujī *to tens of thousands of pupils, took time off to answer a few questions, which I asked of him with enthusiasm.*

Q.- *Gurujī*, what are your observations about the attitude of the present generation towards tradition?

Today, the younger generation has an aptitude to understand the Indian heritage. Unfortunately, however, present day education and the influence of Western ways of living in urban areas has confused the younger generation. The authorities have to give a thought in re-introducing the stories of *Rāmāyaṇa, Mahābhārata* and the *Purāṇa* in regular classes. We need teachers who can bridge the gap, so that the younger generation learns to respect our ancient, rich cultural and spiritual heritage and thinks of what is great and noble.

First of all, it is essential for grown-ups to know that Indian tradition, cultural heritage, philosophical approach to life are not rooted in any "isms". The most freedom of thought and expression as well as universal approach is found in the ancient scriptures. If Cārvāka speaks on a materialistic approach then Vedānta speaks on spiritual approach. How the new generation will know about this freedom of thought unless they are introduced to it?

I would say that they should be introduced to Indian philosophy as well as the epics to know the depth of a right way of living.

---

* Interview by Shodhan Bhatt. Published by the *Maharashtra Herald* on 14th December 1996.

Q.- Do you have any regrets about life?

By the grace of God and my dedication to yoga, I have acquired all things a man usually aspires to. I am definitely contented.

But, I still feel I have not been able to fathom the depth of yoga. Yoga is a vast and fathomless subject. More you dive in, you find that it is deeper than you think. When I began, I never dreamt that I would be considered a world-class teacher. Like a child that tastes seawater and says it is salty, so was I in yoga. But as a sea diver goes deeper and traces the wealth of the ocean, my practice allowed me to penetrate the depth of the oceanic body. Yet the final depth always remains just that little distance further. Finally, as a believer in reincarnation, I continue to practise with the same zeal so that my next life may start with vigour and vitality from where I leave the experience of practice in this life.

Q.- How is it that most Westerners are converted to vegetarianism after taking up to yoga? What are its advantages as opposed to a meat diet?

It was in the mind of Westerners that consumption of meat alone gives strength. When they saw me giving demonstrations and conducting classes for hours without fatigue, it made them re-think.

Since the animal does not speak like you or me when it is butchered, its instinctive feeling is unknown to us. Know well that every living cell has its own feeling. There is an instinctive fear of death and attachment to life in every living being.

Therefore, the fear in the animal at the time of its slaughter is the hidden cause of the development of fear complexes in its consumer. The chemical changes in the blood of the animal react on the mind of the eater. So the mind carries that element of fear.

As far as the sense of purity is concerned, it is experienced only by those who have switched from non-vegetarianism to vegetarianism. The practitioner of yoga vividly experiences the transformation occurring at mental and spiritual levels. That proves the non-essentiality of non-vegetarian food and essentiality of pure, *sāttvic* vegetarian food.

IYENGAR: THEN INITIATED, NOW HONOURED*

It is the bane of mankind that an achiever in any discipline rarely gets recognition in his own homeland or place of birth. But a few lucky ones no doubt get recognised in their own Motherland and one such lucky person is Dr. B.K.S IYENGAR, the 78 year old internationally-acclaimed, yoga exponent who gave a new dimension to the study of yoga. The University of Mysore recognising his immense contribution to the field of yoga conferred on him the Honorary Doctorate in Science. He was in Mysore on April 21st to receive the Doctorate.

Q.- How happy are you to be conferred the Honorary Doctorate?

Though I have been conferred several honours nationally and internationally including the *Padmashri* award, I cherish this honour the most because the fragrance of my birthplace and the grace of Goddess Chamundeshwari have entered into my yogic discipline. I would have died prematurely as an unknown entity but for the grace of Chamundeshwari Devi[1].

Q.- Did you expect the award?

"It is a mystery". I did not know. The credit goes to a lot of Mysoreans and my students who must have moved the idea.

I am proud today since my life took a turn at this place. I was introduced to yoga in Mysore and now I am awarded here.

State of Mysore is my birthplace. I was initiated to yoga here, which gave me a new birth. Now I am honoured by my own people.

---

* Interview by N. Niranjan Nikam. Published by the newspaper *Star of Mysore* on 29th April 1997, p. 4.

[1] Chamundeshwari Devi – A Goddess whose influence is strong in and around Mysore. She is also known as Mahisāsura Mardini.

Q.- Your *guru* Vidwan T. Krishnamacharya was from Mysore. Can you throw some light on this?

My *guru* was a learned person, who in those days travelled from Kashi to the Himalayas, Nepal and Tibet and learned yoga. He was appointed by the Maharaja of Mysore as *rāja guru*.

He was a great scholar and a versatile person.

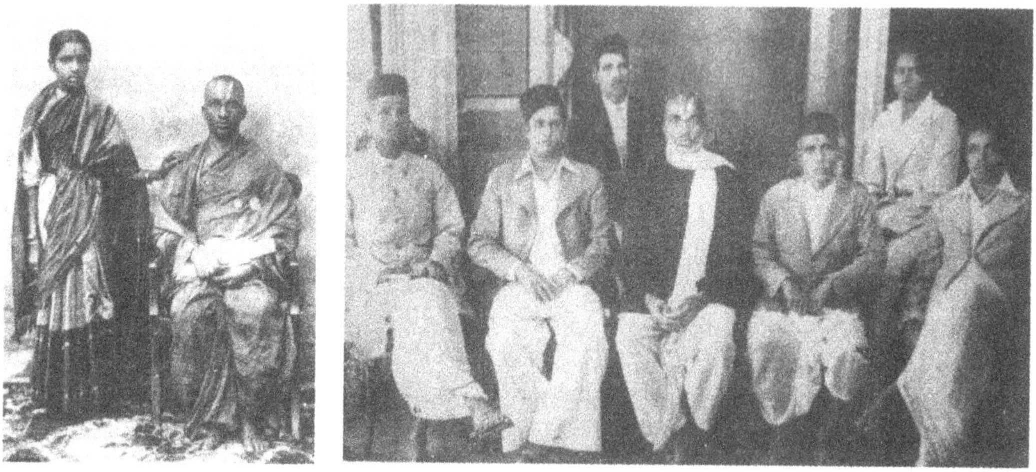

Plate n. 27 – Sri T. Krishnamacharya, scholar and with the Maharaja of Mysore

Q.- Why did you start the study of yoga? Did you find it good enough to propagate?

I was afflicted with malaria, typhoid and tuberculosis. As there were no wonder drugs those days, my *guru* Krishnamacharya, my sister's husband, asked me to come to Mysore, in order to fight these ailments. My *guru* sowed the seed of yoga in me.

Destiny took me to yoga. Except for yoga being patronised by the late Krishnaraja Wadiar Bahadur IV, there was not much recognition to the subject. The awareness of yoga was minimal. At the age of sixteen, I went to Karnatak College in Dharwar and gave a yoga demonstration. There, women wanted to learn yoga from me. This is how my career as a yoga teacher began.

Q.- You never looked back after that?

No! Never! Yoga became my bread and breath. That is how my mind gravitated towards it.

Yoga *sādhanā* is my *pūjā*, worship. The *abhyāsa* of yoga is my *karma*, its *cintana* is *jñāna*, and my devoted practice is *bhakti*.

Q.- How and when did you shift to Pune?

In 1936, I was giving a yoga demonstration in Lingaraja College in Belgaum, when a civil surgeon Dr. V. B. Gokhale who, I am told, operated on Mahatma Gandhi for appendicitis, watching my demonstration invited me to Pune for six months to teach yoga in colleges, which continued for three years. Each college was contributing Rs. 8/- a month for their students.

Q.- Are there many systems of yoga?

Yoga is one. Patañjali codified it in the form of aphorisms. You find the subject of yoga explained in all our ancient scriptures such as *veda*, *upaniṣad*, *saṁhitā*, *araṇyaka*, *purāṇa* and so on.

Just as in classical music there are different *gharānās* to learn under different traditions, similarly, in yoga there are many traditions. Each *guru* imparts the knowledge of yoga in his or her own style. Therefore, one finds a difference in systems.

Often yoga is misunderstood and misinterpreted. Therefore, it is the time to study it from the very base so that the foundation does not go wrong.

Q.- You claim that there is a cure for all ailments in yoga. Is it true?

I am sorry, I have not claimed like this anywhere. The cure for all ailments is nowhere except in the hands of God. But it is true that yoga can cure a lot of ailments. Surprisingly, the yoga I have followed has given good and positive results to many people. Now, it has world recognition.

Sometimes I may not succeed in curing a disease; but the diseased practitioner finds the change within. Yoga in this sense is a boon since it generates the energy, enlivens the cells, revitalises the organs, and uplifts the mind and morale of the sufferer by inspiring him to courageously face the afflictions of life.

Q.- How do we inculcate discipline to follow yoga regularly?

We need determination, will power and will to act. Even if you decide to do so only once a week, you should stick to it. You should not be casual for that day. Sometimes diseases and aches help one to stick to the practice. Laziness is the arch-enemy of practice.

Q.- What do you think of the view to start yoga lessons in schools?

I was the first to promote yoga in schools and colleges of Pune in 1937. The first to introduce yoga in the adult education schemes of the United Kingdom in 1968 and United States of America in 1974.

They wanted me to teach just the physical aspect of yoga and it attracted lots of people to its philosophy. Now, the inclination towards the philosophical aspect is very high.

Yoga is a must in schools. It helps in developing the memory of the child. Remembering various *āsana* is in itself a memory exercise. I am for yoga in schools but the Authorities have to lend their ears for the good of children.

Q.- One main criticism against people like you is that you cater more to foreigners than Indians. Is it true?

In my Institute there are six hundred local people who attend my classes regularly. Four of the weekly classes are remedial classes. Every month we have people from various cities and towns who come to learn for a month.

As far as foreigners are concerned, they have to reserve their seats three to four years earlier. Every alternate month, we allow the entry for 20 to 25 people from overseas. Therefore it appears as though there is a crowd of foreigners. Otherwise this charge is totally unfounded.

However, it is true that many a time I have visited several countries, which attracted them towards this subject and consequently they come to India seeking yoga teachers.

Q.- There are two systems, the Iyengar system and the Pattabhi Jois system, the people say. Is it true?

Both of us have learnt from the same *guru*. So really it is Krishnamacharya's system. We belong to same *gharāṇā*, and therefore there is no basic difference.

Q.- Your message to the people as to how to retain youth.

A sapling can be trimmed but a tree cannot be trimmed. Yoga is the key that unlocks the gates of freedom. Yoga even teaches one how to be friendly, compassionate and joyous over all, and again how to be indifferent to others when necessary.

Whatever my experiences are, I have passed them on to my students and I have not ventured beyond the frame of my experience and knowledge.

I want my brothers and sisters first to begin the yogic practice on health and then move further in restructuring the psychological and moral behaviour and then to the spiritual way of living.

YOGA – A DIVINE EMBROIDERY*

Q.- What is Iyengar yoga? – A common question asked by many.

That is not for me to answer. It is others who call it "Iyengar Yoga", have to answer I am sorry the yoga I practise got this unwanted brand. How can I answer a question that is spread by others? It is not "Iyengar Yoga". It is *Pātañjala Yoga* gifted to us by Patañjali. You may say that yoga as practised by Mr. Iyengar is basically *Pātañjala Yoga*, which is unfortunately termed as *Iyengar Yoga.*

Q.- But there is a difference between yoga practised by others and Iyengar yoga?

Yes, that is because of the inner sight of *Patañjali's,* which I brought out not merely in expression but in experiences of the body, mind and self. The important point in my practice and teaching is the guidance given by Patañjali regarding the interpenetration of attention and touch of awareness of intelligence from the skin to the self and from the self to the skin. The second point is the consciously interweaving together of the physical, physiological, mental, intellectual and spiritual levels of the practitioner. This interweaving and interpenetrating attention that I built up gained ground as time moved on. I am instrumental in attracting people towards yoga, but there is no *Iyengar Yoga*, Iyengar is a mortal person and yoga is an Immortal Universal Subject. I have not called this *Iyengar Yoga*, but others call it so, maybe for the sake of convenience.

It may not be easy to feel the spread of intelligence in the frontier of the body, but many may be under the wrong impression that they feel the spread of intelligence and consciousness covering the frontiers of the extended body with the same length and breadth. The Iyengar method of yoga is like the scale of justice. A scale of justice is considered exact and exclusive.

---

* Interview by Zippy Wiener in the Library of the Ramāmaṇi Iyengar Memorial Yoga Institute, on 28th August 1997.

It should neither be overdone nor underdone. It should neither be too strong nor too dull. In every posture the body, the mind, action and motion as well as each breath of the physical, physiological, mental and intellectual sheaths have to be evenly balanced. In the same way, life energy and consciousness too have to be evenly balanced in the concerned sheaths of man. It is a balance between soma and psyche, or brain and brawn and vice versa. Each and every cell in our system, each and every fibre in our system, each and every particle of the blood current that flows should move in concord and harmony.

When I practise yoga I bring all these things together and I associate my consciousness with all these aspects in each motion and action, so that the divine approach of health coming from deep within is built up. There is a complete concurrence of oneness in this way of *sādhanā*. I try to impart this concurrency in others giving them the right methodology.

While doing yoga *sādhanā*, whether *āsana*, *prāṇāyāma* or *dhāraṇā* and *dhyāna*, it is important to keep one's intelligence alert, active and sharp. For that reason the awareness has to be developed which is known as *prajñā*. When intelligence *(buddhi)* is charged with awareness *(prajñā)* one can hit the target with ease. The body is like a bow, which has to be ready and steady. The *sādhanā* is like an arrow, which is sharpened with intelligence through the practices of *āsana*, *prāṇāyāma*, *dhāraṇā* and *dhyāna*. And the very target is the core of the being – the soul. So I have given the method so that body, mind and intelligence play their role accurately to hit the soul.

I think that many people do not know how to connect the body, the mind and the soul in their practices. They consider *āsana* as a conative action and say that it is good for the body like any other physical exercise. But they cannot explain how the same can be done connecting the intelligence to ignite and discipline the consciousness to reach the Soul. The *āsana* are not mainly the conative actions, but consist of cognitive, mental, intellectual and spiritual aspects. Therefore, the practitioner has to connect and coordinate all the five sheaths[1] of the body while practising *āsana* and *prāṇāyāma*. This I consider as true yoga. On account of my precise presentation and explanation of the yogic philosophy in *āsana* as well as in *prāṇāyāma*, people named it as Iyengar Yoga. I never claimed yoga by my name.

When we point out about ourselves, we know that we are talking about our "self". This "self" is a small self. Beyond this self there is a big Self, which is called "soul". The small self is the conscience keeper between the consciousness and the big Self or the soul *(ātman)*. In order to know and realise the big Self, we need first to know the small self. This small self includes not only the body and mind, but intelligence, I-ness and consciousness *(manas*, *buddhi*, *ahaṁkāra* and *citta)*, as well. We need to see while practising, how to educate, culture and

---

1 *Panca kośa* – five sheaths; *annamaya* – physical, *prāṇamaya* – physiological, *manomaya* – psychological, *vijnānamaya* – intellectual and *ānandamaya* – spiritual sheath.

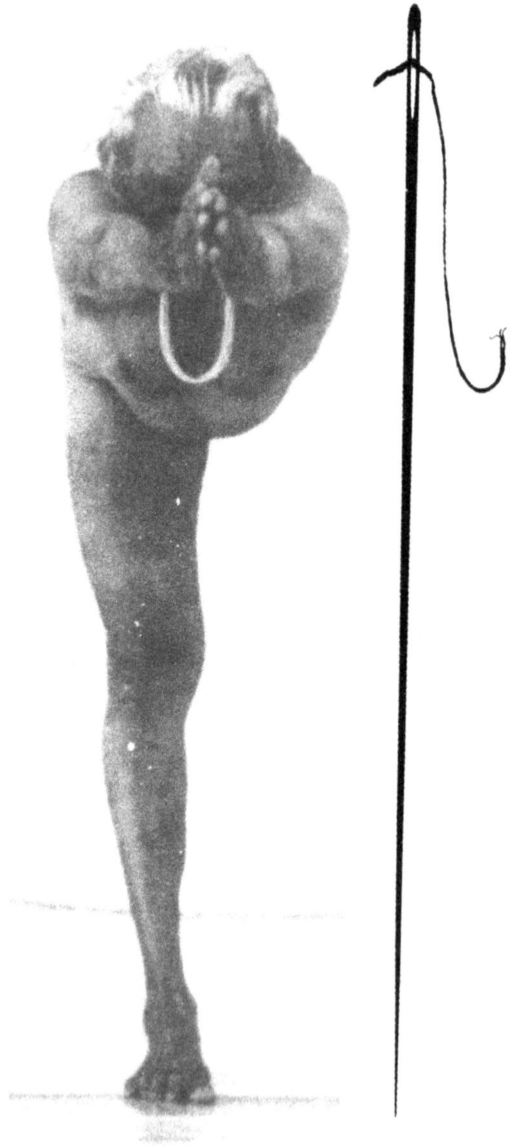

Plate n. 28 – Needle + thread.

utilise these aspects of small "self" to reach the big "Self". Among these aspects of small self the I-ness or *asmitā* is closer to the big Self. Often it poses itself as the big Self – *ātman*. We need to train the I-ness through the consciousness – *citta*. The small self or I-ness is the needle and the intelligence is the eye of the needle. The mind is the head of the thread. In order to insert the thread into the eye of the needle, you sharpen the thread with the hand. If the thread is loose or thick it doesn't pass through the eye of the needle. So you sharpen it by wetting it with water or saliva before inserting it into the eye of the needle. In our body, the nervous system, the cellular system, the fibres, the tendons are like threads. The skin fibres, muscle fibres, bone fibres, nerve fibres are threads. The moment the thread is inserted, the mind pierces the eye of the needle, the intelligence and it disappears. Similarly, in the practice of *āsana*, the mind acts like the sharp edge of the thread, which passes through the intelligence and leads the fibres to sew the body in the right direction.

Then the intelligence takes the lead, the mind disappears or rather it follows the intelligence. The intelligence is the eye of the needle. The intelligence makes the needle to weave the entire body into a perfect cloth.

A weaver through his skill weaves the cloth. Similarly the consciousness as weaver, skilfully weaves the fabric of our existence. I do this in all the *āsana* and *prāṇāyāma* as well as in *dhyāna*.

Q.- What is yoga and how did it come into existence?

First let me answer the second part of the question. I have dealt very well with this question in the first chapter of *Light on Prāṇāyāma*[1].

Nobody knows the timeless, primeval Absolute One, nor when the world came into existence. God and nature existed before man appeared, but as man developed he cultivated himself and began to realise his own potential. Through this came civilisation. Words were evolved with this, concepts of God *(puruṣa)* and nature *(prakṛti)*, religion *(dharma)* and yoga developed.

All our spiritual texts say that at the time of creation of the world, the Creator created yoga. But it remained dormant for sometime as people were moving in the web of pleasure. It is said that God created this world with the first exhalation or the first breath. Probably the first creation was pure, but then, as you speak of today's industrial pollution, or environmental pollution, which destroys the natural resources and natural climate on our planet; similarly, the pollution of intelligence might have occurred in man through temptations that were instilled by the Creator at the time of creation.

God created everyone giving pure, untainted intelligence. He also created the objects that attracted the human beings, and their pure intelligence got tainted and polluted due to attractive objects. Man got involved in creation and not in the creator. The God-created-purity got polluted by the *triguṇa*, namely, *sattva*, *rajas* and *tamas*. *Sattva* is illumination, *rajas* is vibrancy and *tamas* is dormancy. Among these three qualities, *rajas* and *tamas* started tainting the intelligence of the people. Therefore, the subject of yoga also got tainted; the purity of the subject got polluted. Finally, it lost its purity. On account of this impurity and taint, man began to trace the life of purity and went back to yoga. On account of this, the "God-created-yoga" has to take him to the origin – God.

Coming to the second part, I feel it is appropriate to explain the eight aspects of yoga so that one gets the picture of yoga. As I said, the practice of yoga is meant for us to reach God. We started going away from God. He knew that man goes astray soon and created this path of yoga to reach Him. This path is eight-folded, namely *yama, niyama, āsana, prāṇāyāma, pratyāhāra, dhāraṇā, dhyāna* and *samādhi*.

Among these eight aspects of yoga however, *āsana* and *prāṇāyāma* are the exclusively expressive subjects. *Yama, niyama* and *pratyāhāra* can be explained, while the other aspects of yoga, namely *dhāraṇā, dhyāna* and *samādhi* are to be experienced. For these eight aspects of yoga a teacher has to use a method of explanation and expression to feel or experience unalloyed bliss and live fully in the being.

---

[1] *Light on Prāṇāyāma* – Chapter one. Published by Harper Collins, London.

The ideals are not easy to demonstrate practically. One can live in *yama* and *niyama* and through example one can lead the path of ethical practice. *Āsana* and *prāṇāyāma* make one to adopt them practically. The *sādhaka* in his *sādhanā* of *āsana* and *prāṇāyāma* is required to adopt the ideals of *yama* and *niyama* in a practical manner since their adoption builds not only ethical discipline but spiritual discipline also.

When the views and the ways come together through these four streams of yoga (*yama, niyama, āsana, prāṇāyāma*); then comes the state of serenity and tranquillity, which can only be experienced. This can neither be expressed nor explained, but is definitely experienced. This experiencing of an illuminative state of purity, tranquillity and unalloyed serenity is the realm of yoga. Until this experience is felt, uninterrupted practice has to go on to minimise and eradicate the *rājasic* and *tāmasic guṇa*.

Yoga means association. It is the primary way to associate the dissociated human body and human mind or human physiology and psychology. Yoga is the only method to eradicate the human weakness as man looks at objects in a perverted way. Yoga teaches us how to look directly without any perversion, without any imagination, not only from the senses of perception but also from the sense of mind, sense of intelligence and sense of consciousness so that the objects that taint man are completely unveiled.

The real inner core of a human being is surrounded by the evolutes of *prakṛti*. The body, the senses, the physiological and psychological sheaths belong to him. But he gets dissociated or remains careless with these means. This kind of dissociation causes destruction because these evolutes are disarrayed. They remain in a mismanaged state. If he tries to unite and weave his body, senses, mind and intelligence constructively, this construction brings integration. This constructive integration is called *saṁyama*. So from *saṁyoga* (association or conjunction) the progress in yoga changes into *saṁyama*. The moment he begins to feel, "I am an integrated person", he sees no difference between head and heart; whereas in the earlier state he was seeing the difference between head and heart. This is the first experience the practitioner gets. This is how the association and integration in yoga takes place, to bring the head and the heart together at all times.

Yoga teaches how to bring the head and heart from dissociation into association so that they work together with rhythm. When the head and heart are blended and united, then the character of *tamas* and *rajas* fade and *sattva* becomes predominant. When that *sāttvic* quality is developed, one reaches the state of *samādhi*. So yoga means not only union, but from union, integration, and from integration to unalloyed tranquillity and serenity, where the divisions disappear once and for all. These three stages of evolution of the *sādhaka*; association, integration and serenity, are hidden in the eight aspects of yoga called *yama, niyama, āsana, prāṇāyāma, pratyāhāra, dhāraṇā, dhyāna* and *samādhi*. That is why it is called *aṣṭāṅga* yoga.

– Why these eight steps? –

Just now I explained to you and again you are going into the same question.

You know you have an anatomical or skeletal body, a physiological or organic body, you have the mental body, you have the conscious intelligent body and you have the spiritual body as well. This means that our body from the external sheath is tiered with various shapes, various layers. If you go into a cave, at first you have some light but if you go deeper into the cave you are completely in the dark. Like this you can understand the house of the Self, which is deep dark inside the body. You can also guess how many dark caves you have to penetrate to enter in. And if you have to enter into these caves, what kind of brightness, luminosity and brilliance should you have in the capacity of your intelligence. You have to interpenetrate and enter the tunnel of the soul, by crossing these tunnels one after the other. For this, the intelligence has to become sharper and sharper and sharper. If the intelligence is not very very sharp, then you may be penetrating only the physical or the physiological body, or to some extent the psychological body. Beyond that you cannot even speak of the other layers of the body. The deeper the tunnels, the lengthier as well as darker they are, obviously penetration becomes more difficult. One has to struggle hard to go into these various tunnels which are called layers or sheaths in our body using; 1) the intelligence – which is the eye of the needle, 2) consciousness – which is the needle and 3) fibres and nerves or the threads which follow the needle – (consciousness) by passing through it so that it moves from the crown of the head to the soles. This is how the head and the heart are connected. I connect the top to the bottom portion of the body to be one with the soul (the inner being), and to some extent this is what I teach. Because of this specific method of penetration and interpenetration from the physical body to the spiritual body, I make the intelligence sharp and bright in order to unveil layer after layer to cross the dark tunnels. Because of this approach in yoga and by me imparting the same to others, people benefited with the required effect and got transformed in themselves.

So these eight aspects of yoga are required to interpenetrate the five sheaths of our body. The *aṣṭāṅga* yoga is required in order to complete the journey from the body to the soul. You have to cross your own hurdles in the physical, the physiological, the moral, the mental, the conscious and spiritual bodies. That is why there are eight aspects of yoga. I call these eight petals of the yogic flower as emancipation.

– Where does the therapy come in aṣṭāṅga *yoga? –*

I have gone from the physical level to the spiritual level, and having penetrated the darkness of my body, by opening the tunnels for the light to penetrate; the effect of yoga upon various diseases has been revealed and that has attracted people to yoga as a therapy or a remedy.

Look at your own friend; she has suffered with whiplash and blackouts. But in fifteen days what has happened? See how soon yoga affected in bringing solace to her. See, how she came to a normal healthy condition? She was suffering from whiplash for years. Without the depth of experiential knowledge, this interpenetration and interweaving, I would not have succeeded in giving that quick relief to her. While practising *yogāsana* and *prāṇāyāma* from the external to the internal and from the internal to the external, or weaving from outer to inner as well as from inner to outer, from top to the bottom, from the horizontal plane to the vertical height, they are properly connected, co-related, bringing all the threads to the core.

I have used my body, my mind and my intelligence in such a way that the fibres of my body expand horizontally and interweave the horizontal weft with the vertical warp so that it becomes a super fine cloth of the mind, and not a coarse cloth. In order to know the quality of pure cotton cloth, it is measured in 'counts'. The threads of cotton are refined. So more the counts more is the refinement. My method of yoga makes the cloth 100 count or 120 count, and not 80 count or 60 count or 40 count. So I changed the practice of yoga from the coarse cloth of 40 count to 100 count or beyond 100. I refined the texture from the coarse to a refined silk cloth. That is why people are so much attracted to my way of yoga, which is nothing but an exploration and exposition of Patañjali's.

Q.- Some people say "Iyengar Yoga" is physical yoga.

My friend! Please have you noted what I have said so far? One who says that the other does physical yoga, knows that he uses his head, which is nothing but a physical part of the biological brain. When such people analyse from the brain but don't see from the heart, what right have they to call this physical? One who sows the seed of division cannot be a mature person. When such people utter words at these gross levels, know that they live only in their physical bodies; what right have they to say that others are on a physical level? Does this quality of criticizing by such words come from the physical organs or from the soul?

– From physical organs – brain and mouth. –

It shows that their heart needs purging. The person who is fully devotional and spiritual cannot criticize like that. Yoga is a spiritual path. However, only intellectuals in the garb of spiritualism demarcate the practice of yoga as physical and spiritual to misguide the common people.

You say Mr. Yehudi Menuhin's violin renditions are divine. Is a violin a physical instrument or is it something that came from the heavens? Can he bring the divine music without the use of his physical body or his fingers, or the physical instrument such as a violin? Show me any person in the world, who claims to be a spiritual person, without the association to the body and mind. This association is called *saṁyoga*. One has to have *saṁyoga*, i.e. association or union with the body, mind, and intelligence. They do not merely unite, but get integrated. Divinity expresses itself when all these are totally and unconditionally integrated with purity for the sake of the "soul". This is called *saṁyama*.

Can the soul see or speak without a body? Those who say that their method is spiritual and criticize me as a physical practitioner use their soul as an "object". For me it is a subject.

– *What is* saṁyama? –

Patañjali has used the word *saṁyama*. *Saṁyama* is a yogic terminology for the integration of the body, mind and soul. Associating the energies of body, nerves, mind, intelligence and consciousness together to be with the self is *saṁyoga*. Without *saṁyoga*, *saṁyama* is not possible and without *saṁyama* yoga is not possible. Without spirituality all these three are impossible. The practice of yoga is done to have the association, integration and absorption of the body, mind and intelligence to be in union with the soul.

So you ought to understand, that if these people talk this language, they differentiate the body, mind and soul and you should know that they only have bookish knowledge. It does not matter to me. If you know the significance of the scale of justice, then you understand that the scale of judgment is tilted when one criticizes. It is either their totally perverted intelligence or a fallacy, bias or prejudice, or it is unintelligence. Such statements are immature, therefore I advise you to put these thoughts into a waste paper basket. Can the physical part be separated from the spiritual? Can the body be separated from the soul?

– *No.* –

That is why the self is called *jīvātman* – the combination of physical and spiritual entities. *Jīva* means infinite life force. That life force or energy is nothing but *prakṛti*. *Ātmā* is an infinite, spiritual entity. The *jīvātmā* is the embodied self or the individual self. Because of the small self gets embodied in *prakṛti*, the big Self too gets engulfed. Hence the small individual self has to be purified for the big Self. When this takes place, *prakṛti* becomes a noble friend to build up the divine consciousness. If you exist only as soul, then you cannot do anything. Soul is neutral. It cannot do anything. It is lame. Because of its association with *prakṛti*, its movements seem to exist. If *ātman* has to be experienced, then the first requirement is to sublimate the *jīvātman* – the embodied self –, which opens the door for the Self to come out of its prison.

- *Can anybody but you reach this,* Gurujī*?* -

By the grace of God I think I have. I do not know about others. Have you heard me criticize anybody?

- *Never in my life.* -

That is enough for you to understand what is spiritual life and what is egoistic life. Have I criticised any yogi in any paper? But I'm attacked! Why? Because the best form of defence is offence. So this type of criticism is nothing but self-boosting and self-boasting. They have only a copybook intelligence and hence they read the books and speak without experience. But here is a man who does not read books but speaks from his heart! My conscience is clear about what I practise. I want to know whether their conscience is clear or not. If they do not practise, it's their bad conscience that pricks them.

Q.- Can any one show the spiritual yoga without using the physical and mental organs?

I have just told you regarding the tunnels or caves in the body. You have to penetrate those caves or tunnels. Without the instrument – the body – can you penetrate? Can you use some other way? Can you use an arrow without the bow? Without hands can you hold the bow? So this is what one has to understand.

In yoga, the physical body becomes the bow, the mind becomes the arrow and the target is the Universal Soul – the *Brahma*. Understand the body as the bow and use it. In the early days I had to use this body more. Body is not a true friend but a treacherous friend of one and all. You do not know at what time it takes one in a wrong direction. You have to be alert; you have to be attentive regarding its intelligence and its memories.

As far as I am concerned my fingers are pure, my legs are pure, my body is pure, my head is pure, my heart is pure. Whether I reach divinity or not, it is not important to me. It does not matter what people brand me or my practice.

Do you know the story of the donkey and the three men?

– No. –

Three generations of a family, a householder with his father and his son, wanted to sell their donkey at the weekly market. Walking along to the market, a man saw them and said, "Two of you, the father and the son being young can walk, why don't you put the child on the donkey?" So they put the boy on the donkey. After some time, another person walking the same road saw them and said: "Shame, a young boy is riding while the old man is walking. Why not change? The old man should ride and the young boy can walk". So they changed places. A third man saw them and said, "What fools, why not all ride?" So all got on the donkey and the donkey died due to the weight.

This is how the world is. Do anything, people criticise. They go on commenting. Their job is to comment, these are people who love to attack, remark, criticise and give opinions. Their job is not to transform themselves but to play on others. If we give our ears to their opinion and criticism we will perish. Therefore let us concentrate on our practice.

Q.- What is *āsana?*

Āsana is a posture. When you do the *āsana*, then, re-think and re-pose, so that you get the seed of the *āsana*, which is like the base – a vessel. If the vessel is tilted the water spills out. The container should be placed very accurately for the contents to be held fully and evenly. You have to practise each *āsana* in such a way that the container, the body, is very stable for the content to remain steady. That's why after learning the *āsana* if you have to re-do the learnt *āsana*, then you have to re-define it in order to understand the base; so that the blood current in the vessels, the electrical current in the nerves, the chemical current in the organs and the energy current (*prāṇa*) in the *nāḍi* do not get disturbed and flow with potency in a right direction and work with each other in unison. Stability is the real presentation of an *āsana*.

I've used the words "the scale of justice" already: you've got two legs, two arms, you've got two eyes, two ears, two nostrils, there is only one mouth, one heart and one brain. The brain though single shows its division. In the single brain, the functions are allotted departmentally. Physically it is divided into four lobes but even in functions such as thinking, reasoning or decision-making it shows its division and diversity. Even between the eyes and the ears you don't see the singleness. The eyes may get focussed functionally but nerve supplies are separate, and the ears may have capacity to hear but nerve supply for each is separate. Between the two nostrils you find deviation of the septum that causes disequillibrium. The physical heart has four compartments. If the rhythm of the heartbeat goes wrong the four compartments get affected. So while staying in the *āsana* one has to apply this scale of justice and give a proper verdict. However, there is diversity in two arms and two legs. What the right can perform the left cannot and what the left can the right cannot. One eye will be sharp to see and one ear will be sharper to hear than the other one.

The body has these diverse forces. The brain and the heart also have diverse forces. There is unity in diversity and diversity in unity. The meaning of yoga is to join, to bind, to unite. We have to join these "two" to make them "one" and bring unity in diversity. Yoga brings unity and ceases the diversity. *Āsana* is meant to bring unity. It ties the diverse body to a single spiritual heart. It is only the spiritual heart, which is single, and has a single aim.

Q.- Why does *prāṇāyāma* have to be practised? How does it help?

Prāṇa means energy and that energy is produced by the contact or by intermingling of the five elements namely *pṛthvī* - earth, *āp* - water, *tej* - fire, *vāyu* - air and *ākāśa* - ether, with the five atomic energies in the form of qualities namely, *gandha* - smell, *rasa* - taste, *rūpa* - shape, *sparśa* - touch and *śabda* - sound. This you can read from my *Light on Prāṇāyāma* book. As you know something of how electricity is produced, similarly the practice of *prāṇāyāma* generates and develops currents of energy that protect the life force that exists in the doer. Among these five elements: earth, water, fire, air, and ether; if you observe, only water and fire are the two that are "contra"-elements. If there is a fire what do you do? You put it out using water. Other elements act as supporters. Earth creates space for it to burn more. Air acts as fuel and ether spreads the fire. Only water can bring the fire down and it is only fire that dries the water. That is why I say fire and water are the two elements of the system that are opposite. The other elements are all friends.

With the practice of *āsana* and *prāṇāyāma* we fuse the elements of water and fire, which generate energy. The river that flows has current. Can it produce electricity unless it turns into a waterfall?

- *It can't.* -

Similarly, though the normal breath has got some current (energy), it does not generate as much as it should generate for the entire system to be positively healthy. This is the reason why we sometimes say, "I am healthy", and sometime say, "I am not keeping fit." For example when you do *Viparīta Karaṇi*, the blood pours like a waterfall from venous blood vessels towards the heart for purification. If you do *Paschimottānāsana* you allow the blood to spread latitudinally to reach the side body. The arteries are not forced to pump. Similarly, certain *āsana* keep the mind pensive and reflective while others make one dynamically positive. As the electricity has positive and negative currents, similarly the practice of *āsana* and *prāṇāyāma* too produce positive and negative currents. That's why various *āsana* and *prāṇāyāma* are practised, so that the blood gets filtered and re-filtered. The blood's contents are transformed into a very high quality. What you call in today's language as R.B.C., W.B.C., haemoglobin or hormones, etc. are improved quality wise. In olden days these were called "pearls of blood" *(ratna pūrita dhātu).* Though new names are given to the same thing it must not make any difference. The concepts are the same but the words are different. The various *āsana* and *prāṇāyāma* help the flow of blood by creating certain banks so that it may be blocked in certain parts. As doctors tighten the tourniquet at certain areas to control the blood circulation, *āsana* work in the same manner. When you do *Marichyāsana*, or *Paśāsana*, what do you do? You do not allow the blood to circulate in certain parts and you change the blood flow from these areas to move where the gates are opened for circulation to take place or saturation to take place. When you release the pose, the blood spreads and is supplied to the dried area. This is the way in which the energy is produced by the *āsana*.

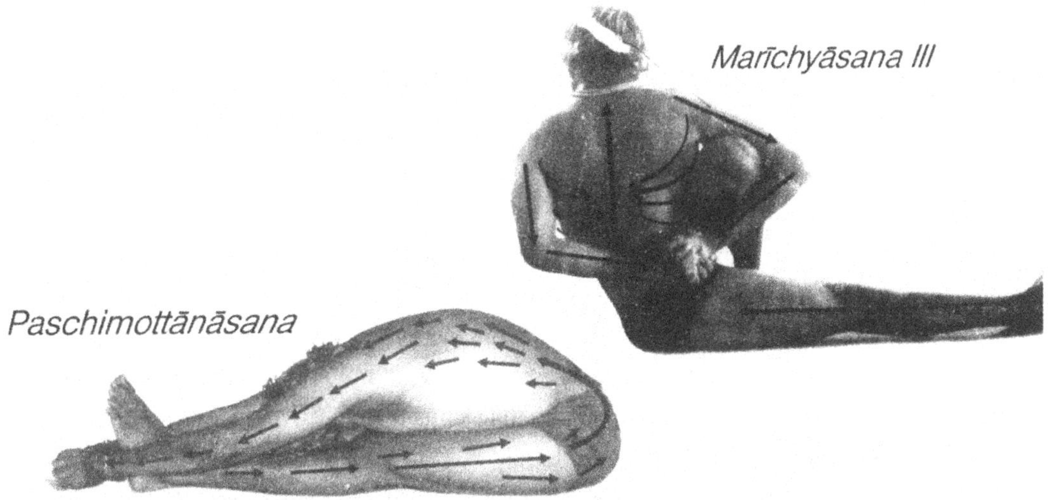

Plate n. 29(a) – Blood flow in *Paschimottānāsana* and *Marichyāsana*

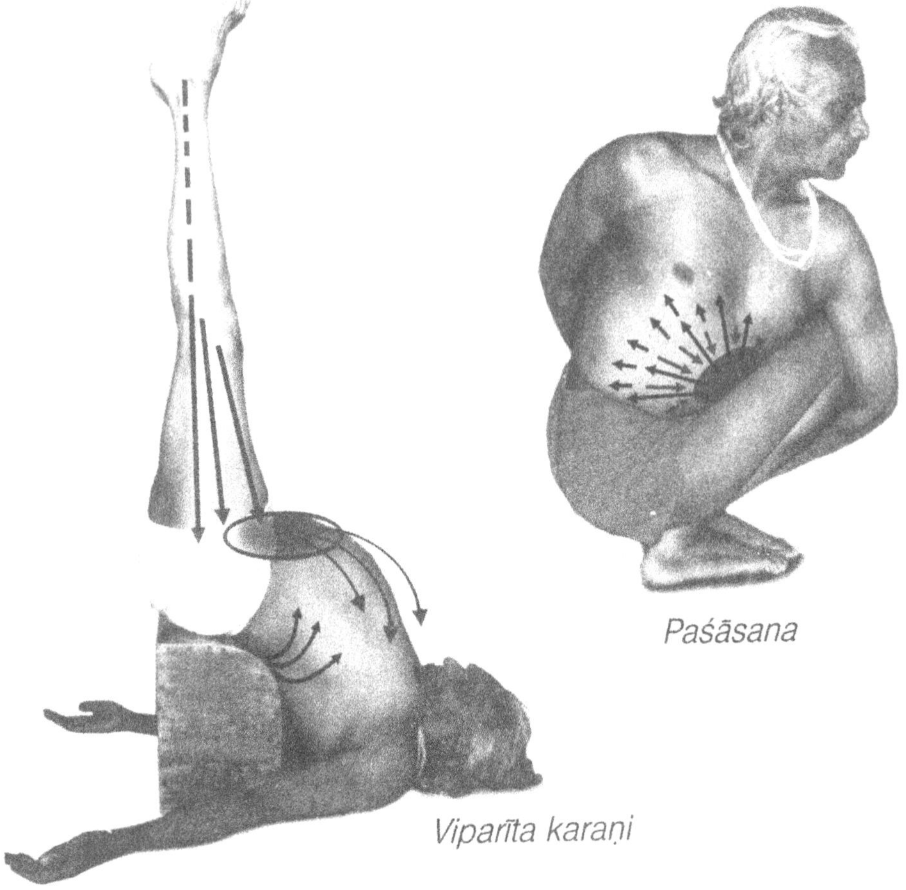

Plate n. 29(b) – Blood flow in *Viparīta karaṇi*, and *Paśāsana*

Once the energy is generated, then how to maintain it without wastage is *prāṇāyāma*. That is why *prāṇāyāma* is given. More than the generation of energy, *prāṇāyāma* helps to protect or save that energy which is generated from the practice of *āsana*. The *cakra* in the body are like storing places that keep on supplying energy to the various parts of the body as well as the mind and intelligence when needed.

Prāṇāyāma acts as a tanker in order to store the energy. The earned energy, generated by inhalation, is maintained and used by the system through the practice of *prāṇāyāma* known as *kuṁbhaka*. The unwanted, polluted or poisonous air has to go out. This is known as exhalation. When the cellular system of the body absorbs the energy, then it releases what is not wanted and this goes out in the form of exhalation. If the urinary system is blocked you cannot pass urine. Whatever force you may use it does not pass. So a catheter is used. When the drainage system gets blocked, you need special hosepipes to pierce the blockage and clear it. Similarly, the blockages that block the liver, spleen, pancreas, heart or brain are cleared by *āsana* and *prāṇāyāma*. The fungus grows on the periphery and then goes inside. These are like the blockages in the gutter. As you flush the drainage system, *āsana* and *prāṇāyāma* flush them through blood circulation. That's why various *āsana* are given so that the body may be flushed from impurities. Some may be fully blocked and some may be partially blocked, and at some places it may flow easily, at other places it may not flow easily. *Āsana* are meant to remove the blockages in the system so that when you do them the energy that is drawn in can be spread to feed the cellular system. Through the practice of *prāṇāyāma* the generated energy is maintained, retained and what is not needed by the system is discarded.

Patañjali explains the effect of *prāṇāyāma* at a spiritual level. He says, "The ignorance that covers the intelligence is removed and the mind becomes clear for meditation."[1] This too is a flushing process of the intelligence. Everybody speaks of meditation – "Instant meditation," like fast food. Yoga Meditation too is treated like fast food. I'm sorry to say that such people who run after meditation say that I don't teach meditation while others are teaching meditation. It's like hankering after fast food, which has no nourishment and no food value at all. That is why in order to develop that concentrated attention, *prāṇāyāma* is given to maintain energy. Without energy there is no concentration. The way I do my yoga, my physical body gets married and united to the spiritual body within. The marriage of *prakṛti* or nature with *puruṣa* or soul, is the effect of yoga. Hence I say, "I am a perfect yoga practitioner." You may call it pride. But know that it is a genuine pride.

Practice of yoga is like the embroidery work done by using skin fibres, muscle fibres, nerve and bone fibres along with breath, mind, intelligence and consciousness using as needle and finally you see a beautiful embroidery work in the form of *āsana, prāṇāyāma, dhāraṇā* and *dhyāna,* ultimately converting into a Divine embroidery.

[1] *Tataḥ kṣīyate prakāśa āvaraṇam* (*Y.S.,* II.52).

THE YOGA OF INTELLIGENCE*

A life dedicated to yoga and a method whose virtues are praised by hundreds of thousands of occidentals are the trademark of maestro Iyengar, considered by many to be the grandest living yogi of our time. Mental sharpness, flexibility and corporeal strength accompany Iyengar's eighty years as if ageing had forgotten him. And despite the admiration of so many or that his figure is on its way to being converted to myth, he continues to consider himself a yoga student who still has much to learn. So he confesses in the exclusive interview conceded to MAS ALLA DE LA CIENCIA (Further Beyond Science) with the motive of his recent visit to Spain.

In the Centre of Yoga Iyengar of Madrid one breathes a festive atmosphere. More than two hundred followers of this yoga system fill the small practice room anxiously awaiting the arrival of Bellur Krishnamachar S. Iyengar, the practically legendary Hindu yogi whose method has extended throughout the Occident, revolutionising the practice of yoga like none other.

ETERNITY FRIGHTENS US

After a long wait he enters the room with decided steps and an ample smile, which show the contrast between his perfectly white teeth and his sallow skin. He is not a tall man but tremendously corpulent and vital; he belongs to that category of persons who involuntarily occupy much more space than the physical contours of their bodies. Seeing him it is difficult to remember that in a few short months he will be eighty years old. The living example of what he predicates, his shining eyes and childlike enthusiasm give his words the flavour of authenticity. "If it weren't for my daily practice I would not be alive", he repeats on more than one occasion.

He is not an easy person to interview although he is very suggestive. He possesses the agile verb and sense of humour, which emanates from his wide vital experience. His words, pronounced with the resonant voice of a much younger man daze in such a way that even though his replies are different from the questions the interviewer feels no frustration. Impatient, Iyengar does not like to repeat himself and demands attention and mental clarity from those

---

* Interview by Concha Labarta in Madrid on October 1997. Published by the Spanish magazine *Mas Alla de la Ciencia*, January 1998.

who surround him. He exercises the role of maestro with ease but one senses that he would be willing to change to discipleship the moment the opportunity to learn something new presents itself.

"A professor can only light the lamp of intelligence", he affirms, "but it is the student who must keep the lamp alight using the fuel of his conscience and the wick of his consciousness so that the light shines always". No mystic halo surrounds him; Iyengar is a practitioner and an untiring worker and he is proud of that: "With the practice of āsana *confidence replaces doubts and fears. One is closer to God because one fears nothing. This is the spiritual value of the* āsana. *You have to practise to resist the fear of eternity that appears in front of you and makes you tremble. In that moment you will understand how much the* āsana *can help you to come face to face with the divine."*

Iyengar has accomplished that everyone present is entirely concentrated on his words. He responds precisely to the technical questions of some of the students. With one of these questions he offered the occasion to verify his penetrating knowledge of human anatomy. A question passed to him in writing (the author anonymous for the moment), a student was concerned with the arrhythmias suffered when practising breathing exercises. "Those who experience this type of problem tend to be persons with long necks, thin but wide at the hips", described the maestro who then asked that the author of the question come forward. Upon verifying that the person's constitution was exactly that described by Iyengar, a murmur of approval went through the room. Energetically applying himself to correcting the posture, adapting it to the person's physical condition, one sees how Iyengar is really enjoying himself; his explanations are so profuse that the translator can hardly keep up with him. Realising how he is converting the reception into a practical class like those he directs weekly in Pune, his native city in India, he returns to his role as orator with an impish smile on his face.

In 1940, twenty-two year old Iyengar without schooling or possibilities of finding work decided to use yoga – the only thing he knew how to do – to survive, realising public demonstrations to attract future practitioners. But, as he confesses, that it did not satisfy him so he decided to concentrate on the inner essence of yoga, studying the ancient texts and passionately practising ten hours daily until he outlined his system which today triumphs throughout the world.

Precision, intensity and dynamics are what characterise his method. These qualities develop what he calls "the intelligence of the cells", the only intelligence capable of maintaining the house of the soul or the body in ideal condition to seek spiritual fulfilment. For Iyengar any division of man or of yoga into body, mind and spirit is fictitious. These aspects are all so inextricably united that it is impossible to evolve in one of them if the others remain still. For the yogi working one's body is an absolute necessity: only he who has a healthy body and who functions at his maximum potential is prepared to face the voyage of evolution. In order that no one be excluded from this possibility, always searching, Iyengar has invented supports – imitating the ancient practitioners who hung themselves upside down from trees – so that even persons with physical limitations are able to execute the postures and enjoy the advantages of yoga.

Today he continues to personally attend to his classes, dedicating himself with total concentration on his students as well as having supervised the Spanish version of his latest book titled Light on Prāṇāyāma *(edited in Spain by Kairos and considered the essential guidebook for those interested in yogic breathing) and periodically visiting his yoga centres in Europe and America. He affirms that with experience his body's intelligence has refined itself to such a point that it is possible for him to pinpoint the connections between nerves, muscles, bones and tendons which many newer yogis have impudently copied. As a result of this precise state of physical and mental refinement, he is able to penetrate the human body, from the outermost to the innermost, and illuminate it with the light of intelligence and consciousness. Explaining that only in this way a yogi attains his maximum expression: "Your practical experiences and mine must be integrated into a universal state of unity without division. I have probably been sent here to ignite and enlighten you, so that your practice becomes more internal so that this internalisation leads you to the hidden nucleus of being, what we call ātman. I hope with all my heart that all who practise will arrive to this state". "In yoga there are no miracles" – affirms Iyengar – "only spiritual evolution." And under the auspice of his words as a yogi Iyengar shows us one of his radiant smiles. "Yoga does not generate supernatural powers but evolution. Evolution however, for an ordinary man can seem to be supernatural", maintains Iyengar.*

Q.- For someone who decides to practise yoga there are many methods and schools in the market. What is it in your system that makes it different from others?

I would like to make clear that yoga is one like God is one. Yoga is not a subject for marketing. One cannot buy yoga or sell yoga, though there might be differences in approach. Therefore, one has to use one's discrimination.

I do not distinguish between physical, mental or spiritual yoga. The container is the body and the content is the soul. In the same way differently shaped pitchers give different shapes to the water they contain. I try to present yoga in a manner that even though the container changes, the content remains the same. I teach the way of practising yoga to all in a way that the conscious perception of intelligence expands by itself, so that there remains no difference between the frame of the body and the content of the body that hides within. There remains no disparity between the body, mind and soul. There must be an intellectual involvement, a conscious perception and total attention so that no part of the body – the outer as well as the inner – remains untouched by the effort. Others teach in a compartmental way; I teach in a global way.

As you ask me about my system, I can say that it is meant for one and all and is a whole system. It touches all aspects of our existence.

Q.- How do you respond to the criticism of those who say that your system is excessively physical?

This is a kind of brainwashing. Those who brand my practice of yoga are only seeing the postures as physical; this is their expression, according to their understanding. Obviously their idea is not going to disappear that quickly; because they do not know what to see. They, themselves, do not see the involution of mind, involvement of intelligence and vastness of consciousness. They do not see the journey from the skin to the soul that exists in my practice. If you see my practice or even the photographs of my *āsana*, you will notice that there is unity and sobriety in my expression. For example, when you see others practising the same *āsana* or see their pictures in magazines, their bodies express Herculean muscles. Such muscular expressions today are called "Power Yoga". Yoga does not demand muscular power. It demands mental power. It does not demand muscular control, but mental control. It demands a total integration from inside out and outside in, which is known as *saṁyama*.

When they do the *āsana*, they do them as a show off, but I do them with gracefulness and inner beauty, using the body as an instrument. My body does not appear as Herculean or robust. Even if one calls it physical expression, the muscles express humbleness and not physical prowess. Yoga demands loveliness, elegance, beauty, charm, gracefulness and nobility.

– But doesn't emphasising the role of the body discourage those who don't believe that their physical aptitudes can meet the demands of your metho i? –

This is again just an imagination. The body is the first avail ıble instrument, which many may not know how to utilise for a spiritual journey. It appears as I demand physical exertion but factually I only demand physical discipline. There is a diff ence between exertion and discipline. People think that they have to exert themselves and workout with their bodies. They have not to exert for workout, rather exert to get tranquillity. There is no need to torture the body, rather the demands and commands the culture of the body. I practise yoga accordingly, to culture the frame of the body as well as its contents.

Some insufficient translations of original Sanskrit texts say that a *haṭha yogi* is a man who realises certain penances and uses his body at its maximum level in a way that seems like torture. But that is a wrong expression at the origin, and a seemingly false statement. Scriptures are not asking us to torture the body. They show the methodology of withdrawing oneself from the outside world so our cells turn about with mind to look within. This cellular discipline seems to be hard and exhausting. The ancient texts say that in those *āsana* which appear extreme, if the practitioner consciously maintains a state of tranquillity, he is considered as an authentic *haṭha yogi*. I experiment in my practice to find out whether this is true or not. As the yoga texts speak, I see if the nucleus of my being maintains this state of tranquillity. It is devotional, not torturous.

- Understood, but what do we do with the natural limitations of each person? Nature has not given everybody the same flexibility... -

Can everyone who likes to paint become a Picasso or all cellists become Pablo Casals? Do we criticise these great personalities for their maestro-ship in their field or should we look to them as beacons so as to learn from them? My recommendation is that you should try; if you don't attain it, blame your limitation and not the essence of the subject. This is what I am doing and it is for you to take it and learn or leave it.

Your mistake is that you are looking at only the flexibility factor of the body. Flexibility is not the parameter. I was very stiff once upon a time. I did not practise to break the calcification of my joints, but the calcification of the mind. As you say, everyone has natural limitations, but who puts these limitations? Is it not the mind that puts these limitations? When you do not want to practise, then you say you are stiff. You are unprepared and you find excuses to escape from the fact. People want not only readymade, but also undisciplined freedom. Freedom in a sense for you may be no efforts, no involvements, and no inclinations. So it is the mind that needs flexibility. It needs to be bent. The calcification of the mind is built by the ego. Before the body says "no", the mind says "no". It is because of latent laziness, inertia, non-willingness and non-incitement. In order to practise yoga the mind has to gravitate very strongly towards the Soul, which nature provides in all.

Q.- You know that many people are drawn to yoga seeking a miracle be it mental or physical curing. Is this justified? Has yoga no limits?

There is nothing like a miracle in yoga. There is only the spiritual elevation or evolution. My academic performance in school was very poor. I never got beyond 30 percent in any subject. It was what is called a scholastic failure. Nevertheless in the subject of yoga I found my mental faculties opening and from that development and evolution I began teaching. How could this happen to me? Is it not a miracle? Even today I continue practising the same way as I did decades ago. Isn't that also a miracle? I, who had been completely given up by the doctors, am still alive. Is it not a miracle? Caught in the jaws of death, have I not created a kind of miracle in yoga?

So a miracle is not something that happens out of nothing. Yoga has a cure for physical and mental problems. But one has to generate through one's own efforts in order to have the miracle happen.

Now, as far as the limitation in the curing process is concerned, then medicines too have limitations. The question is not of limits in a subject. The question is about the practitioner's limitations. One needs to put extra efforts in the practice in order to eradicate the impediments such as wrong *karma* – wrong actions, wrong thoughts and so on. The practice of yoga brings basically the change in eradicating hindrances, obstacles and impediments. When water does not flow to reach the plants, the gardener removes the obstructions and makes a smooth channel for water to flow; so does the practice of yoga.

Q.- Isn't yoga losing its true essence in its contact with the Occident similar to what has occurred with the martial arts and other oriental disciplines?

I do not think so. I am visiting the west since 1954. Many of my students are honest, sincere and dedicated to yoga, but some with a commercial mind knowing that there is a market to make money in yoga. Numerous charlatans are there who go around saying that they have practised and discovered something new. Such inexperienced people proclaim that they are creative masters in yoga. But a creative artist has to have a mature intelligence, which does not arrive at the call. One has to reach a certain state of stability in practice as well as in intelligence for creativity. This alone and not any other is authentic creativity and hence I am sure that the essence of yoga will not be lost.

I'll give you an example. There are so-called maestros who say that relaxation is attained with the method of tensing your fist shut and then opening it. If a man is able to tense the lobes of his brain in the same way as his fist, then perhaps he would understand the idea of relaxation as some yogis speak of. This type of propaganda on relaxation is painful to hear for a practitioner like me. In *prāṇāyāma* or the breathing exercises some affirm that you have to inflate your abdomen; which will contract your chest in the process, despite the fact that this claim of theirs cannot be found in any ancient yoga texts. This is tricking people. If we puff our abdomens, then the internal organs prolapse; it is a crazy way of teaching that I can't do because I'm not crazy.

Being a universal subject, the applications of yoga cannot differ whether one is Oriental or Occidental. Unfortunately, some people adopt such crazy ways just to please, attract or cajole the enthusiastic aspirants.

Q.- Your body is capable of realising the same exercises as decades ago. Does that mean that yoga has stopped the process of ageing in you? How do you experience the passing of years?

Nothing but practice. I do not practise to stop my ageing process. I just do it. I have not stopped my practice. I do the practice of *āsana, prāṇāyāma* and *dhyāna* regularly. Perhaps I do certain things better than I used to do earlier. My practice is my prayer, my worship, my aim and my life.

There are yogis who when they reach a certain age don't particularly continue *āsana,* claiming that their spiritual evolution is such that they don't need to come down to physical practice. The real reason, which people don't know, is that the yogis can't do the *āsana* any more. I continue practising them because it's the *āsana* that has brought me to this level. According to modern science, I know that at my age, I should have a lot of health problems. Have you seen those athletes who have won medals in the Olympics and years later after their retirement they can't even walk? Thanks to yoga, I still practise and maintain myself. The mind is the enemy. If the mind says, "I can't do it" and if I believe that, then I am lost. If I reach ninety and continue to maintain this rhythm then I will sustain it. What I will never do is to say to people that I have reached such a level that I don't need to practise any more. Rather I say I cannot repetitively do more, but I study the behaviour of the mind more by staying in *āsana* longer than before.

Q.- From where does this tremendous enthusiasm come at your age?

Simply I say, by my continual practice. Age cannot be the problem coming in the way of practice. One needs to have strong will power in one's practice. I have will power and positive faith, and courage and vigour in practice. The keenness in practice keeps me enthusiastic.

A human being is easily affected by advancing age, the approaching disease due to age is a known sign death is close by. Though I have no fear of death or disease, I do not want to be callous. I do look if some unknown sickness or disease is attempting to take hold of me; if I find some weakness or detect the disease, then immediately I take preventive measures by bringing the appropriate changes in my practice. I take care that the nine doors of my body are not soiled. We have nine doors in the body – two eyes, two ears, two nostrils, one mouth cavity, anus and urethra. All these nine doors throw the toxins or waste matters, out These also are the gates through which the diseases enter in. The practice of yoga brings control over the body, senses and mind keeping all the dirt and dust away.

I aspire to be an example for others, that people be stimulated and think, "If Iyengar does it why can't I?" If I abandon my practice, how can I be an example to my aged students? To maintain the fire of yoga burning in them I have to continue my practice.

Q.- You have spoken about tracing illness in your body. How do you manage to do something like that?

With yoga one cultivates a great amount of intellectual sensitivity. If this sensitivity is lost in some part of the body, that is sickness. It is a difficult theme to explain. We yogis say that two rivers exist in our bodies: one is the conscious intelligence and the other is *prāṇic* energy. The function of the conscious intelligence is attention and awareness, and the function of energy is to feel that it is flowing abundantly everywhere in the system. When we practise *āsana* this conscious attention and awareness, with the flow of energy, should be perceived with absolute clarity in every point of the body.

In yoga if you practise too little it means that there is no water in the well of the body; if you practise too much then the well overflows. With the *āsana* we learn to maintain the circulation of the blood in such a way that it reaches the minutest parts of our bodies. When blood circulates you feel a sensation of warmth in the area. To bring the circulation to an area you have to transfer the attention of your intelligence so that it reaches there. When conscious perception and intelligence go hand in hand then you experience the life flowing in those areas of the body and feel a healthy mind and a healthy body.

It also depends upon how you practise. In each *āsana* you need to check the right and left sides of the body. In each *āsana* there has to be a perfect balance, firmness and equality as well as even action. You have to feel this also in *prāṇāyāma*. This way of practice brings new awareness and sensitivity. This sensitivity that comes to the body makes us aware of problems and if we practise, paying attention to its queries, then yoga keeps us free from illness.

Q.- And what if despite everything you were to become ill, would you seek treatment with an occidental doctor?

Here, I am speaking of myself. Why should I go to a doctor if I know how to cure myself? Many of the famous doctors in India come to me for treatment! Let's suppose that I have a fever: never would I be so crazy as to do backbends; on the contrary I would do those *āsana* that cool the body. Yoga is as much a science of health as it is a philosophy, it covers all aspects. With yoga the body develops its potency so that it can defend itself against any sickness. If everybody practises for 20 or 30 years then one may come across a state of non-illness. In case one is afflicted beyond one's capacity, the modern medical science is well advanced and hence I say that those who have not got that faith and will power can try other treatments.

Q.- There are several fads that are always associated with yoga. One of them has to do with what to eat. Does one have to be strictly vegetarian to practise yoga?

I suggest to my students to eat when hungry and to avoid eating too much or too less and not to eat when not hungry. Sickness is inevitable when one cannot digest what one eats. I do not say that one should eat only fruits or vegetables. What is possible or accessible to the common man in that geographical area is his food. For me, assimilation is more important than choice of food. Having come from a poor family, it would be wrong on my part to speak on dietetic recommendations. I only say that what is available to you, eat with pure mind joyfully.

However, it is true that vegetarian food is easy to digest and assimilate. Do not have in mind that vegetarian food is a fad. It is its simplicity. For a non-vegetarian it is difficult to become a vegetarian. If one advises vegetarian food, he may simply run away from the yogic practice. Therefore I do not advise, but I am certain that one who practises yoga, the change or transformation occurs in him. They change their food habits on their own. I want yoga to go into their system rather than ideas.

Q.- Another cliché is the question of sexuality. Does one who practises yoga have to abstain or practise a certain kind of sexual relations?

I am not an ascetic. I'm a family man. Yet I am practising yoga. There is a difference between the sexual relations in married life and sexual relations in certain other situations. I do not know in what sense you are asking the question. Yoga is a discipline through which the practitioner has to train himself to cleanse and purify his or her consciousness. Yoga is not against married life but against sex life. Married life disciplines the sexual behaviour of the couples. It controls free sex or extra marital relations. Married life disciplines one for a healthy life. Yoga recognises this discipline. So the question of abstaining from sexual relations does not arise.

Yoga guides the *sädhaka* to follow his conscience and not renunciation.

Q.- The supposedly supernatural powers that are said to accompany a yogi, are they the result of the awakening of the body's intelligence of which you spoke?

It is not the supernatural powers but the evolution of a practitioner. It's true that a yogi's evolution might appear to be supernatural for a common man but they are very natural achievements or accomplishments of a skilful yogi.

Prudent practice of yoga helps one to understand and conquer the five elements, five energies, five senses of perception, five organs of action, mind, intelligence, consciousness and conscience of the body, and when this happens the so-called supernatural powers naturally surface. So when I speak of awakening of the body intelligence I encompass all these aspects of the human being.

Q.- How would you advise a follower of your method to plan his regular practice of *āsana*?

In the sixties, when I wrote my book *Light on Yoga*, I outlined a course of 300 weeks (more than five years). I had in my mind my own practice and measured, according to my dedication, the possible time it would take to learn, but I never thought of practitioners at large. I didn't think that people who follow my method could dedicate ten hours a day that took me to come to that level. Now, as a mature man, I realise I should have divided the course into 900 weeks. At least that much is required to this measured control of *āsana*.

Actually there are no prescribed rules. Only one who practises has to establish his own sequential series of *āsana* to maintain rhythm and exhilarative feelings. There are many yoga books without a healthy sequential practice. The sequential series given in my book offer protection in their practises. Don't forget that practice of *āsana* is subjective. If a series of *āsana* causes you difficulty, then you have to change the series. When the series and the execution of *āsana* are perfect, then the intelligence expresses itself with joy of lightness and illumination and shows no sign of fatigue or wrongdoing or faulty actions.

As I tried to give a sequential method in *āsana* practice in *Light on Yoga*, I also gave a sequential progressive method of practice of *prāṇāyāma* in my book *Light on Prāṇāyāma*.

MASTER UNFOLDS THE SECRET OF WHAT YOGA IS*

Born in 1918 in the south of India, in order to improve his precarious health he was initiated into the practice of yoga at 16. His brother-in-law, the famous yogi Krishnamachar, was his guru. Since 1937 he has lived a life consecrated to yoga in Pune, where he has taught such distinguished personalities as the philosopher Krishnamurti and the violinist Yehudi Menuhin. His method of yoga, taught in *some 200 schools, is renown in the Occident.*

Bellur Krishnamachar Sundararaja Iyengar speaks with passion and laughs heartily; one notices that he enjoys his long life. Soon he will turn eighty but he continues practising āsana *and* prāṇāyāma *daily. And when something is not right, like someone who takes a pill from the medicine desk, he prescribes himself certain* āsana *and* prāṇāyāma.

Congregated around him are students of Madrid's Iyengar Yoga Centre. They have received him pronouncing the syllable om, *which in chorus acquires the prolonged sound of a Tibetan horn. Except for a small altar presided by the God Hanuman and the Sage Patañjali in one corner, the room resembles a gymnasium; in it are rungs, a balance-beam, ropes... and not it vain. One of the* gurus *– maestros – who most has contributed to the extension of yoga in the Occident, Iyengar's method is based on physical effort.*

Not knowing exactly what yoga is, I approached yogi Iyengar and he replied to my queries.

Q.- Can we consider yoga as a sport?

No. Yoga cannot be considered as a sport but it is the mother of sports. For all the sports it could be a base as well as a supplementary and complementary method.

Athletes do not use their bodies one hundred per cent. Depending on the sport certain parts of the body are developed more than others. In yoga all the areas of the body are attended to. This activity does not build up musculature but rather teaches how to strengthen and use

* Interview by Teresa Ricart in Madrid on October 1997. Published by the Spanish magazine *Muy Interesante*, February 1998.

the muscles in an active way. Besides, in sports the lactic acid always accumulates in the articulations, which produces fatigue, aches and pains in the muscles and the joints. Yoga improves circulation, which eliminates the lactic and uric acid that is why athletes who practise yoga do not feel tired; it accelerates them and prepares them to play with more energy and enthusiasm.

Yoga develops the skilful actions required in every sport. It provides stamina, endurance, quickness, suppleness, and required stability as well as mobility. A sportsman always wants to improve his or her performance. *Āsana* assists them to re-tool those parts that create doubts in the mind by re-adjustment and re-alignment of the weak parts which hinder them.

Moreover, the attention, concentration, strong will power, awareness and the total involvement they need can be achieved by practising yoga. It also guides in the art of relaxation and recoupment for mental composure. That is why yoga is considered as a base or foundation for any sports or athletics.

Q.- Then can yoga be considered a kind of gymnastics?

I have said what yoga is and can do. Yet it seems your mind is fixed and cannot be beyond the frame you have in mind. What you see is the *āsana* that is performed by this body is beyond that frame of gymnastics. Yoga is a disciplined way of living. By following this discipline you channel your physical, moral, mental and spiritual energy. Yoga derives from will power, where you train, trim and tone your inner strength. Yoga is a methodology that helps in uniting the body, mind and intelligence.

It is not meant to develop a Herculean body. These days people do some *āsana* and call it "Power Yoga". A yoga practitioner does not need the muscular or Herculean power. He needs enduring power, tolerance and the inner mental power.

Yoga is not done to show off muscles. It is not done to show the power or the flexibility of the body. Even in the most difficult *āsana*, the quality of elegance in each and every fibre of the body without tension is to be expressed.

In yoga, the skin fibres, muscle fibres, nerve fibres and every cell are well attended. This science is a guide to work on intense penetration from body to self and from the self to the body.

Instructed by the famous yogi T. Krishnamacharya, B.K.S. Iyengar began to teach yoga when he was eighteen. Since then his method is imparted in more than two hundred cities throughout the world. In recognition of his work in 1991 he received the Padmashri Award, the high distinction of civil achievement given by the president of India.

Q.- What is it that your disciples seek when they come to you?

Ninety-nine per cent of people, including those who say they are interested in the spiritual aspects of yoga, really confess to me of their physical and mental weaknesses and ask me for remedies. Why did Krishnamurti, one of the most famous philosophers of the 20th century, come to me? Because he had many problems. So people who live and lead a spiritual life have to come to the physical level to keep their body healthy, as they find the hindrances coming to them and distract their spiritual way of living. The body is the vehicle of the soul, and without freedom in the body, there is no salvation for the soul. That is what one has to know whether one is an intellectual, an athlete, a politician or a doctor. One has to be healthy so that one can proceed further for better living. One should not be satisfied with physical health, but must proceed and arrive at spiritual happiness. This depends on each person. Yoga is very democratic, it is tailored to the needs of a person who practises it.

I have disciples of all categories. Some come to seek health, some come to get rid of pains and diseases. Others come to have psychological relief and freedom from stress and strain. Some come purely as aspirants; as the knowledge deepens, the experience also gets deepened. So the pupils come to get health, peace of mind, a balanced state of mind and in search of the soul.

Q.- If yoga is not equivalent to gymnastics, is it equivalent to a religion?

I do not know why you are jumping from one pole to another, which have no connections. I do not think that it is a religion as one normally sees it. Yoga protects, sustains and supports. This is the tripod of religion, and in that sense it is religion. The practice of yoga makes the religious person a better religious person. So do not compare it to any specific religion. It makes a human being a better human being.

The practice of yoga is a guide that leads man to a higher level than where he is. Yoga is the union of the body with the mind. When an *āsana* is correctly done, experienced and felt, the dualities of body-mind and mind-soul disappear. *Āsana* and *prāṇāyāma* help to draw the veils aside so that the intellect can see with total clarity. They are the means that facilitate the progress of each individual's evolution.

Q.- In your opinion is the practice of yoga compatible with the occidental way of living where body and spirit have traditionally been so separate?

If Occidentals think that the body is separate from the spirit, the Orientals gave a thought that there is a connection between the body and the spirit. All men and women of the world want peace of mind: happiness, health and to improve their lives qualitatively. Oriental and Occidental are geographical divisions and yoga does not make such divisions. Undoubtedly, it is an oriental science because the Orientals began to work in this field in an epoch in which people could not communicate as they do now. This lack of communication then must have kept the Occidentals away from the subject. Now the world has come closer and yoga is receiving renovated interest in the Occident. Society today has become enormously competitive and people's nerves cannot withstand that much pressure and therefore find it difficult to maintain a balanced life. As the practice of yoga strengthens the nervous system and keeps the body healthy in the midst of all tensions, it has become congenial for the Occidentals to take this art now, though people like you see the body and spirit as separate.

Spirituality for Occidentals is something beyond their capabilities as if it is supernatural. That is why they separated the body from the Self. Yoga particularly connects one's body, mind, intelligence and consciousness to the core (Self). The interest has enormously increased and many in the West feel its compatibility.

According to yoga, the very core of the being is pure and sacred. All of us are basically pure at the root. The soul is never polluted. It is the body, mind and intelligence, which gets polluted with wrong thinking and actions. Yoga is that through which the body, mind and intelligence are purified and consecrated in order to co-operate with the core of the being that exists within.

Q.- Does the practice of yoga imply leading a life of asceticism?

Yoga does not say to mortify the flesh, nor encourage the philosophy of denial or to live precariously. One's needs change with the times. Renunciation does not mean to escape from the competitive society of today. Each person must analyse his needs and live with happiness and contentment. I prefer to follow my conscience rather than so-called renunciation.

Yoga does not enforce asceticism. It helps in training one's mind, behaviour and character to accept the right thing and deny the wrong. It gives a new vision to discard whatever is perishable and accord with what is imperishable, i.e. the core of being.

Q.- What is the relation between what we eat and yoga?

Food is not only the builder of the body but also of the mind. We all know that a proper diet is required to get strength. It is a known fact that calcium for bones and proteins for muscles are required. The hormonal glands are built up on these bio-chemicals and the brain functions on glucose. Yogis of yore realised that even the mind and intelligence need a proper, balanced, clean and pure food. In this sense, food and yoga have a great relation.

Personally I am not a food fanatic nor am I a fanatic of yoga but a disciplined human being. My yoga is designed for the common man. My advice is that when you see the food and your mouth gets filled up with saliva, then think that that food is your right food. What brings sickness is when your tongue does not segregate saliva but you eat. Also when the mind dislikes that food, know it is unpalatable to the body.

The beauty of yoga practice is that the body rejects that food which is unpalatable and delights in what is congenial.

Q.- Before, yogis hung themselves upside down and their postures seemed to be like contortionists. Do Hindus have a different anatomy than ours?

How can the Hindus have a different anatomy than that which exists now? Anatomy does not differ but geographical conditions and food habits may change the structure of the body and not the anatomical truth. Fortunately, yoga fits for all. *Āsana* is one of the aspects of yoga. They are not contortions of the body. Flexibility of the body might be one of the aspects. But I have spoken sufficiently on the values of *āsana* and no repetition is needed again here.

You see the Indians sit in the lotus position with ease. It is not because they are more flexible but because they sit on the floor all their lives. The anatomy of the body is similar whether one is Occidental or Oriental. Because of cold conditions here, you do not sit on the floor like Indians and you think you are made up of stiff bodies. Today many Westerners do cross legs more easily than many so-called sophisticated Indians.

Q.- How does one begin in yoga?

You are coming to the point with this question again. Religion, age, flexibility are not the qualities of eligibility to do yoga. Everyone is welcome in this field.

One begins yoga with physical discipline. The body is the first instrument that has to be disciplined in order to channel the energy. That is how the practice of *āsana* begins. We think we know the body but we don't. Therefore, we need to know this God given first instrument of ours. One has to begin the practice of *prāṇāyāma* through which the channelled energy is felt in the vital body. However, the practice of *āsana* and *prāṇāyāma* begins to show a remarkable effect on mind, which is the mirror of our behaviour, character and nature. Here, the mind begins to change for good and one begins to change one's attitude. Slowly, one transforms oneself in moral and ethical disciplines and then proceeds to quieten the consciousness. This is how the yogic journey begins.

Q.- What happens if a student does not attain a correct yoga practice?

Can you all become Picasso or Paul Casals? Everyone has to practise yoga correctly at his or her own level. For instance, you go to primary school and learn the alphabet or basic mathematics. Later you go to higher education. Similarly, yoga too takes one to build up the art of living in a right way. Precision gives precise effect but no wrong happens. So my advice will be to go in for correct practices so that no bad effects result.

Q.- What is the true role of a *guru*?

The role of a *guru* is to guide and uplift the pupils higher than their own level. But this guidance is different from a professor who guides in an academic discipline. First of all, a *guru* has to be his own critic because the art of yoga is completely subjective and practical. Remaining as his own critic, he has to improve himself. Then, he must know the problems and difficulties of his students and from there he should lift, help and protect them to get liberated from their problems and difficulties. Then he uplifts them delicately to the level that he as a *guru* has attained.

– Thank you very much for replying to my queries and clearing up my doubts. Now, I understand that yoga is neither sports nor athletics nor gymnastics. It is neither religion nor asceticism. Thanks for convincing me that it is purely a self-culturing and self-disciplining process.

YOGA, THE MENTAL EDUCATION*

Visiting Paris at the moment, B.K.S. Iyengar, 80 years old, explains to Le Figaro *his contribution to this millenary discipline.*

As fit as a fiddle, an emblematic figure of discipline starts a tour in Europe. Coming from all over the world, the disciples of this eighty year old Indian sage, who is dressed in white with a red line on his forehead, won't miss the rendezvous Saturday, Sunday and Monday at Park Vincennes to listen to their guru's *voice. There are around a hundred teachers in France and a thousand adepts, who affectionately call Mr. Iyengar* Gurujī.

Q.- What is the difference between your method and other teachings?

Yoga has existed for centuries. It is not my method but a system that evolved centuries back. All I have done is to improve and deepen the thoughts of my ancestors to express for today's people. I started learning yoga at the age of fifteen. Two years later I was forced to be a teacher. As a young man, I started to teach and became the first to gather men and women together to practise in my classes. I tried to study yoga through books, but they weren't of any help. But they left me to think afresh. Presentations of *āsana* in books did not show proper connections between the techniques and illustrations of the *āsana*. So I experimented with *āsana* to bring awareness of sensations in the *āsana* practice. I succeeded in connecting the body with the mind and mind with various parts of the body, which took me years of practising ten hours a day to experience this. Each *āsana* is a phase with its inner sensations. It is by the grace of yoga I could share with my students elaborating this rational and schematic practice.

* Interview by the French newspaper *Le Figaro*, published on 18th November 1997.

Q.- What famous people have you won over by your method?

I do not claim that I have won famous people through my method. A human being is a human being. I do not see difference. But I am happy to say that I have attracted not only famous influential people but also the ordinary public towards this subject.

Q.- What does yoga bring to those who practise it?

I can say what yoga has done to me, but what can I say of those who practise? Yet I say that it brings bliss and wisdom. This yoga covers moral, intellectual and spiritual work as much as its physical value. Like a kite player plays with the kite, we use the body as a kite. The fibres, tendons and ligaments act as strings. The brain is the controller of the string. When the somatic action is done well under the supervision of the intelligence, yoga establishes mental peace. Women are often overcome by emotional problems. Yoga helps bring improvement in the secretion of the hormones to preserve their sensitivity and emotional stability. Yoga helps men, who often show arrogance, to sublimate their ego. This yogic discipline balances one to find harmony even if one is caught in the ups and downs of life.

Q.- Is this discipline not more sleep inducing than a source of energy?

It seems your questions suggests that you have no idea of yoga. It induces sleep in those who need the sleep and builds up others to channel their physical and mental energy. The yogic discipline generates energy in the body, mind and intelligence. In the beginning the effort is there and therefore a beginner may need more sleep to recover from that effort. It is like children eating food to build up their bodies.

As one gets acclimatised through practice, sleep lessens. Through the practice of *āsana, prāṇāyāma* and *dhyāna,* the nerves connecting the brain and body awaken themselves with a new, self-generating energy. This energy is distributed properly and precisely not only to the body but also to the mind and intelligence.

Often, the beginners tend to go to sleep in *Śavāsana* because of the quietening sense in the nervous system. I would say that "sleep" is a phase the practitioner faces in the beginning. Yoga is not a steroid. One has to face the "sleep-phase", and then the newly generated energy begins to circulate.

Q.- Can we consider yoga as a therapy?

Actually and honestly it is not therapy, but it does act as therapy in many ailments. In India numerous doctors have sent me patients that they couldn't succeed in treating. Yoga helps those people suffering from cervical lesions, hearing troubles, glandular problems, pain in the spinal column, diabetes, blood pressure and so on.

Therapy is a by-product of yoga. One may give a programme of *āsana* and *prāṇāyāma* for different diseases. However, while practising, the application of our body and mind – the physical and mental instrument – has to be there in totality for higher development of the intelligence and consciousness.

Q.- Do you continue to practise this discipline?

Absolutely yes! There is no end to the discipline as learning goes on. It is not only a life-long process but it becomes a life itself.

I am still practising. I have not limited my practice. Yoga is my life. How can the question of discontinuity arise in me, when it is my life elixir?

Q.- Yoga can also lead to skids: Gilbert Bourdin taught it before dedicating himself to the mandarin sect. How can one distinguish between a true yogi and a quack?

Yoga creates intense energy. Often the practitioner walks on the edge of a cliff. But when the mind has reached a certain intelligence, one should not fall. But who knows it maybe possible to slip and lose hold and fail to maintain the progress.

While teaching *āsana, prāṇāyāma* or *dhyāna,* I see whether the mental body is reconstructed morally, intellectually and spiritually. That makes one a real yogi who won't skid or have a fall. The practice of yoga has to be within the compound wall created by *yama* and *niyama* – the moral and ethical principles.

Q.- What message would you like to transmit to Westerners?

I'm sorry to say that we neglect so much our interior environment. We are more and more concerned about the exterior environment and with healthy food. Yoga permits health not only in the body, but also in the mind and intelligence.

Therefore yoga is a universal art as it concerns all human beings on Earth. Only, it has to be adopted by one and all for the health of physical, moral, mental, intellectual and spiritual joy on the global level.

IYENGAR LOOKS BACK*

At age 79, one of the world's greatest yogis reflects on more than six decades of practice.

The first time I heard the name Iyengar, I was still a newcomer to yoga. In college on the East Coast, I had dabbled in kuṇḍalinī *classes with a turbaned Texan, which ended abruptly when he eloped with an undergraduate. After graduation, in Santa Fe, I had sweated through some Sun Salutations with a visiting teacher at a local massage school, which left my body vibrating with energy like a plucked guitar string.*

But then I dropped in on a yoga class that bore no resemblance to anything I had ever encountered. Twisted into what felt to my untrained body like an awkward windmill, with one hand on the seat of a metal folding chair and a sandbag under my back heel, I was squeezing a wooden block between my legs as a fellow student tugged on a canvas strap lashed high around one upper thigh.

"The top of the back-leg femur bone tends to roll in," my teacher was explaining. But Mr. Iyengar says that the top of the femur bone should roll out, while you draw in the skin of the top inner thigh."

At that moment I was too preoccupied with trying to locate my femur (let alone roll it in the opposite direction from my skin) to inquire about the identity of Mr. Iyengar, whose name she had pronounced with the reverence with which my Catholic school nuns had referred to the Blessed Virgin Mary. But after class, I asked, "So who is this Iyengar guy, anyway?"

My teacher just looked at me with blank astonishment, as if I had professed to have never heard of the Beatles.

As I soon came to realise, for tens of thousands of students worldwide, the name B.K.S. Iyengar is virtually synonymous with haṭha yoga, *the branch of yoga that emphasises physical postures* (āsana) *and breathing techniques* (prāṇāyāma) *as primary tools for spiritual awakening. His classic* Light on Yoga *is the illustrated Bible of* āsana *practice, the ultimate reference manual; when teachers refer to the 'traditional' way to do a posture, they're usually looking to no more an*

---

* Interview by Anne Cushman. Published by *Yoga Journal,* issue 137, December 1997.

ancient text than this. His precise approach to āsana and prāṇāyāma – solidly grounded in Western anatomy and physiology – has revolutionised the way yoga is taught in the West, with even non 'Iyengar' teachers profoundly influenced by his principles of alignment and therapeutics.

"Unless freedom is gained in the body, freedom of the mind is a far cry," Iyengar has said. "It is through the body that you realise that you are a spark of divinity." Iyengar Yoga emphasises rigorous instruction in the nuts and bolts of the postures – presented (at least by Iyengar himself) with an almost military precision. The point, says Iyengar, is to awaken intelligence in every cell of the body, so that even the skin becomes conscious. In the process, the mind becomes anchored in the present moment. "If you cannot see your little toe," Iyengar asks, "How can you see the Self?"

Iyengar at Home

I first saw Iyengar in 1990, from the back of a packed auditorium, when he gave a talk and demonstration of therapeutic yoga in San Francisco. As he barked out orders like a general, I watched in astonishment while my own august teachers scampered around the stage on their hands and knees to fetch him blocks, sandbags, sticky mats and blankets. I saw him again at a national convention in 1993 – but again, only from a distance, as a Zeus-like figure who would descend on classes to hurl inspiration, insights, and occasional thunderbolts at teachers and students alike.

So I was a bit stunned at how easy it was to approach him for an interview at his Ramāmaṇi Iyengar Memorial Yoga Institute in Pune, India, when I passed through last year researching a guidebook to Indian yoga centres and āshrams. Arriving at the Institute – a modest building in a quiet residential neighbourhood, with a statue of Iyengar in Naṭarājāsana near the entrance – I presented my card to an attendant who promptly ushered me straight to the dim, cave-like library where Iyengar sat behind an immense desk, perusing a copy of the Yoga Sūtras. Dressed in a crisp cotton kurta, he regarded me with amused benevolence and amiably consented to an interview later in the week. "First, you come watch my medical class tomorrow," he invited me warmly. "Then you will understand better."

But this avuncular demeanour evaporated the next day, when I dropped in on the medical class, a special class for people suffering from ailments ranging from heart disease to chronic depression. (Iyengar is famous for his ability to alleviate and even cure conditions that medical doctors have despaired of). The bright, airy practice room was jammed with fifty to sixty people in an array of supported postures: draped over bolsters, suspended from wall ropes, strapped to wooden horses, buried under sandbags and immense iron disks. From my perch in a corner stairwell, I watched as Iyengar, his immense chest and torso swelling over his *shorts, darted through the room with the intensity of a sheep dog corralling an errant flock: growling, barking, offering lightning-quick adjustments with a tug here, a slap there.*

Catching sight of me, he strode over. "You people! You say that Iyengar yoga *is only physical! But where is the spiritual person who does not have a body? Show me that person! Where is he standing?"*

I meekly admitted that I couldn't produce such a being.

"You say that singing is spiritual. But without the body how can you sing? Tell me that!" He glowered at me. "You do not understand anything." he concluded, and walked away.

This kind of transformation is vintage Iyengar – he can go from sage to samurai warrior faster than you can say Adho Mukha Śvānāsana, *a transformation that his students say is just a device to prod students into awakening. He's famous for deflating egos – thereby leaving a space where awareness can arise. "I am a fanatic when I am practising," he told me cheerfully as we sipped chai together in our interview a few days later. "But when I finish my practice, I am just like an ordinary being."*

Interviewing Iyengar was like interrogating a river in full flood. A question or comment would barely be out of my mouth before he would be responding in a torrent of anecdote, opinion, and charm.

Q.- What first drew you to the practice of yoga?

Actually, I never knew the word *yoga* and what this subject was for me. It's only a coincidence that in 1934 my *guru* – my sister's husband – went to Lonavla. On the way to Lonavla he stopped in Bangalore to visit us. He asked me, "Why don't you be with your sister in Mysore until I come back?" Mysore has lush gardens and palaces, which for any youngster is attractive. I thought of seeing the Royal City of Mysore with my own eyes and I agreed to stay with my sister.

When he returned after visiting Lonavla and Mumbai, I said to him, "I should go back to study." Instead of sending me to Bangalore, he told me to join a school there, as the syllabus was the same throughout the State. For me there was no difference whether I stayed with my sister or my brother. I had lost my father when I was young. It was a hard job for any joint family to bring up children not their own. My brothers had their own children, and their desire naturally would be to bring up their own children, not me. So I joined the school in Mysore.

He didn't teach me yoga for nearly six months. Then one day he said, "Why don't you do something, go! Do yoga." But he never taught me what to do.

Finally one day he called me: "Do this, do that, do that." But my body was just like dry wood. He tried to teach me a few *āsana*. But my body was not able to bend at all. He said, "Your body is so stiff, only do what you can do". That's how the beginning was made.

My *Gurujī* was called by the Maharaja of Mysore to give a demonstration in front of the All-India World YMCA Conference, which was held in Mysore. That I think shook him a bit, because there were none who could do the advanced *āsana*. So he called me. For three days he broke my back, and said, "You have to do this in a demonstration." Only three days he taught me. And the demonstration was in a week's time.

This is how I got initiated into yoga.

Q.- How many poses did he teach you in three days?

Only backward extensions. My body was not extending forward. Bending forward was a painful process. Fear set in as I had very little instruction to do the *āsana*. I was an orphan and was treated like a slave. Fortunately, what he had taught me, I presented. He was very impressed and complemented with these words, "I never thought that after training you for only three days, with your stiff body, that you would do it."

However, I earned pain, which continued for months later.

Q.- How old were you at that time?

About fifteen and a half years.

Q.- Did Krishnamacharya teach you *prāṇāyāma* as well as *āsana*?

I was suffering from influenza from birth, then malaria, typhoid, and then tuberculosis, one after the other. My lungs had gone weak. My breathing was laboured. So what *prāṇāyāma* could one teach? Hence, he said that I was not fit for *prāṇāyāma*.

My body was not made for yoga, but there were some exhibitions in town wherein we had to give demonstrations. So my *guru* made me do a few *āsana* as a preparation for demonstration. If there were no demonstrations, probably he wouldn't have taught me, and my line would not have been yoga at all. But destiny made me gravitate towards yoga.

Q.- And did he teach you yoga philosophy at all?

Honestly, nothing! I learned everything on my own. If you ask me, his grace was there. Every word of what I am teaching today is my own perspiration and inspiration. But my *Gurujī* is the seed, for which I am grateful.

Q.- How did you begin teaching yoga yourself?

In 1936 it was my *Gurujī* who made me teach at Dharwar and Hubli. When I said, "I know nothing," he said, "Do whatever you can manage to do, but teach!" Perhaps that was not only his order but his blessings too.

Then, in 1937, I was called to Pune by one Dr. V.B. Gokhale, who had seen my demonstrations in the north of Karnataka. Though I had no expressive muscles. He was impressed by my performance. He asked, "Why is your body not developed?" I explained to him about my poverty and my diseased body. I was left untreated for a long time. He was astonished and said, "As a surgeon I have not seen anything in my life like what I am seeing in your presentation. It is unbelievable that such diseased body can perform any number of *āsana* in this way".

Three months after my 1936 demonstration in Belgaum, he retired and settled in Pune, and went around the colleges of Pune for the introduction of yoga to the students. The college authorities promised that they would experiment for six months with a yoga teacher. I was invited to teach for six months.

Thus, I came and began teaching in the colleges of Pune, and also at the Deccan Gymkhana Club. Most of the people were not interested, but some came for health. The colleges of Pune and some top-class schools and the Deccan Gymkhana Club joined together, collecting six or seven rupees a month from various institutions to pay me sixty rupees (about two dollars) salary per month.

This is how I started to be a teacher in yoga.

Q.- Was the path smooth or had you any opposition?

The so-called recognised yogis were dead against teaching yoga enmasse. The end of my teaching came on account of these people who opposed me. They said that it couldn't be taught at all in public. I was teaching 30 or 40 people at a time. So the Educational Institutions, on the advice of the yoga authorities of the day, closed the classes. Yet the classes went on for three years in all the Educational Institutes of Pune.

Then some of the students wished to do and some for health's sake. It was a challenge that I had to face. Though the Institutional authorities stopped me from teaching, these students kept continuing, so the classes went on privately.

Q.- At the same time you must have been working on your own practice.

Yes! I was working on myself with my own practice but in a different way. I was so slim, and people were laughing at me, saying, "If you do yoga, the result of yoga will be like this man is." I had no flesh. If I had some flesh on my body, probably that would have given me some hope. But I had to suffer because I had no flesh at all. People could count my ribs easily.

In the classes, when I was teaching, I would perform with the students. These students were well nourished, they were not only elder but also muscle bound and taller than me. However, while doing *āsana* my body was not sinking or collapsing, but they used to get tired easily. So I used to say: "Hey, see my body, see your body – why do you pride yourselves when you are all collapsing? I am not collapsed! I have no muscles. But see, you are tired and I am not." As their teacher, I was the youngest compared to all those students.

I was teaching many classes, one after the other. I was doing with every class the jumpings *(vinyāsa)*, standing *āsana* and all.[1] By continuing this way, I built up some muscles and endurance. The students were sweating but I could practise without sweating. That created interest in the people to learn yoga.

Most of the time my practice was with my students in the classes. However, I used to work alone on backward extensions and arm balancing.

Q.- Were the poses you were teaching at that time the poses that are now in *Light on Yoga*?

Not really like *Light on Yoga*. As I was not fully matured, I say I was teaching in a crude, clumsy way.

---

[1] See the article in *Aṣṭadaḷa Yogamālā* vol 2, "*Vinyasa Yoga*".

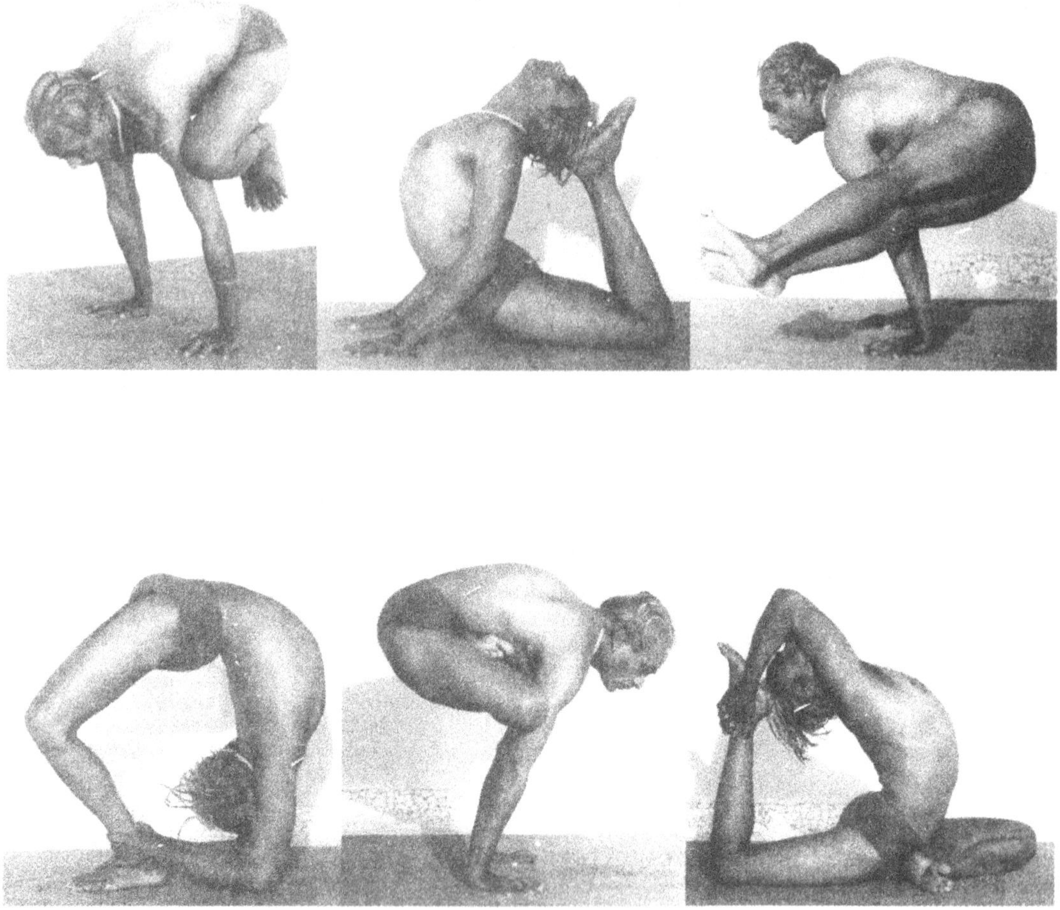

Plate n. 30 – Backward extensions and arm balancing

Q.- There are a wide range of poses that you teach now, and that are in *Light on Yoga*, which are not in the *Haṭhayoga Pradīpikā* or other ancient texts. Where did they come from?

No books have presented those *āsana*. My *guru* had some drawings with him. I had seen those drawings – yoga on the ropes and on trees. It was a hand-written book. In it I saw some of the *āsana*. And I had a book in Marathi, which is about 100-120 years old. That also represents some difficult and complicated *āsana* in drawings.

Undoubtedly, the variety of *āsana* was there. Though one cannot find them in a book, one certainly finds in the drawings as well as in the temple's sculptures. You need to visit ancient temples to see the sculptures in these postures.

When I was teaching in the college the students did not like the same thing to do over and over. Their indifference to repetitions gave me a chance and made me think and create new *āsana* with new ideas on the subject.

Q.- Your approach to *āsana* is famous for being very scientific and anatomically precise. How did you develop this precision?

Doctor V.B. Gokhale, who invited me to Pune, was a great help. He used to give talks, and I used to demonstrate. Secondly, I could not speak on yoga as I did not know its philosophy. Doctor Gokhale said, "The body is known to me. You leave it to me for explanations. Being a medical man, he used to explain the human system very clearly as I was presenting. It was a real good combination of two of us to make yoga popular; I was really happy, and while he was explaining I started learning the anatomical terminologies and functions as well as their physiological explanations. This helped me a great deal in developing myself in the subject.

Q.- Another technique that sets apart your approach to yoga is your extensive use of props such as wooden blocks, sandbags, ropes, etcetera. How did you develop this approach?

My *guru* was using the wall ropes, two on top, two in the middle, and two at the bottom.

In those days, diseases which medicines or surgery could not handle directly were coming to *yogaśālā*, where *Śīrṣāsana, Sarvāṅgāsana, Halāsana, Pūrvottānāsana* and forward bends were taught with the help of these ropes. In 1937 the principal of Ferguson College of Pune, Shri Rajawade, who was 85 years old, was suffering from dysentery. And Doctor V.B. Gokhale asked me whether I could help him as he was unable to stand or sit.

How to make him do yoga in that condition was the question I had to face. By helping him I learnt the first lesson of how to teach such people. I started teaching *Trikoṇāsana* making him lie down. You can call it *Supta Trikoṇāsana*[1]. I had to lift his chest and turn it to the side so that the intestines get some movement. Since he could not spread his legs, I used to insert a walking stick between his two legs to keep the legs apart. This is how I learned to create props for getting benefits. I started treating the patients one after the other, just by instinct.

[1] See plate 7, 8, 9 and 10, *Aṣṭadala Yogamālā*, vol. 1.

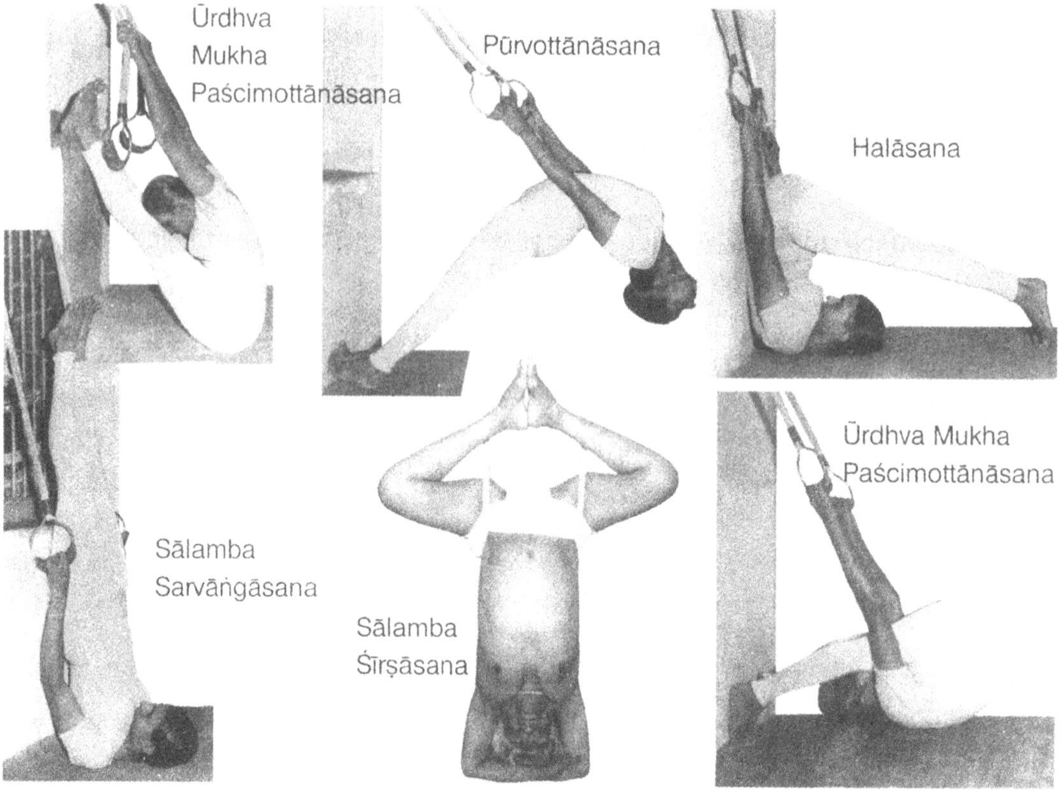

Plate n. 31 – *Āsana* with the help of a rope

Secondly I was practising myself. I was not doing *Hanumānāsana* as I had a tear in the hamstrings. Even simple *āsana* like *Baddhakoṇāsana* was not coming. In those days, workers used to dump big stones on the roadside for road construction. Nobody would object if one picked them up. I used to bring such heavy stones to keep on my thighs to learn this *āsana*. This way I used to pick up stones, iron rods on the wayside and carry them home, which would be useful for my yoga.

You know road rollers that flatten the roads? On the front wheel I used to do backbends, because my body was not doing this on its own. So if I saw a machine on the road, I used to go to do backbends on it! Then I used drums. Because of this practice, people used to call me a mad cap. I was! Because I couldn't do the *āsana* independently, so I was always thinking of how to do so and I was finding means to learn. This way I found ways of using blocks, weights, sandbags, to learn and to show the accuracy of *āsana!*

My props became my *guru* and taught me how to use the body. I could sense that I did better with supports to master the *āsana*. These supports helped in certain areas to get a better action and at the same time the sense of ease. Thus props helped me to teach well and to create a quicker healing process.

– Your approach proved very popular with Western students. –

Yoga became very popular in the West only after 1968. In 1954 not even one student was willing to come to a class. At London airport in 1954, when I told them, "I am a yoga teacher," they said, "Do you swallow pound notes? We can't trust you, you have to be screened because you yogis walk on fire, chew glass, and you may also swallow our currency."

It took me several years to build up classes in England – it was not so easy to come to the masses. I had to cajole people to come. It was a hard task to open a class. I did so in 1960 and do you know how many people came? Three or four. But I never lost heart.

Then fortunately in 1971 Mr. Peter McIntosh, the physical director of the London Adult Educational Authority, wanted to replace their callisthenic exercises with some other type of physical work that would be more effective. He was a friend of Mr. Menuhin. One day he asked Mr. Menuhin, "What are you doing?" and Mr. Menuhin said, "I stand on my head to keep myself fit. My teacher is here, if you want you can meet him."

So, Mr. McIntosh came to my class at Sloane Square in London with his advisors. They saw my classes and were pleased. Mr. McIntosh wanted to introduce yoga in the Adult Educational Scheme with a condition that I should teach yoga without using any philosophical terms. I consented to teach introducing the benefits of yoga for the health of the body and contentment in mind. McIntosh was happy with my promise and showed his willingness to introduce yoga to Inner and Outer London Educational Authorities. Again some scientists, doctors and members of the Educational Board watched my class and they opined, "He teaches with language which is of the ground reality. So we have no objection at all." That's how I won.

Then the problem came – the media started writing unfair comments on my stand. They wrote that yoga is a philosophical subject, a spiritual subject, and unfortunately the physical aspect of yoga is taught in England. I asked Mr. McIntosh, "Could I speak on the spiritual level? If you permit me I can do that." He said, "No, I don't want it. You should teach purely on a practical level only."

See, people say that yoga is a spiritual subject. I say it's a physical, physiological, physio-neurological, neuro-psychological and psycho-spiritual subject. You cannot separate them at all. A layman can understand only from the known, not from the unknown. So I have to start from the known – the body, to move towards the unknown – the Self. Before this introduction, people never even knew the basics of yoga. They knew the effect, the high goal of yoga, but not the starting point.

Q.- You continue to receive criticism for focusing on the body. Can you comment?

When you have to educate a child, how do you do it? Tell me! Do you educate from the soul? Do you educate them in maths or teach them with fruits and flowers? You bring them and show the fruit, do you not? This is how the knowledge has to come. That is what I am doing.

People can criticise me. If I had not worked with so much zeal, would yoga have become so popular? The seed of yoga was sown in America by Swami Vivekananda. He introduced the subject. But what happened later? When I came in 1956, still nobody knew it. Even my demonstrations were banned after Swami Yogananda collapsed when he stood on the stage to address. Now open any book, you see *āsana* postures. From where did this understanding come? Who was it that introduced yoga, house to house? To criticise is easy but only I know how I had to struggle to take it to every household.

Coming to the point, if you are a raw student of yoga, you know nothing about philosophy, you know nothing about the mind. In case you come to me, what I do is, I try to build you up from the base using the body as your instrument to guide and build up gradually towards the higher aspects of yoga and life.

Again, when I ask you to focus on the body, is it an external focusing or do I take you towards internal penetration of the body? Unless the mind comes in contact with the body, can you interpenetrate or can you move the body well without the involvement of the mind?

I care for the needs of those who come to me to learn and criticisms do not affect me or my approach to yoga.

Q.- You have said that for you, the physical is spiritual.

I have not said anywhere that physical body action is spiritual. I only said that the body is the instrument to help one to progress towards the spiritual. The cells have their own intelligence, the cells have their own memories. They carry imprints. With yoga you are culturing each and every cell. You are culturing each blood cell, as well as bone cell. So I say, the gateway for spiritual life is *āsana* and *prāṇāyāma*. If those gates are not open, there is no difference between a man who says, "I am meditating," and a person who is sleepy.

The body and soul are not separate. We cannot separate them. You cannot think without the body. Brain, the so-called thinker in you, is still a part of the body. How can you separate the brain and the thinker? It is true that the body or the brain survive on food. Body survives due to the presence of *ātman* (soul) as well. If soul is absent, that body does not need food as it is declared dead.

The soul gives to the body the *chetanā* – the vital, conscious energy, and the food taken from outside is absorbed by the body because of the *chetanā*. If the body is without food and starving, then it dies. No more will the body be friendly with the soul.

For the practice of yoga, we too need the body and the soul. The soul in our body is called the embodied soul – *jīvātman*. The *āsana* and *prāṇāyāma* are the internal food for the spiritual life. As you need food to maintain the body alive, for your worldly presence, you need *āsana* and *prāṇāyāma* for its spiritual presence. If the physical body is nourished with food, the spiritual body is nourished with *āsana* and *prāṇāyāma*. With the practice of *āsana* and *prāṇāyāma* the cellular body is intelligised, cultured, purified, sanctified, rather spiritualised for yogic practices. With physical food, it merely keeps alive for *bhogic* practices (sensual enjoyments).

In philosophical language, I feed my body with *āsana* and *prāṇāyāma*, so it survives for spiritual practices. My body is for spirituality.

Q.- Then how do *āsana* and *prāṇāyāma* relate to the other limbs of yoga?

Though Patañjali has used the word "limb," one is interconnected to the other. You cannot do *āsana* and *prāṇāyāma* unless your nerves, your cells, your mind, your intelligence are treated as an integrated whole. You cannot practise them making your mind to run hither and thither. *Yama* and *niyama* have been given by Patañjali to discipline and educate the cells, cleanse the cells, change the physical and psychological behaviour of them for its inward journey. For a newcomer in this field, the saint Kabir says, *Mana jāye to jānede, mata jāne de śarir* – In the beginning if the mind runs after outer attraction, let it go, but don't allow the body to follow. What great wisdom it conveys. The tendency of the mind is to run after objects. One may find difficult to shackle it, but body is the first instrument available, it is perceivable, so control it. The body shackles the mind. When you say the body, your cells, your nerves, including your mind and intelligence, come under that! If you walk zigzag on the road what happens? Tell me.

– Here, in India, you get run down by a rickshaw. –

In your country you get hit by a car. You meet not only an accident but perhaps death too. Is it not?

– Yes. –

In the same way, how do we know that the energy in our body is running in the right direction or in an exact way?

- We don't know. -

These *āsana* are given to us so that the energy is made to flow where it has to flow. Not only that, but we are able to face the turmoils, we can face even the invisible fears. If we cannot face the visible ones, can we face the invisible ones? Have you got that strength?

- No, because we don't know them. We can't see them. -

Exactly. The principles of *yama* and *niyama* have to be followed so that the invisible, unpredictable, unknown fears are avoided and eradicated.

So when we speak of ethical growth, *yama* and *niyama* come in the picture. These principles have to be adopted by the body for its ethical growth. For example you go into *Trikoṇāsana* on the right side, you are very attentive there. But on the left side you don't think at all.[1] So on the right side you overstrain, murdering the cells and on the left side, you under stretch and starve the cells. People say, "Mr. Iyengar is aggressive," right? But if Mr. Iyengar is aggressive, he is equally aggressive on the right and the left. If he is non-aggressive, he is non-aggressive equally on the right and left.

I am not an aggressive practitioner, I am an attentive *sādhaka*. I want to learn how each and every part is to be interconnected. Even if I stretch my finger, I want to feel how far the intelligence flows inside. I spread my consciousness everywhere. That is why my practice is whole, attentive and intensive. While teaching others, if I have to make people aware of this method, it looks like aggressive teaching, because people want to be slow, dull and lazy. They do not want to be awakened. They do not want to be rectified. Rectification is denied. As I bring that needed attention, it is wrong to interpret it as aggressive teaching. When I bring this attention in the practitioner does it not convey to you that I am introducing the other aspects or limbs of yoga.

Q.- By developing that awareness in your *āsana* practice, does it begin to extend into your life?

---

[1] See plate n. 3.

Yes, of course! It is not only extension but expansion of lifes force. This has to come automatically but gradually to all those who do with observation and attention. Each one wants his cells to feel the tranquillity, not the brain alone. The very approach becomes rectitudinal, honest. In this thinking, the very thought process changes. It is how one has to begin to expand equity and equanimity in the consciousness.

Q.- And what about the limbs of meditation – *pratyāhāra, dhāranā, dhyāna* and *samādhi*?

Does not this attention, extension and expansion in *āsana* and *prāṇāyāma* convey the principles of meditation? Can one do an *āsana* without meditation? An *āsana* without meditation becomes an exercise. An *āsana* with meditation brings poise, pensivity and serenity. Patañjali says, *Deśa bandhaḥ cittasya dhāraṇā* (*Y.S.,* III.3) – i.e., one can concentrate inside the body as well as outside the body. Vyāsa mentions both ways in his commentary. Some may be teaching outside the body, but with the *āsana,* I am teaching one to concentrate inside the body. What difference does it make? Vyāsa mentions that one can concentrate on *mūrdhani, nābhi, hṛdaya* and so on. I teach *āsana* in such a way that each mental part and each cell of the body becomes the object of concentration.

When my *gurujī* came to Pune for my 60th birthday, he advised me, "Now you should stop all these *āsana* practices and do only meditation." Respecting his words, I stopped for three months. What was the effect? I lost everything of what I had earned in my *sādhanā.* Three months break took me years to come back to get the lifeful feeling. I realised that my *āsana* practice is not merely physical. It cleansed me again internally and I realised that that itself is meditation.

Like the water finding its level, if my intelligence finds its level and spreads in this entire body, is it not meditation?

A beginner demarcates all the limbs of yoga as separate entities. But at a later stage, the practitioner does not think of these as separate limbs. He treats them like the petals of a single flower. While practising each *āsana* or each breath, the body cooperates with mind, and mind with the body in order to go towards *pratyāhāra, dhāraṇā* and *dhyāna.* Without the introduction of these, *āsana* is incomplete. With all these sheaths of yoga the practice culminates in oneness.

Q.- So there's no need to withdraw from the world and be a *sannyāsīn* to reach the highest stages of yoga?

Do you mean to say that all the *sannyāsin* have withdrawn from the world? In fact they are more attached to the world than an ordinary man like me and you. It is the inner education that is required. Whether you put on saffron garb or dress in a simple *dhoti*, the dress does not make you *sannyāsi*. An aspirant strives to search the hidden inner attachments in order to liberate himself from them. For you my *āsana* practice seems to be a physical practice but fortunately, for me it is a total freedom from the body. My senses no more require any entertainment from the external world. *Vairāgya* (desirelessness) being the highest stage of yoga, one does not need the change of garb.

In my early days many *sannyāsi* allured me to take *sannyāsa*. Probably, seeing my practice, they might have thought of exploiting me under their command. I preferred to stay away since I wanted to lead life that is common to all. Though I am a family man, I lead my life with *tapas*, *svādhyāya* and *Īśvara praṇidhāna*. When I am doing any part or petal of yoga, nothing remains in my heart except meditativeness.

Q.- Does the idea of God or Spirit have a role in your approach to yoga?

It is very subjective and close to my heart. Being subjective and personal it does not need any explanations. Without God, there is no yoga. I need not declare or beat a drum about it. God is invisible and all pervading. God is within the body as well as outside and He is everywhere.

It is a force that has no form but keeps me practising. It is not my will power that makes me practise, though people say I have a strong will power. The inner voice forces me to do yoga and that force wants me to be always in yoga, and that I consider God.

Q.- Do you think that a practitioner needs to have some sense of Spirit in their practice?

Whether one believes in God or not is immaterial. One believes in one's own self, is it not? If each one of us is true to our own selves, then everything is possible. Forget about God. But one certainly has faith in one's self. That is enough to charge the inner spirit to do yoga.

Even if one does not believe in God, yoga makes ghim a perfect man. Patañjali, anticipating those who do not believe in God says that by supreme attentive awareness through yoga he is lead towards the fragrance of virtue and justice.[1]

---

[1] *prasaṁkhyāne api akusīdasya sarvathā vivekakhyāteḥ dharmameghaḥ samādhiḥ* (*Y.S.*, IV.29) –The yogi who has no interest even in this higher state of evolution, maintains supreme attentive discriminative awareness, attains *dharmamegha samādhi*: he contemplates the fragrance of virtue and justice.

He neither involves himself directly nor induces or abets anyone who inflicts any affliction upon him or through him on others.[2]

Q.- Have you felt your own practice changing as the years go on?

I won't say changing – no. My practice is not changing. It is transforming. It is becoming subtler and finer. The change is impermanent. There can be constant changes occurring, and one may progress or regress in those changes. In me, only progressive transformation is taking place.

Q.- What sort of transformations are you finding now?

Clarity, precision, the feel of the inside body. Even my toe – if it's slightly wrong, I know my toe has gone wrong. Can you know that in your practice? Tell me.

- Not usually. -

You can see me when I am practising, I will tell you which knee is out, which calf muscle is in, which toe, nail is stretching straight and so forth, as my presentation appears perfect. You cannot perceive these defects, until I say and you look.

This I consider transformation. The light is coming from within to those areas. In the early days there was no light, it was all darkness.

All these years I practised yoga to get maturity in my body and mind. Now I am practising yoga after maturity. Then I was seeking. Now, I am seeing. Even if it is a small or petty mistake, it reflects on one at once. Being a raw student, you may not understand. As you go on practising, one day this illuminative light also may dawn on you.

For me, previously it was all crude, now the subtle things surface. In the earlier days I used to think like you, "This muscle is not working, that one is not working." Today my cells speak to me. My mind speaks to me. I perceive the movement of my energy, of my mind, of my intelligence. Not only do I observe, but I am with myself – I am there. This is concentration and meditation. A hunter hunts in the jungle, I hunt within me. A searcher wanders in a wonderland; I wander within myself.

---

[1] *tataḥkleśa karma nivṛttiḥ* (*Y.S.,* IV.30) – The comes the end of afflictions and of *karma*.

For outsiders, *āsana* seems to be contortions. But what I see is vastness of my consciousness in these contortions. It is not my body that extends but the mind that expands. When I do *Tāḍāsana* or *Kapotāsana*, my intelligence in the body expresses *Tāḍāsana* in *Kapotāsana* and vice versa.

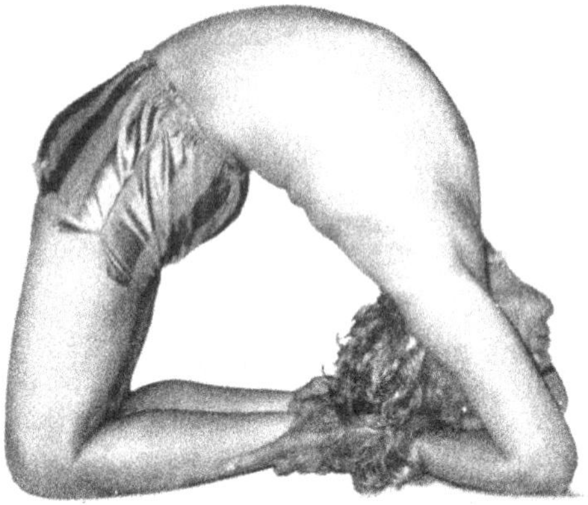

Plate n. 32 – *Tāḍāsana* in *Kapotāsana*

When people see me doing the most difficult *āsana,* they say, "He just does *āsana*." But what am I seeing inside is unknown to them. They cannot see that. A saint may meditate. Can you see his meditation? Do you know what he does? He says that he is seeing God, then do you see what he sees? How do you know what I see when I do *āsana?* Do you know how I penetrate within myself? Do you know how I penetrate the opaque body so that it becomes transparent? Not only each and every part of my body but my mind, intelligence and consciousness become transparent to me. This transparency reflects the very being. That is the transformation.

Q.- Do you still find challenges in your practice?

Yes, the challenges have to be there, but these challenges today are quite different. Previously I used to challenge the body, now the body challenges me. Nature plays its own role. The body hasn't got that strength which it had years ago. So I have to fight. Earlier my mind was demanding the body to do in certain way. Now the body says what the mind has to see and feel in the *āsana.*

At this age I am a bit at the precipice. The body is giving way. If I surrender to this weakness, I am lost. If the slightest idea comes to me that my body cannot take it, I am lost in yoga. So I am practising with more zeal than before.

Q.- But the body inevitably grows old and dies. Isn't there a point where we have to focus our practice on something beyond the body?

That's what I am doing! I have not lost the grace in my practice. Even though my *āsana* may not be as good as they were, the grace is even more now, as I create the road in my inner body for the intelligence to move in that road. Not elsewhere. I also keep the consciousness steady without allowing it to fluctuate in the *āsana*. So I focus on the consciousness and not on the body.

The difference between you and me is that by knowing very well that the body becomes old and dies, you neglect to maintain it in a good condition, but still you do not mind fulfilling all its desires for food and sensual enjoyment. I know well that body decays but I do not stop my practice, I am using the body and maintaining it in good condition, so that I can go beyond the body, which you cannot see.

Q.- Suppose you reach the point where you can no longer do the physical practice at all?

After explaining so clearly the indepth, the values of *āsana*, I am surprised that your mind cannot go beyond your fixed ideas. First of all, what do you mean by physical practice? Do you mean to say that when I do *āsana*, I do it only as physical practice? What fantasy! I do not do so only for the body. It may appear to you as such. I go beyond. In fact, *āsana* takes me beyond my body consciousness. Otherwise, at the age of 79, whose body can perform *Ūrdhva Dhanurāsana, Kapotāsana, Vṛśchikāsana?* If I, think the same way as you, that *āsana* are only physical practice, the body might have given way long back. For me *āsana* practice is a melody. The body at this age can no more hold the physical strain. Why don't you think the other way round that in this aged body the *āsana* are established the way Patañjali explains; with stability, comfort and ease?

Secondly, why should I give up before the body complains? I have had some accidents, years ago. I couldn't even lift my hand. Because my shoulders were injured. I had dislocated my arm, and my hip was injured in an accident. So these things do happen. Injuries come. I had to combat the pain. I had to do my *sādhanā*. I overcame diseases at early life when I had T.B., malaria, jaundice and more. I had injured myself while teaching yoga and helping others. Pain, injuries, accidents and so on are part of life. Ageing too is a process. All the time you do not remain young. But yoga is not only a part of life but life itself. It is my very breath.

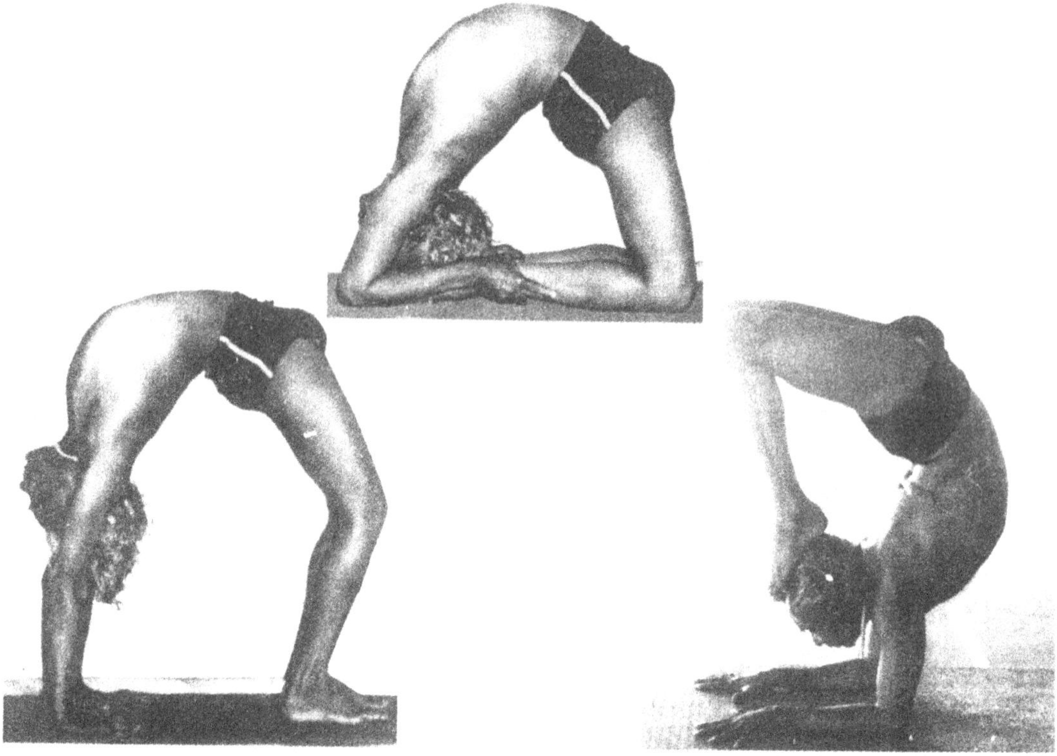

Plate n. 33 – *Ūrdhva Dhanurāsana, Kapotāsana, Vṛśchikāsana* at the age of 79

The mind may play a trick and say, "No way, oh! it is a painful process, so forget and rest". But if I do that, I am lost. Have I to listen to the soul or to the body and mind? Even if the body wears out, I say that worn-out body should keep doing something in order to be independent in life. I don't want to be in a sterile and stagnant state. Many saints, *sadhus*, yogis, when they can't walk, can't stand, say that "Now ours is spiritual practice". In which way do you label them as spiritual practitioners? For invalidity or incapability? Please give a thought to this.

Sādhanā never ends. We are not the deciders to declare that now the practice ends. Our body, mind, intelligence, consciousness, all these need to be kept intact for the soul to be revealed.

Q.- But what is the ultimate aim of all this *āsana* practice?

Though I have already answered the question, please know that when I have no aims to achieve, it does not affect me. I practise for the sake of practise. First of all, though *āsana* and *prāṇāyāma* are separate aspects, they are complementary and supplementary to each other and both generate the inner hidden energy. The human energy has facets such as moral, physical, vital, mental, intellectual and spiritual. This energy helps to reach the cosmic energy. I want my inner energy to be in contact with that cosmic energy. You see only my *āsana* practice, but I see whole of yoga in my *āsana* practice. My mental and inner practice will not be known to you. You cannot perceive it.

As a matter of fact, I am practising *āsana* and *prāṇāyāma* to have a divine health till the end. Health is *prajñā*. I want *prajñā* (awareness) running in all the spheres of myself.

Patañjali says[1], "The conjunction between the seer and the seen is the cause of pain. Avoidance of the union between them is the remedy to be free from pain." Later[2] he says, "The moment the purpose of nature for the emancipation of the seer is accomplished, nature's relationship with the seer comes to an end. However, the vehicles of nature continue to function for and affect average seers and ordinary people. For one who is able to perceive his own form, the conjunction of nature comes to an end. This is the divine union or the divine health where soul and body unite or where nature merges in the *Puruṣa*. Like body merges in the soul, nature merges in the Universal Force. For others, the conjunction continues." This means pain continues for others. However, what he further mentions is most important, that is why I am doing *āsana*. "The purpose of the conjunction of the seer with the seen is for the unfolding of the inherent powers of nature and spirit, so the seer discovers his own true nature." Now I have given the quotation from the *Yoga Sūtra* of what my practice of *āsana* means. My body intelligence is guiding my intelligence in understanding the meaning of *svādhyāya*, i.e., self-generating *jñāna*. If I don't know the subtle part of nature, how can I know the subtle seer? That's why I am doing regular practice – so that nature teaches me. The inherent power of nature gets unfolded by the practice of *āsana* and *prāṇāyāma*. The body, senses, mind, intelligence, consciousness, I-ness, all these are the aspects of nature. The seer is the soul. In yogic terminology the nature is called *prakṛti* and soul – *puruṣa*. *Puruṣa* and *prakṛti* are united. This association or fusion is for both good as well as bad. It can be used by us either for a right purpose or wrong purpose. The body can be used for a right purpose in order to follow the path of emancipation. This is what *āsana* is doing for me. It can be used for sensual enjoyments or fulfilment of desires. The practice of *āsana* refines this tool – the body – so that we begin to use it for a right purpose – a higher purpose – a spiritual purpose.

The body is the gross vehicle whereas *citta* – the consciousness – is the subtlest vehicle of nature. When the consciousness becomes absolute, then it transforms into a seer. That means it has crossed the threshold of nature to embrace the seer.

---

[1] Second chapter, *sūtra* 17.
[2] Second chapter, *sūtra* 22 and 23.

We use yoga as an instrument to convert and accept nature's qualities in the favour of the Self.

- And this is something you experience in your practice? -

This is what I am saying to you since the beginning. Yes, I do experience. That's why I am able to explain the transformation that is occurring in me. I keep the nature of the body, mind, intelligence and consciousness under control so that the seer witnesses nature. That's why I am able to do difficult and advanced *āsana* even today, due to that friendliness between the body and the seer.

I am drinking the fruit of nature by the practice of yoga so that I see the seer.

I have seen, I have experienced, but I can't explain. The experienced seer cannot be explained. If I say that I have seen the seer, I am telling you the untruth. If I say I have not seen, then too I am telling a lie. It's only an experiencing state, that's all. The moment I come to express it, you know that the seer has gone back. It's the mind, the consciousness which speaks, not the seer. Seer cannot speak. Seer only experiences.

If the cosmic intelligence exists everywhere in the universe, then the individual intelligence also has to exist everywhere. Our intelligence spreads easily for objective knowledge. I see whether the same intelligence can spread for the subjective knowledge too. I like to feel whether it is existing in the frontiers of the human body. For that reason I am doing *āsana* and *prāṇāyāma*. Even if God comes and tells me, "Give up the *āsana* practice," I will say, "No, I will not give it up." Whatever transformation has to come in me, it has come to me through my own practice. That's my God who has taken me to this level. As I said, I could not speak one word in English. I was not knowing the philosophy of yoga. *Āsana* alone taught me everything to come to this level. How psychology works, how the mind works, how the intelligence works, I have learned through this. So my *āsana* are my God. I can't leave it.

Q.- You are sometimes criticised for being arrogant.

Because people have not found weaknesses in me to speak about. So naturally they want to find something and say, "Oh, Mr. Iyengar is a very hot headed man." If I am so, then I ask them to present that yoga so that my arrogance may cool off. Sometimes I say jokingly people in the class, "God has permitted me to show off vanity."

I feel that showmanship of vanity is wrong without mastery on any subject. If I have perfected in one thing, why should I not show vanity? I will show you each and every part, including the nail, where it goes wrong. Is the nature of truth and honesty an arrogance? Truth and honesty cannot withstand untruth and dishonesty. I am truthful and honest to my practice. I do not do practice for showmanship. If I do wrong, I admit it. There is nothing to hide. My practice is direct worship. My arrogance is towards pretension and hypocrisy. As far as the practice of yoga is concerned, if anyone pretends, I cannot tolerate that. One cannot and should not cheat the people under the name of yoga.

For those who call me arrogant, it is as clear as the day that they are more arrogant than me. May be, my presence makes them nervous and say behind my back. If I am in the class, my presence is enough for my pupils to do far better than they normally do. Whether I look at them or not, they do better. They say immediately that there is a vibration in the class. If I am not there, they feel something is missing. Whether I teach, or don't teach, the vibration is there. Students say, "Mr. Iyengar must have walked this way. Something happened to me in my body," And it's true since I have passed that way!

Calling me arrogant is nothing but want of their understanding, so let us forget about it.

Q.- And where do you think that vibration comes from?

My body is singing, ringing yoga. So naturally one has to feel the bell of yoga ringing when I walk by.

– So I suppose after all this exposure, I should go home and practise right away. –

Naturally! That will teach you automatically! Why should I say no? Then you will realise what power it gives. One day you too may experience what I have experienced. So right away go and practise.

– I hope so! Thank you very much for answering my queries patiently. –

EVOLUTION IN *SĀDHANĀ*[*]

Q.- People look at you and admire you at the age of eighty, still full of health, energy, vitality and spirit. This is a clear sign of what yoga has done for you. Could you please tell us something about the difference in your practice, over the years, in your thirties, forties, fifties, sixties and seventies?

You should know that evolution in practice goes on as one refines the interior body and learns to sharpen the intellect through sensitive transformations, which occur in *sādhanā*. This intellectual development and refinement develops tremendous conscious understanding to feel and see different perspective transformations that take place in attentive practice. After years of *sādhanā*, what I see is that the inner body and the inner mind automatically become more attentive than before for further development in toning and culturing the various states of consciousness.[1] In the early thirties, I was struggling to do the *āsana*, in my forties and fifties I began consolidating them. Actually in the early years I was seeking and searching in my practice and bringing the missing things and thoughts and link them in each *āsana* for the cognition of the intelligence. I was studying the missing things, changing the various grips in the body, at different times measuring the wrong and right tensions and vice versa. It was like a fluctuating body in a fluctuating mind. All these were there for years. Sometimes, I began to touch the zero tension. This way I worked for the imprints to remain permanently in my head and heart.

---

[*] Interview by Gabriella Giubillaro in Pune. January 1998. Published in *Yogadhārā*, LOYRT, Mumbai, 2000, pp. 79-85.

[1] There are seven states of consciousness which are; emerging consciousness *(vyutthāna)*, restraining consciousness *(nirodha)*, peaceful state of consciou sness *(praśānta)*, creative consciousness *(nirmāṇa)*, one-pointed consciousness *(ekāgra)*, breaching or fissured consciousness *(chidra)* and divine consciousness *(divya)*.

Also there are seven states of awareness, these are: awareness of the physical body, awareness of energy flow, awareness of the collection of experiences, discriminative awareness that filters these experiences for perfect judgement, awareness that illuminates consciousness, unbroken flow of awareness to trace the source of consciousness, and awareness of surrendering oneself into the Cosmic Being – *Paramātmā*.

The matter of studying the *āsana* and *prāṇāyāma* to become a perfect *sādhaka* was not explained or taught by anybody. I studied the effects of *āsana* and *prāṇāyāma* explained in the yogic text books and created techniques to define the *āsana* with the general available explanations, the movement of the in-breath and the out-breath as well as the fluctuations and oscillations to feel those effects.

The body has its own mechanisms and the intelligence and the mind too have their own. I had to unify all these for a right focus on all the facets of body. This is actually the body-mind language, which I do not think is the right terminology to use for the intelligence of the body. The body language is an outer expression and the language of the mind is an inner expression. Intelligence of the body rubs with the intelligence of the head and heart. This is an unknown phenomenon. Only yoga practitioners will be able to understand it. There is a vast difference between body language and body intelligence and its wisdom. The body language is an expression of failures or successes. These things were there in my earlier presentation. Body language is a kind of exhibitionism or showmanship. While giving public performances I used to make each part of the body express itself as an individual entity. This is known as body language. You may call it as the ego of the body. After expressing the ego of the body I used to feel that there was something more than body cult or language, which is the inner quality of a man as a whole. I call it a psycho-philosophical expression. I do not know if there is any terminology for this. It is a difficult point for me to explain. But I began to work in unison so that both the content (mind, ego, intelligence and self) as well as the container, body, express together.

Everybody knows that the body is a part of matter. Our ancient science declares that mind also is matter. If the body is a gross matter, the mind is a subtle matter or one can call the mind a finer matter. These differences in matter took me a very long time to realise in a practical way. It is very easy to talk about such things but to experience the elements of matter moment to moment in *sādhanā* is very difficult. These differences surfaced in me after I reached the zero state of tension in *āsana*. Now I say that my physical, mental and intellectual maturity is on par with each other while doing *āsana*, *prāṇāyāma* and *dhyāna*.

In the case where one thinks that he or she is intellectually matured, and the body does not respond and send messages while in practice, then one should humble that arrogant intelligence which proclaims itself as mature. As long as one does not recognise the good or bad, the right or wrong, then that practice is of an immature quality. When it comes not only from the intelligence of the body but also from the intelligence of the heart and head, then I say that the feel of harmony is intellectual maturity. Before reaching this state, all efforts should be considered as nothing but manual physical pressures, where unevenness remains predominant.

In my earlier practices the balance of the mind was also uneven. I could not express these uneven sensations and pressures between the body and the mind.

When I had even extension of body and mind in each *āsana,* I had a set-back in 1979. I met two scooter accidents in that year which limited my movements a great deal with uneven feelings. They opened my eye of knowledge – *jñānacakṣu.* Probably if I had not met with these accidents I would not have penetrated the inner body – I use the word the inner body – with ease and comfort. For me, the inner body is where the physio-psychological body ends and the mental body begins. I could feel the organic body with ease, but beyond the organic body I was feeling the empty spaces, and to penetrate those empty spaces required truly a great amount of discipline. Not only that, but a great amount of saturated attention with observation was needed. While observing one has to reflect again and again attentively on adjustments so that in the re-adjustments one does not disturb the other established parts that are already in an attentive "zero" state of action. I began to feel this new experience in my practice after the accidents. Probably these accidents were a blessing in disguise by God for me to re-learn.

Perhaps I could have jumped miles ahead in my practice if the accidents had not occurred. Sometimes destiny plays and disturbs one's determined practice and goal, tempting one to give up making further efforts. Destiny almost made me give up the practice, as the movements were very painful. My determinative power did not give up practice. Only, after the accidents I had to begin again as a raw beginner and pursue yoga with persistence. I re-tried and re-tooled myself. My inner body was still aching but the determined perseverance ignited me to come out from my mind's weakness and strengthen and heal the parts of the body that were injured. Even at eighty-one, I can say with confidence that I am bringing out the best. Just now, you said that I am keeping very well. The quality of keeping up the well being of my earlier days was definitely on the physical plane, which I was using with great intensity for recovery.

Today my well-being is not from the physical level but from the intellectual and spiritual levels. In old age, it is natural for the body to decay first. As the elements of matter decay, the gross body too decays before the subtle body decays. When the gross body goes on decaying, the mind gives way and the inner body too decays. In order to keep the mind in fine tune, I have to tone and keep the gross physical body expressing the dynamic vibrancy latent in the cells by attending to each and every fibre of my body. It is a sense of well being in the very life force of man.

Glamour is purely the external expression of the body. My practice of yoga has brought glamour to my inner body, to my cells, fibres, tendons, muscles and organs. This glamour is nothing but refinement in practice and experience. Refinement of self comes with intense work with the internal body and mind. I continue to maintain the inner glamour without allowing arrogance to surface and accepting the deterioration that comes with age. With my intense devoted practice the natural process of deterioration is slowed down and arrested. My yoga practice is now aimed at transforming the glamour into glory.

I did not pay attention to external beauty as I was sick and looked ugly even in my youth. I paid more attention to the inner life force and inner lifeful sensation, which to me is inner beauty. Today, I do not think of my age as eighty-one when I practise. The very thought of age can become the enemy in one's practice. People remind me of my age, but while practising I am beyond my body and its age.

The moment one thinks of old age the mind takes shelter for escape and the body fails. Whenever the body expressed its failures, I started to enthuse it for work by rejuvenating and recouping the part of the body that remained dull. The moment my mind says I am eighty-one, the mind naturally wants to give way. Then I am lost for yoga. Hence, I work and struggle to find out where the mental blocks are and each day I work to remove these blocks and go ahead with my practice without thinking of my age. I keep in my heart the will to work in order to maintain this extreme refinement in my body and sharpness in my intelligence. If in my practice my skin contracts, I feel my mind too is contracting. If part of my body is dull, I know my mind is dull in that area. At this age these are the observations that take place, but very few pay attention to these. I am grateful to God for giving me the wonderful gift of sensitivity of mind, intellect and body.[1] I am working in such a way that even now I maintain that quality, because nature – *prakṛti* – shrinks, fades and deteriorates as one ages, but I am not allowing it to shrink so that my mind may not become small or petty. If my mind shrinks, my courage also shrinks and the ageing tells upon me.

Q.- Is it a struggle?

No, I do not think that it should be termed as a struggle, because I love practice. I am comparing the duality that arrives at this age. Where the body says I cannot reach, practice helps me to reach there. Having seen ageing people the mind entices with thought, "Why do I want to strain myself so much? I have worked with discipline, but often my mind says forget everything and enjoy life." I say, "No," to the mind. In order to be honest to my conscience I practise. Even to day my goal is to reach the space in the ethereal body, beyond the organic

---

[1] The gerontologists may say that one should not think that one is old. Old people are also advised to keep their mind occupied in some leisurely activities. At the age of eighty-one to make the body bend in advanced *āsana* like *Śīrṣāsana*, *Kapotāsana* and *Vṛśchikāsana* and to stay longer in the *āsana* is extremely difficult and challenging. This requires mental language flexibility, stability, compactness and balance. *Gurujī* talks about the courage of the mind, but for other old people courage at the body level is difficult to maintain.

body. Now, I say I am not struggling but educating the channelled mind to move consciously, everywhere in its frontier – the body. I am educating myself when I stretch my body. I create an internal stretch, which is impossible for others to see. I am bringing my Self, the inner being, close to its envelope, the skin. I practise in order to keep in contact with the innermost body, so that the outer body does not feel its age and it is brought to be one with the soul.

Though ageing and death is certain, practising yoga keeps me away from this idea of age and death. Practice brings the diminishing body in contact with the eternal soul. The eternity of the soul does not remain as a mere ideology any more as I experience it practically.

This union is a very complicated thing. Many people may not easily understand. Know that I do not stretch the body today, which I used to do in my thirties and fifties. Now I stretch the intelligence in my body to expand so that the intelligence stretches my body. Today I make the intelligence to trace and reach the body everywhere. That is why I say I was a seeker in the beginning. Being no more a seeker, I see and stretch my intelligence and make the body to stretch on its own. If I stretch my body I may feel the signs of fatigue, because the body feels the strain, the mind feels the exhaustion. Now I work with the intelligence so that I support the mind in the body and spread the Self everywhere. Previously, I was making my body and mind as the major important means in practice. Now, they are secondary and I move my intelligence firmly with the Self. The Self (as content) expands in my body and the fluidity of my inner body expands the solid body. In the early days I was using the solid body to make it fluid. Today it is not so, it is the fluid I make to come in contact with the solid body. It is a very subtle and sublime practice, which non-practitioners perhaps may not understand.

Q.- Once, I heard you say that you now understand what happens to the body when it becomes old, could you explain what happens?

This is also a new thing. If you see a youngster's body and if you see an aged person's body, the top ribs shrink in an ageing person. Because when we are full of life, the top chest is made broader than the middle chest or the bottom chest. Look at a skeleton. There you see the contraction is on the top. This fact was guiding me, it made me to watch how the energy of life gradually shrinks from the extremity towards the interior body and then towards the innermost body, which an ordinary mind cannot easily grasp. When shrinking takes place, the life force does not reach there. When the life energy starts contracting, the top ribs get narrower and narrower, leaving no room or space for the energy to occupy. The sternum gets dried, and the energy is felt in a very low ebb. The dryness in the sternum, which sets in, indicates that the life energy is not reaching and goes on shrinking the sternum. This made me to think and practise so that the life energy reaches and stops shrinking in the sternum. This I learned very recently.

You have seen me today doing a lot of backbends. When you do backbends you complain of backache and pain, you will be surprised to know that at this age backbends did not bring me pain but dryness in the sternum. I do not get pains or aches like you, but I feel dryness and shrinking sensation in the sternum while doing backbends.[1] This is how I have learned how old age sets in. The sternum is known as a dry area, where energy recedes. Even a doctor will tell you that this area is a bony structure and movement is very little. One does not feel the dryness in the sternum at a young age. With years of practice, it was an enigma, a mystery for me with this feel of dryness and shrinking. This is how I know that the old age had set in and again with my determinative practice, I eradicated this dryness and shrinkage.

You know that sometimes the strong athletes die earlier than the common man does. They overwork and dry out. They do not know how to recuperate and do not know how to keep the dry areas wet. Even today when you see my backbends, I do them more in the area of the cervical spine than the lumbar or the thoracic dorsal spine, because the dryness is only on the top region of the sternum. While doing backbends, I used to rub my hands on the sternum. This is what this age taught me, and warned me to be careful as dryness and shrinking has appeared in the sternum. Because of my sixty years of practice, my developed sensitivity and intelligence guided me. This shrinking stopped at the sternum.

At the time of ageing, the new understanding, the deep penetration, the fresh courage is required. I think my recovery from this dryness at the sternum may act as a guide for you all to be careful and face such situations.

Q.- Once I heard you saying that once you used to practise for teaching and now you practise for yourself.

If I have to teach I have to be an extrovert. Hence, I have to work on myself a great deal. An introvert cannot teach. My practice time then was meant to learn the art of teaching. As you know from the story of my early days, the art was not well known. I had to practise well in order to present this art in public. With respect to the public, one has to show them what they do not know. Naturally, I had to learn both exhibitionism and inhibitionism. I was giving public demonstrations as well as teaching. Both teaching and demonstration needed glamour in the

[1] The dryness has dissappeared by 2002 through persistent effort and attention on the sternum while practising backbends.

expression. I had to create attractiveness in my presentation to win people towards yoga not only on the physical level but also on intellectual and emotional levels. I was making each fibre, each tendon, each cell express its presence in the *āsana*. I am not sure whether anyone presented the *āsana* the way I was presenting. Each *āsana* has its own profile. I used to trace the profile of each *āsana* and present by expressing from the profiles. This way I used to bring attention in the audience to make this dry subject attractive and tasty. Gradually, my presentation attracted millions of people who are now practising, for which I am grateful to all of them. From my efforts of seventy years what I got is unimportant, but what yoga carried the message to the mass was something, which I say is a great success in my life.

People came to me with their physical and mental problems. Obviously, I had to practise to see how *āsana* can be effective to give relief to the patients. I had to do lot of searching to find ways in my own practice. What yoga did not give me, I began giving that to others. See how far it has spread now on account of my early works! For example, in 1989, I was invited by the Ministry of Health to visit Russia to introduce an unknown subject there. Now there are a dozen or more centres in Russia. See how much yoga has spread there! I think my practice has opened the eyes of the masses. If I am not benefited, it does not matter much to me. I am happy that the grace of yoga is on my students who have benefited and are benefiting. I had to struggle in yoga from A to Z, but my students need not struggle so much as they have got a good foundation already. Even if a small percentage of my way of practice is taught, one sees the benefit of yoga taking place.

I teach less these days because I want my pupils to come up. I do not want the yoga that I practised to die with me. I see a lot of learned people do who not allow their ardent students to grow under them. If I am the trunk, the branches are my pupils. They have to be kept in an even, fresh and trim condition. That is why I give chances to all the youngsters irrespective of place or gender to progress in yoga. That is why I have stopped teaching to encourage teachers like you to carry on.

This is the stage in which by closing the windows of knowledge from the senses of perception (which go outside), I reverse them to see what is inside and make it more glamorous. I am using the word 'glamorous' because the Western world is very much attracted to this word. That is why I want to show that, that glamour should shine from within in such a way that the others can see and feel that person is totally within and without. With this in mind I am doing more and more to find out whether further refinement can be made to become supremely sensitive so that I can impart that also to you all.

I am still practising so that the impressions *(saṁskāra)* may remain in the heart of the soul, so that if I am destined to be born again, I may start yoga from where I ended, with more enlightenment than at the time of death.

I do not want to die as a stopper. Many must not have had the courage to face the difficulties coming in old age and had no courage to accept the truth. They might have expressed with a double face that they have reached a certain spiritual level in order to cover up their weaknesses or to save their self-honour. I want to be true to my conscience and hence I continue the *sādhanā*.

I am a liberated Soul; I have experienced what is freedom. I have experienced the quality of what freedom is. I do not think of liberation while I am practising. My mind probes on what yoga can further reveal through practice. My mind is still open. As it is open, I am seeing the *āsana* now as a seer. I am not searching. As a seer I am seeing, and seeing as a seer. Who knows if God gives me next life, if people like you are made to do yoga again you may be searching for a good practitioner? You may find me again to learn yoga! Therefore, I am practising yoga for the knowledge that has not struck me so far but may strike in my next life. So, I do not stop my practice. Let that light, which may not be coming now illumine me in the course of several lives. Please do not think that what I am saying is my selfish motive. For me it is not. On the other hand, I say that even if I do not get illumination, in my next life I may re-start from where I stopped in this life. If I stop my practice before my life ends, then I may have to start as a beginner in my next life. Therefore I am practising so that my consciousness will be in that same point of yoga to start in my next life.

Why do people say that in old age one should have hobbies? My profession was yoga and now my hobby is yoga. A hobby means to keep engaged in other activities, to avoid monotony. So, I converted my professional yoga into a hobby to find out how much more it can exhilarate my heart.

YOGA: A WAY FOR ARTFUL LIVING*

Desikachar: *As I spoke to you earlier, uncle, two years ago, in Madras, we had a* Healing Conference *and seven healing traditions participated in that conference over a period of seven days. The conference included; Acupuncture, Tibetan medicine, the physician of the Dalai Lama was there and his assistant. Of course it included modern medicine, allopathy as well as* āyurveda *and yoga, something where they don't use antibiotics. There is an organisation in America called* Common Way, *which works for cancer, and was also included in it.*

The conference was a very good occasion. We were all very much together. And then the idea came that maybe a book could be brought out about these healing traditions. The title was Awakening the Body, Mind, Spirit.

Uncle, this conference was organized by an American Foundation called the Aperture Foundation. *The* Aperture Foundation *was originally doing some photographic exhibitions in places like Philadelphia, they went on to present certain issues such as poverty. Then they began to bring some biographies on spiritual people like the Dalai Lama. Now they are going into this question of healing.*

When the topic of yoga came they asked me to be in charge. I insisted that this topic won't be completed without your most important contribution to yoga, I insisted on this. So the managing director of this Foundation asked me whether I can do this. I said I can go to Pune and request my uncle to share his experience in the field of yoga. He was very happy, so I have been in correspondence with you and finally I am here now in Pune after nearly thirty-seven years.

I am very grateful to you for allowing me to ask some questions like a layman. Please I am very much a layman, definitely in front of you, and you must forgive my silly questions.

---

* Interview by T.K.V. Desikachar. *Guruji's* nephew, T.K.V. Desikachar, is overseeing the aspect of Yoga in a future publication, a book to be called *Awakening the Body, Mind and Spirit.* For this reason he had traveled to Pune to interview his Uncle. The interview was realised in the Library of the Ramāmaṇi Iyengar Memorial Yoga Institute on Saturday the 21st February 1998 and continued on Sunday the 22nd February in the Main Yoga Hall.

Q.- The first thing that I would like to ask you is, how to understand yoga in today's context where you have made it so popular? How is it that yoga is accepted all over the world today, even when it is coming from the *Vedas?* How did you manage to make it so popular?

You know, first of all yoga has got all the three aspects essential for today's intellectual standard namely, art, science and philosophy. For me philosophy is neither *jñāna,* nor acquired knowledge, but filtered experiential knowledge.

Undoubtedly, the origin of yoga is found in *Veda.* The moment we say *'Veda',* it is equated with Hinduism. I do not believe in calling it Hinduism. For me it is *sanātana dharma* – eternal religion – as it expresses what is good for the whole of humanity. *Veda* basically teaches the ways in the art of living and life as a whole. Life has to be designed artistically and lived with an artful approach. The nature of creation is a beauty made by God. As nature attracts us, art too attracts us. The nature does not differentiate or change according to religions. Nature does not ask us to which religion we belong. I got inspired by this quality of nature and I took the Art. Art also, like nature, is impartial. I took it as a Universal Culture and went on demonstrating *āsana* wherever and whenever the occasion arose and opportunities came. I developed the artistic quality and aesthetic value of each movement of each *āsana* and attracted the audience not only by educative expression but by presentation towards yoga.

Secondly, when I began teaching, I did not use *yama* and *niyama* as disciplines, but fitted them to be within the frame of each *āsana.*

Patañjali appears to be a great mind reader. He studies the hidden instinctive mental and intellectual weaknesses of humans, which are violence, untruth, stealing, incontinence and greediness. Respectfully he uses the opposite terms to these above five mental and intellectual weaknesses to cross over towards non-violence or non-cruelty, truthfulness, non-covetousness or non-stealing, celibacy, and non-grasping or non-attachment to greed.

For example, violence – *hiṁsā* – is physical, mental and intellectual, which works in all. Similarly, we are susceptible to be dishonest. Covetousness and greediness are ambitions to gain fame and make quick or easy money. Even the patenting of ideas has brought the civilized and sophisticated intelligentsia into the art of stealing. Similarly immoral trafficking, free life, free sex, have brought HIV and AIDS. By this, one can understand why Patañjali insisted on *brahmacarya* – celibacy, which is not renunciation but a controlled sex life. These five aspects of *yama* are meant to control that mind which goes with the current of the sensual objects. Hence, Patañjali introduces *niyama* to counteract these instinctive weakness of mind and intellect.

Niyama is a method to discipline and channel the mind to put a restraint on it. *Niyama* speaks of cleanliness and health, contentment, determination, study on life beyond worldly pleasures and to be humble within oneself so that the mind and ego are subdued to take one towards God. Callousness on health, discontentment, unhappiness, are some of the means that take one away from the true art of living.

In my demonstrations and teachings, I kept away from traditional explanations of *yama* and *niyama*, but emphasised on human values and how they should be respected in today's life-styles. Obviously, one cannot enforce moral values on traditional language. So, I had this strong feeling that I could introduce those principles of *yama* and *niyama* indirectly in the practice of *āsana* as the explanations through *āsana* appeals to one and all universally.

To follow *yama* one needs deliberation –*pratipakṣabhāvanam* –, whereas *āsana* could be brought directly into practice to bring the mind into a quiet, passive state. *Āsana* practice not only keeps one organically healthy but also free of the instinctive weaknesses of the mind and in its place builds confidence.

We are made of five sheaths or *kośa*, namely, *annamaya, prāṇamaya, manomaya, vijñānamaya* and *ānandamaya*. Among these we are familiar with the first three – *annamaya, prāṇamaya* and *manomaya* – physical body, organic body and mental body. The physical body and the mental body are connected to each other through the organic body. The *āsana* work directly on the organic body, which produces life-giving chemicals. We can say *āsana* act like alchemy to produce nectar *(amṛta)*. While doing *āsana* certain actions produce the nectar or elixir of life through fusion. But today the deep effects of *āsana* are lost, due to the attention mainly on the external and anatomical body, .

I began to practise yoga for gaining health and I took health as the main source in the art of living. My ill health taught me that health is very important for mankind. I do not think any religion has negated health. I took health as a universal religion and this aspect remained supreme in my mind. Life is dynamic. It moves like an electric current but nowadays we treat life casually. We do not pay respect nor think of protecting life which has been given to us. Health has to be acquired through physical discipline, organic discipline, mental discipline and intellectual discipline. Then the subtle ethical disciplines begin to set in. These changes convinced me of the importance of *āsana* and it stuck to me like a leech to carry these ideas in all classes whether it was for men or women. After all, the individual self is inside the body and, as such, the body becomes the envelope of the Self. This feeling enlightened me regarding the importance of *āsana* to protect the envelope. The yogis gave many *āsana* because Life is vibrant and dynamic but not static. Therefore the *āsana* done ten years ago, if done without paying attention to the dynamic movements of life today, they will not have any effect on body, mind or self. As life is like an electric current, health is also like an electric current and hence the *āsana* should be electrifying the life force.

First of all, is it not important to know one's own body before one talks of God?

We have hundreds of muscles and joints, hundred thousands kilometres of blood vessels, sixteen thousand kilometres of nerves in which the nervous energy flows and various organs like lungs, heart, liver, spleen, pancreas, intestines, glands and so forth. All the various systems and sensory nerves (connecting to the skin), and the motor nerves (connecting to the spindles of the muscles), all of which have to work in unison.

Here, the age-old science of yoga plays a very vital role in making the systems of the inner body to work in concord, harmony and balance. *Āsana* are like flying a kite in the body. The self is the holder of the thread and that thread is intelligence. That is why various *āsana* are discovered for the thread of intelligence to grip and interweave according to the extension and contraction with unison. From this one can gauge the value of *āsana* as well as health.

The interior body is very dark. In order to know the body, the performance of various *āsana* with awareness lights the light of intelligence to feel and penetrate the dark caves inside the sheaths of the body. Hence, *āsana* lights and enlightens the intelligence for it to move and penetrate the subtler layers of the body.

The inward journey is from body to the self. The body is perceivable, yet it is less known. When perceptibility is wanting, can we conceive it?

So, I began introducing through *asana* the ways to trigger the intelligence to feel and experience the body. Here the question of alignment struck me. Most people practise *āsana* on the theme "as the wind blows so the leaves move". Today the practice of *āsana* is such that people move the body as it directs and forget to pay attention to correct it along with the other layers of the body.

When I speak of alignment, it means we have to balance the energy and intelligence evenly throughout the body so that the life force is maintained ever-green and ever-fresh by the practice of *āsana*. We have to develop through alignment to enlighten the intelligence in all *āsana* as each *āsana* distinctively beams different rays of awareness and attention on the intelligence. For example, the flow of intelligence in *Trikoṇāsana* is not the same as in *Pārśvakoṇāsana*. It is not the same in *Vīrabhadrāsana, Sarvāṅgāsana* or *Śīrṣāsana*. Each *āsana* has its own diamond cut facets of light. We have to understand these various facets of light that flash in each *āsana* to present them with precision as a gift to the Self. This needs attention, observation and awareness both in intelligence and consciousness. It is the *prāṇic* energy that acts as a powerhouse for the intelligence and the consciousness to work and hence, they depend upon *prāṇic* energy.

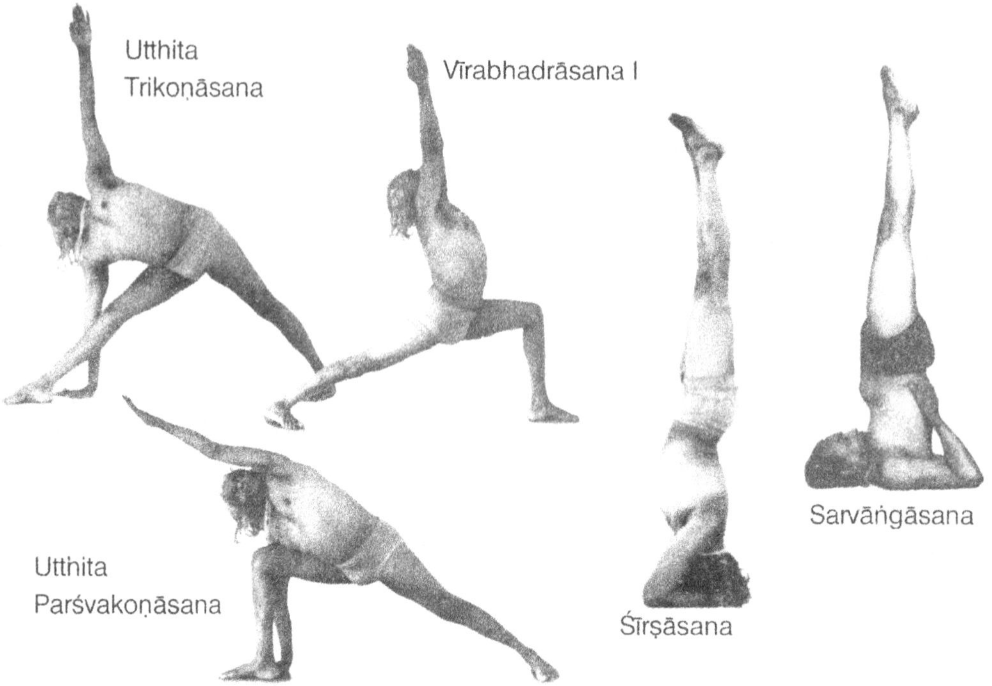
Utthita
Trikoṇāsana
Vīrabhadrāsana I
Sarvāṅgāsana
Utthita
Parśvakoṇāsana
Śīrṣāsana

Plate n. 34 – Flow of intelligence

When we are practising the *āsana* the energy wets certain areas, dries certain areas, rinses certain areas. After rinsing and releasing, the energy is made to withdraw from the focused area to spread to other places. If the water runs like a brook, it becomes ferocious and disharmonious, while in a river the water runs smoothly within its two banks. Due to our behavioural patterns of standing, sitting, walking, sleeping or exercising, the *prāṇic* energy flows like the brook. Therefore, I learnt to do the *āsana* aligning with rhythm the bones, joints, muscles, fibres, tendons, nerves, mind, intelligence and consciousness with full attention.

As your question was on various disorders which the body succumbs to and how yoga heals, I am explaining in length, though the question appears simple. Because I cultivated to observe and align all the ingredients of the body from the skin to the self, I could make the subject not only popular but educative also. Let me go into alignment. Alignment is of several types. It could be physical alignment, muscular alignment, alignment of nerves, alignment of fibres and tendons, besides the alignment of the intelligence, consciousness and self. Many see *āsana* only as physical alignment and therefore they have lost the opportunity to savour the flavour of the *āsana*. The intelligence has to understand the body language, which means not only communication but also of communing with the body. No doubt the body has its own memory and intelligence, which has to be tapped by the intellectual intelligence.

Everybody calls man a psychosomatic animal, so the actions of psyche on soma and of soma on psyche, have to be studied. It's a two-way avenue but many people take it as a one-way avenue. We all say that we are psychosomatic but we often feel the sensations from soma to psyche as well: Therefore the *āsana* were invented, built up and developed to awaken the qualitative memory that is hidden in each cellular system, in each fibre, to guide the brain how it has to react. In our science we call them *karmendriya* and *jñānendriya. Karmendriya* are nothing but the efferent nerves, and the *jñānendriya* are the afferent nerves. They communicate between themselves as they are the windows of knowledge and action. When we are practising *āsana* we have to see how the five *jñānendriya* react to the five *karmendriya* and how the *karmendriya* react to *jñānendriya.* In modern terminology, how the motor nerves – *karmendriya* – and sensory nerves – *jñānendriya* – respond to each other. Their functions should be such that a friction between the two is not created. There should be room or space between these two, so that with the action and reaction, there is reflection and re-reflection. There has to be a parity of the sensory nerves and the motor nerves as they act through and interact between, the body, mind and intelligence. Only then is there equanimity or *samatvam.* A perfect reflection, parity or samatvam between the motor nerves and the sensory nerves is the primary target to attain *samatvam,* firmness and contentment in *āsana* – see II.46 – without that how can there be any paired reflections, or re-reflections between body and mind, mind and intelligence? One will only end up with refractions. Through the reflections and re-reflections between –the *karmendriya* and *jñānendriya,* refraction is eradicated and the mind and intelligence assimilates the ripeness of the *āsana.* This is the essence of the *āsana;* firmness and contentment, without contortion or distortion.[1]

In our *āsana* practice, we have to see whether the sensory and motor nerves are coordinating with each other or not. If this coordination comes, then our intelligence understands the vertical extension of attention, which is its quality, and the horizontal expansion of awareness, which is the quality of the consciousness. When this experience sets in, then consciousness, intelligence and energy are evenly coordinating in concord. Mind belonging to the *tejas tattva,* observes how they function on the gross elements of earth and water.

The five elements are *pṛthvī, āp, tej, vāyu* and *ākāśa.* Each element has its own characteristic, its own way of functioning and reacting. In *āsana,* the *annamaya kośa,* the outer body as a *ghaṭa* or pot, has to have firmness and solidity. The *prāṇamaya kośa,* the organic body as fluid, has to remain soft but vibrating. The *manomaya kośa,* the mind as *tej* or fire, has to function as a medium to charge them with mobility, stability and sensitivity. Up to this feeling, the *sthūlendriya* get involved in *āsana.*

---

1 See *Yoga Sūtra* II.46 – *sthira sukham āsanam.*

The *vijñānamaya kośa,* belonging to the element of air or *vāyu.* It is connected to the *sūkṣmendriya* which are the intelligence and the consciousness. The intelligence and consciousness has to energise and make the *āsana* lively. This live wire (intelligence) is the connecting wire between the body and self. The *ānandamaya kośa,* belonging to ether or *ākāśa* as space-connector, acts as a transmitter, establishing close contact between the body and self, i.e., *pṛthvī* and *ākāśa.*

If these two subtle elements *(vāyu* and *ākāśa)* are involved in the practice of *āsana,* then all the five elements get totally involved, drawing attention inwards *(antarlakṣya),* and with eyes kept open for outward attention *(bahirdṛṣṭi).* This alignment envelopes all the vehicles of *prakṛti* (nature) to be in communion with the *puruṣa (ātman).*

When we are doing the *āsana* there are two main directions. One is going away from the central body, that is from the bone, and the other is from the muscles towards the bones. The muscle fibres are like the wings of a bird. Can a bird fly with one wing? So while practising *āsana* we have to see whether both wings of the muscles, the inner edge and the outer edge, the inner bank and the outer bank, maintain space between them with equi-distance to the bones and bone marrows to act and react. That is known as physical equipoise or the awakening of the body. The use of the muscles in *āsana* is to create actions in the body so that the mind gets the imprint and then sends the message for the intelligence for right readjustment. This is awakening the mind. This is what I did in my learning. Then I connected the intelligence and consciousness to align with the āsana, thus awakening the dormant self to become active. I used all these alignments in my demonstrations to attract people towards yoga and in my teaching to ignite interest towards insight.

I built up on this understanding by the grace of your father, who allowed me to find out the hidden wisdom of *āsana* by myself. I practised as if I were doing on the sharp edge of a razor and found out through aligning my mind, intelligence and consciousness vertically and horizontally along with the stretch of the body. I used this skill in my public performances and in teaching. That is how yoga gained tremendous popularity.

Q.- You have explained the concept of art beautifully, I must give my respects to you. Now, I would like you to explain why you also believe that yoga is a science because it is something that is said repeatedly, that it is a science.

See! Science is an inquiry; art is an answer to an inquiry. Science is prescription. Art is description. Science is theory. Art is practical. *Jñāna, vijñāna, prajñāna* are the three aspects, which go in an ascending order in every art and science. *Jñāna* is just to know. It is just a way of acquiring knowledge. *Vijñāna* is *viśeṣa jñāna,* special, specified, where knowledge is tested by experimentation. *Prajñāna* is *prakarṣa jñāna,* exalted knowledge with wisdom. It is the experienced knowledge that is filtered and refiltered to reach the ultimate. Often one says, "This is my experience". It's a casual statement. But how many people have filtered the same experience thousands of times to come to that state of *prajñāna,* which is unoscillating wisdom?

The wisdom is experiential knowledge or *prajñāna. Prajñāna* surfaces after being critically tested and ascertained through the process of *jñāna* and *vijñāna.* Patañjali coins this *prajñāna* as *viveka-khyāti, vivekaja-jñāna.* Patañjali has not used the word as only *viveka* but added *viveka-khyāti* (glory of knowledge) and *vivekaja-jñāna* (exalted wisdom). It is nothing but ripeness in experiential knowledge, which does not waver at all. He uses another term for *prajñāna* as *ṛtaṁbharā prajñā.*

The first step to reach this exalted state of wisdom is inquiry. And here lies that yoga is a science. You have to go on trying and retrying with trials and errors on the subject. Experimenting with trials and errors is science *(vijñāna).* When the trials and errors come to an end, it is *prajñā.* When this *prajñā* is put into a subjective experience, one eradicates faulty experiences. Then it becomes error-free. To reach this error-free state subjectively is *prajñāna.*

Now, let me talk on art. Patañjali says, *pratyakṣa anumāna āgamāḥ pramāṇāni (Y.S.,* I.7). Here, he defines *pramāṇa vṛtti* on a valid, experienced, verified, correct knowledge. *Pratyakṣa* is direct perception, *anumāna* is closer to imagination. It is inferred and proved with thoughtful imagination. *Āgama* is to collaborate with experienced persons or scripts to know whether one's experience in doing is right or wrong. Art is dependent on these three wings namely, *pratyakṣa, anumāna* and *āgama.* There is no artist in the world who can claim that he is an artist without these three pillars. He perceives directly the forms of art. Then he infers to put it in an artistic form. Afterwards he refers to the legacy of the ancestors. Patañjali too begins yoga in art form by following *pratyakṣa, anumāna* and *āgama.* I am proud to say that I followed all the directives of Patañjali to experience, facing trials and errors *(anumāna),* without accepting the things straight away. In *pratyakṣa* I repeatedly re-examined my own perception to find out the truth, but I did not take things for granted. Then I referred to *āgama pramāṇa* or *ṛṣis' pramāṇa.* When my experience almost came close to the essence of the *ṛṣi's* teaching, I got the confidence that I was near the perfection of the art.

Patañjali speaks of *prayatna* or persevering effort (II.47). Of course *prayatna* is needed. You have to put in effort after effort in order to get the best essence. When the best of the efforts is reached, *śaithilya* or the effortless state comes automatically. The regimental force and effort that is used in the beginning to learn transforms on its own into a natural force. This is effortless effort. A master musician sings effortlessly. Does it mean that he did not put in his efforts in the beginning? Will he sing accurately without the scientific knowledge of *rāga?*[1]

Like the rhythm and melody of the music, Patañjali speaks of the artistic presentation of *āsana* by *rūpa lāvaṇya bala vajra saṁhananatvāni kāyasaṁpat* (III.47), meaning "Perfection of body consists of beauty of form, grace, strength, compactness and the hardness and brilliance of a diamond". This is completely an artful *sūtra.* He explains that there should be *rūpa,* there should be form, there should be *lāvaṇya,* there should be grace. There has to be *bala,* firmness. A painter may take a brush and paint so easily that for onlookers it seems that he has done it with a light touch of brush on canvas. But if you ask him, he will say that even to show the loose clouds in the sky while painting needs a light but firm touch. Then he speaks of adamantine discipline. It is 'freedom in discipline'. *Vajrasaṁhananatva* means experiencing and living in the freedom that is real.

As he explains artistically, yoga is an art, and when I practise it as an artist and then I try to explain the subjective experience objectively. Because the subjective experience needs technical terms to explain, then it becomes a science. What I have experienced in an artful way, I explain in a scientific way to my students to experience what I have experienced.

Yoga first creates the views, then it says *krama anyatvaṁ pariṇāma anyatve hetuḥ* (III.15). It means transformation takes place according to the sequential changes in *krama.* As one tries various sequences while practising, it means experimentation, and hence it is a science.

That's why I say, yoga conveys description as art and prescription as science, because if I know the *āsana* I have to explain. In order to explain I need a technique. Without technique, one I cannot explain.

- Very good, Sir. -

Technique is needed. A technique with which we build up. For example, when we breathe, whether it is the in-breath, the out-breath or the retention, there must be a methodology for that. Therefore you have to study what is right and what is wrong. If you do wrongly, what happens? If rightly done, what is the effect? If there is a mistake, what defect does it bring? I think with these practical clues, the art is converted into a science, where we say: "Don't do this, do this; don't do that way, do this way". And here, it acts as a science.

You must have read *Man the Unknown*[2]. Man the Unknown is an easy terminology. But does man know truthfully and honestly his own body? The one, which can be known, one does

---

[1] A musical scheme of five, six or seven notes composed logically which forms the basis of Indian classical music.

[2] By Alexis Carrell.

not know. Man has landed on the moon but he has not landed in his own body. What yoga teaches is to land on the self. The *ātmā* – Self, which is the Sun. Sun never fades. Consciousness in us fades like the moon. We can land on the moon, i.e., we can land on the consciousness, but we cannot land on the Sun. When attention of intelligence and awareness of consciousness fuse together, then we land on the sun and experience *ātman*. That is *ātma-sākṣātkāra*.

– And it is then a philosophy. –

Philosophy is *vedānta*[1]. It comes at the end. It comes at that moment when the vertical attention and horizontal awareness meet together. When this happens, the soul exists now here and everywhere and at that state one forgets the body but loses even the idea of seeking the soul[2].

As the eyes can see all things but cannot see themselves, the Self becomes the first person and so the feel of it disappears.

Q.- Uncle, we are Indians. Sitting with you is like coming home. You have succeeded, making this teaching understood outside India, where the culture is so different, where the value system is so different. How did you do that?

I had lot of problems in the early days. If I go and think back to the hardships I underwent, I feel that it was an amazing feat. I laugh at it now. You know, when I went to Europe for the first time, I was asked, "Can you chew glass? Can you swallow acids? Have you swallowed currency notes?" and so forth.

For example, my first public lecture-demonstration in the West was in 1954. It was in the World Fair, held in Lausanne, Switzerland. At that time our Ambassador was Mr. Gundevia, who was my friend who had arranged a demonstration for this World Fair. I was very happy being my maiden show in the West. When I was about to go on the platform, the police officials came and said that I could not give a performance unless checked. Then I was questioned, "You are not allowed to use a razor or a sword, not even match box with match sticks". That was the understanding of yoga in 1954. Though it hurt me, I stood in front of officials with my underwear and said, "Search me". Even Mr. Gundevia was upset. Mr. Sen, Consul General was

1 Literally, Veda means knowledge and *anta* means end, i.e., end of knowledge is *vedānta*.

2 *Viśeṣadarśinaḥ ātmabhāva bhāvanānivṛttiḥ* (*Y.S.*, IV.25). For one who realises the distinction between *citta* and *ātma*, the sense of separation between the two disappears.

also upset. When nothing was found, then the authorities allowed me to demonstrate. There I talked on the philosophy of the body. From then on, I spoke on the philosophy of the mind and soul in later demonstrations.

The *Yoga and Health* magazine was attacking me saying that my yoga was purely physical yoga and it had nothing to do with philosophy. In 1971, the Education Department, under the control of the Government of England, wanted to change the callisthenic system in order to awaken and alert the body consciousness. They wanted something that could stir the life in the body. I think it was Noel Baker, the leader of the Labour Party, then a hockey player. He had broken his hipbone. He came to my class. I helped him and he got rid of the pain in his hip. He could walk better. When discussions were going on, he, Yehudi Menuhin, Lord and Lady Coleraine were there. Mr. Menuhin spoke to them that he would send his children to Mt. Everest if Mr. Iyengar were to take them. "He is the best one you can think of", Mr. Menuhin opined.

Then they, along with the Education Board, attended my classes. Doctors too came to see. The first question they asked was, "Can you teach yoga without using any philosophical terminologies?" This was a big challenge. It is very difficult for an Indian to speak on the subject, which is basically philosophical. Then I thought that if I hesitated, it would be a failure on my part and I would not be able to popularise yoga.

So I thought of culture of the body and culture of the mind would be easier to convey the essence of life than philosophical terminologies.

In India, yoga was a neglected culture except singing of its greatness. The *Kālidāsa* says, *śarīramādyam khalu dharma sādhanam* – body is the main source to do righteous *sādhanā*. But when we come to *śarīra,* we neglect it completely. To achieve the four aims of life *(dharma, artha, kāma* and *mokṣa),* the body is the base for all actions. We neglected, though the *Veda* have said that body is the foundation for worldly as well as spiritual achievements.

According to Patañjali, yoga has a code of discipline, *atha yoga anuśāsanam* (I.1). I started explaining that indiscipline is the negligence of duty *(adharma)* and discipline is duty *(dharma).* So I changed the vocabulary to make them understand from their perception that yoga means a discipline. So, I began teaching the culture of the body and how the mind has to penetrate the movements of the body. They all realised that what I was saying was comprehensible. This way of explanation made yoga become very popular. Then it spread to America, Africa, Japan, Europe and Australia and became a household word.

Q.- One more thing. If you had to define yoga today, how do you explain it, which is acceptable to Indians as well as others, how do you define that?

Everybody knows that yoga means union. The word *saṁyoga* is used in the context of the union of *jīvātmā* with *paramātma*. *Saṁyama* is the methodology where the union of body, mind and self takes place through perfect health on these three sheaths. *Saṁyama* and *saṁyoga* are synonymous terms. Without *saṁyoga* there is no *saṁyama*. Without *saṁyama* there is no *samādhi*. Therefore, today, we have to emphasise *saṁyoga* – the union of body, mind and self, as the definition of yoga.

There is disunion and disconnection between body and mind, mind and soul. We don't know where the body ends and mind begins or where the mind ends and the self begins. They are interconnected but we demarcate.

According to Patañjali's *saṁyoga;* the four parts of the brain, namely *vitarka* (analysis), *vicāra* (synthesis), *ānanda* (bliss) and *asmitā* (pure consciousness) (*Y.S.*, I.17), have to be united with the four parts of the heart, namely *maitrī* (friendliness), *karuṇā* (compassion), *muditā* (gladness) and *upekṣā* (indifference to I or me or mine) (*Y.S.*, I.33), and this is yoga. The four functions of the brain and the four functions of the heart make each individual's body quite different, though the muscles, joints, length and width of the circulatory and nervous systems are almost identical. Therefore I feel the union of the head with the heart and the heart with the head is yoga, which transforms the practitioners to be good human beings to treat each other with equanimity.

The structure of each *āsana* has its own anatomy, whereas the body has its own anatomy. The anatomy of *āsana* has to fit according to the anatomy of the body. My presentation of the *āsana* may not fit into that of somebody's body, so I have to think in what way the structure of the *āsana* has to fit into that person's anatomy in order to bring his body to be in union with *āsana*. This way of presentation is *saṁyoga* to me.

The different bodies, different minds, different structures of the muscles, different movements and levels of freedom in the joints, have to be thought of to make them work unitedly. When association builds up, integration takes place.

When this integration takes place between the body and the mind, the real discipline to cultivate the mind begins.

It is not possible for everybody to have the *ātma-darśana*. Even a man like Arjuna had to beg Lord Krishna to bless him with a divine eye. We are in the process to develop that *saṁyoga* and *saṁyama*. When we reach that level, then *samādhi* is possible.

Here, *samādhi* does not mean trance but the total absorption in action and reception from the bottom of the soles of the skin to the apex of the head. There has to be oneness like that of the river when it has joined the ocean. As life is a flow, awakening our body is to allow the river of the body to flow to enter the ocean, i.e., the Self and rest there. It means that here the macrocosm and microcosm unite. If macrocosm is *mahadākāśa*, the microcosm is *cidākāśa*. Both *mahadākāśa* and *cidākāśa* i.e., outer space and inner space becoming one is yoga. This is *samādhi.* Today in order to make the *sādhaka* to understand this union, I say body is *tāmasic,* mind is *rājasic,* self is *sāttvic.* The *āsana* and *prāṇāyāma* remove the *tāmasic* quality of the body and make the body as vibrant as the mind and later, through *dhyāna,* take the vibrant body and mind to dissolve in the illuminative light of the *sāttvic* nature of the self, and that is for me yoga.

- Well, nobody can complain because you are not bringing God, prayers, rituals or traditions and all that... -

Q.- Another question comes to me. The West doesn't accept teachers. Unless a person has a teacher, there is no way he can appreciate yoga.

A teacher, no doubt, is a helping hand for those who seek knowledge. One can cook food and invite guests. The one who prepares food may request the guests to eat but cannot force it into their mouths. Similarly, the teacher is there to give a helping hand but cannot force the subject.

I said earlier that whatever I have learnt it is by the grace of my *guru.* Also on account of his frightful commands. I had to suffer a great deal with body aches and failures. Nothing came to me with ease. I had to find out whether I was balancing rightly between the little toe and the big toe or, like the scale of justice, whether my body and mind, mind and intelligence and intelligence and self were evenly co-ordinating or not.

In the court, the scale of justice is held by the Goddess of justice with blind eyes. It indicates that the justice should be done clearly without favouritism. So one has to work on all aspects of yoga judiciously.

The teacher can only guide and the rest depends on the calibre of the students. If one finds a teacher, I say he is very lucky, because the teacher who knows the techniques and intricacies of the subject can guide and blend the student. If a teacher is not available, then to learn will be definitely hard, which takes a longer time than with a teacher's guidance.

Today the *guru* has become a rare product. Secondly, the modern *guru* goes according to the taste of the students. It has become almost a puppet game. If the students complain, the teacher adjusts to the wishes of his students. That means the pupils are corrupting the teachers and they get corrupted. As all arts are pure, teachers have to give the students the best. If the teacher is very good, the students need not undergo the trials and errors as the teacher saves them from wasting their time. These good teachers can build them up constructively.

- Good. -

But I do know that the Westerners do not accept or respect a *guru* as Indians do. Our moulded *saṁskāra* is not the same with their moulded *saṁskāra*. But in recent years, there is change in the West. In earlier days of my visits to the West, they were calling me 'Iyengar', not even Mr. Iyengar. Today, they call me *Gurujī*. You go to any of the Institutes in the Western countries, they ask you to leave the shoes outside.

So by example, they have learnt. Most people are now vegetarians. In the 1950s I was called a grass-eater. Today, vegetarian food is available in Western countries. So in the 1950s I lived only on coffee and toast.

– I have seen you drinking coffee. –

Today you see all my students have become vegetarians. They have learnt on their own to cook vegetarian meals. I say, by example, they cultivated these habits. So, if a teacher is available, they should make the best use of him. If a teacher is not available, then they have to work from *anumāna*, then *pratyakṣa* and then *āgama*.

Q.- Uncle, I have one more delicate question. You see, you do better than I do. But still I want to discuss. We have to clear certain things for this book. See, you have until now, in almost one hour, you have not used certain words that are to be used otherwise you are considered that you don't know anything about yoga. For example you have not used the word *kuṇḍalinī*. If you don't use the word *kuṇḍalinī* it is like you don't have a passport. So how to understand that you have been able to confine clearly this concept of body, mind, etc., without this terminology.

First of all, we must know that any journey is from the known to the unknown. But today, many people are jumping on the unknown as a mystical practice, which attracts them. But, honestly, I feel that one who starts from the unknown point is lost. Even the medical scientists had to study the body from its known end. They dissect the inner body from outside the dead body. In early days treatments started at a peripheral level. As the science developed, one came to know the functioning of the body, inner organs and various systems. Yet, there are many things that remain unknown.

It took a long time to know the glandular system of the body. We know that the hormones are produced and secreted into blood vessels in order to get circulated in the body. How they are produced is not yet clearly and precisely known, but that they govern the physio-psychological body, is a fact.

Similarly, we have a spine and the science talks about plexuses in the spine. The plexus are the centres of the network of nerves with which all our physical and mental functioning are related and connected. Why I referred to these two systems is because they are related not only to the well-being of the body but of the mind, intelligence and consciousness as well. For instance, if your digestion is affected, you may suffer from acidity, constipation, diarrhoea or any of such diseases related basically to digestion. But if you think a bit further you know that because of this small physical upset your mind loses its clarity and sharpness to some extent. Such is the close relationship between the body and mind. This can give you the idea how much the glandular system and nervous system are related and by which the mind gets affected.

When we come to our science I am very proud to say that we had developed the knowledge of the body more than modern science had discovered.

Our *ṛṣi* and yogi had reached the inner depth after knowing the physical and physiological body where they could visualise *citta, pañcakośa, pañcavāyu* and *saptacakra,* which is unknown and non-perceivable by naked eyes or on electronic devices. These are beyond the perception. Similarly, *kuṇḍalinī* is also a divine life force in the form of energy which is non-tangible, non perceivable, yet existing in everyone as *citta, pañcakośa,* etc. Some people are physically strong, some mentally, some intellectually, some emotionally and some spiritually, as all these depend upon *vāyu, citta, kośa* and *cakra.*

As a yoga practitioner, I say that *cakra* are within the spinal cord and plexuses are outside the spine. However, in order to understand *cakra,* one has to strengthen oneself on the physical, moral, emotional, mental, intellectual and spiritual levels before going into *cakra.* In all there are seven *cakra.* Though all yoga texts speak of *saptacakra,* Patañjali says slightly differently.

They are the seven *cakra,* which can only be known by a person who has got *saptaprānta bhumikā.*[1] You have to connect the *saptaprānta bhumikā.* There are sevenfold or seven forces in the spiritual body as *cakra.* These *cakra* are the seven *prānta* of which Patañjali speaks. He wants that conscious *prajñā* should be there, and how it has to be brought in the seven facets of the *cakra.*

The *mūlādhāra* at the base (*mūla*-root, *ādhāra*-base or support) is the abode of storing the reactions of actions *(karmāśaya)* (*Y.S.,* II.12). Maybe, *mūlādhāra* acts as the black box of an aeroplane which records all the details. When the plane crashes, the black box is searched, which throws the light on the causes of the accident. Similarly *mūlādhāra* may enlighten our accumulated imprints of past lives.

Svādhiṣṭhāna is the abode of one's own – *sva*-one's own, *adhiṣṭhāna*-abode. A human being has two types of hidden tendencies in him. One pulls him towards *bhoga* – the enjoyment of pleasures – and the other pulls him towards *apavarga* – freedom from pleasures or

[1] *Yoga Sūtra* II.27, also see *Astadāla Yogamālā* vol. 2, 'Physiology and *Cakra*' and '*Cakra, Bandha* and *Kriyā*'.

emancipation. Both the tendencies oppose each other moving in opposite directions – downwardly bondage or upwardly freedom. If the *karmakośa* is found in *mūlādhāra*, *kāmakośa* is found in *svādhiṣṭhāna*. Patañjali refers to it as *sva-śakti* (*Y.S.*, II.23). It is the power of *prakṛti* in which I-ness triggers since one is on a precipice to decide which way one has to move.

Maṇipūraka is *nābhi* (navel). The infrastructure of the network of the body is found in the navel. The root of all the nerves is the navel. The nerves are the connecting bridge between the body, mind and self. The area of the navel is the abode of root-mind. When *svādhiṣṭhāna* gives direction to mind which way to go, the chemistry of the body gets affected. If the mind says, "Bondage", our actions, tendencies, behaviour and character take their patterns, which are ready to follow bondage. If the mind says, "Freedom", all these factors mould into different patterns. This is *kāya vyūha jñāna* or the perfect knowledge of the disposition of the human body (*Y.S.*, III.30). The navel is a very vital area where the vibration of the mind and the movement originates for speech. I said that *mūlādhāra* and *svādhiṣṭhāna* are *karmāśaya* and *kāmāśaya*. They have great connection. So many *āsana* were discovered by yogis to have effects on the various sheaths of the self. For example, backbends were given to awaken the physical energy. The backbends, what we call as *pūrva pratana āsana*, are meant not only to straighten the crooked and curved tailbone but also uplift the core as they bring alertness and make us active to remain lively.

In III.35 Patañjali speaks of Self residing in *hṛdaya*. The *hṛdaya sthāna* is nothing but the seat of *anāhata cakra*. *An* indicates not. *Āhata* means to strike. If you strike a drum, sound is produced. But in *anāhata* the sound is produced without striking it. *Āhata* means also injury. The chest is the area of biological heart as well as spiritual heart. When you are emotionally upset, depressed or have a guilty conscience, the spiritual heart begins to sink. Some of the *Upaniṣad* recognise *sūryacakra* and *manascakra* between the navel and heart – between *maṇipūraka* and *anāhata*. It is very significant. Sun and moon signify heat and cold, *piṅgalā* and *iḍā*, soul and consciousness, whichever way you may say. Patañjali says that by *saṁyama* on the region of the heart one acquires the knowledge of contents, functionings and capacities of consciousness *(citta)* (*Y.S.*, III.35). By doing backbends we awaken this energy. *Mūlādhāra* leads towards *karmaśuddhi*, *svādhiṣṭhāna* towards *kāmaśuddhi*, *maṇipūraka* towards *kāyaśuddhi* and *anāhata* towards *cittaśuddhi*. Today we are living in an unhealthy society created by us alone. Unhealthy competition, egoistic competition, demoniac ambitions are the invitation to cardiac diseases, injuring heart. If consciousness is pure, conscience is clear.

Patañjali coins *kaṇṭha kūpa* as *viśuddhi cakra* (*Y.S.*, III.31). Its place is in the pharyngeal area or throat. *Vi* stands for speciality. *Śuddhi* means purification. It is a place of special purification. The throat is a very complicated area, a lively cross roads, heavy traffic, busy square, as you find in the city of Chennai. Physiologically it is a bridge between brain and brawn, head and trunk, organ of speech, wind-pipe, food-pipe, all are crowded here. It is a meeting place of two types of desires - desire of worldly enjoyment, which is called as *bubhukṣu vṛtti*, or desire, and emancipation, which is called as *mumukṣu vṛtti.* The noose of disease, worries, fear, physical and mental suffocation, anxieties, will always be around this area. An average man like I and you commonly get affected at the throat. Patañjali refers to *kanṭakūpa* and *kūrmanāḍī,* which is nothing but *viśuddhi* area (*Y.S.*, III.31 & 32). Anger provokes restlessness and irritation at the throat, affecting the *viśuddhi cakra.* If there is purification here, then not only hunger and thirst but also desires get arrested. *Kūrmanāḍī,* which exists at the pit of the throat, gets stabilised.

Then comes *ājñā cakra. Ājñā* literally means command. The command is the attribute of will power. See, will is superior to intelligence. You may be intelligent, but if you have no will power, what will you do? What is superiority complex? It is the other end of inferiority complex. When there is superiority complex we need to bring the ego down, and when there is inferiority complex we need to uplift the I-consciousness. In spite of having intelligence, if we lack the will power, then we need to lift the I-consciousness from *svādhiṣṭhāna* to *ājñā.* At *svādhiṣṭhāna* we are on the precipice of *bhoga* and *apavarga.* Here, at *ājñā*, we are on the precipice of *vinayatā* and *ahaṁkāra* - humbleness and ego. To surrender the ego by retaining the will power *(icchāśakti)* and by sorting out ego for non-egoistic mentality is the function of *ājñā cakra.* Above this is *soma* (moon) and *lalāṭa cakra. Soma* is the hypothalamus region and *lalāṭa* is at the top of the forehead region. *Soma cakra* not only keeps the body temperature under control but the temperament as well. *Lalāṭa cakra* and *mūlādhāra* have internal relationship. *Lalāṭa* controls destiny. Destiny is nothing but the result of our own *karma* done in the past, or even previous lives. If *mūlādhāra* is the root of *karma* (*Y.S.*, II.12), then *lalāṭa* is the fruit of *karma* (*Y.S.*, II.14). According to our own *karma* the destiny is written. We get pleasant and painful experiences as these are dependant upon our own *karma.*

The last one is *sahasrāra*, the thousand petaled lotus in the brain. As I said the black box is at *mūlādhāra*, which throws the light on imprints of past lives, I would say that *sahasrāra* is the white box, which throws the light on the ultimate future -emancipation. On *lalāṭa* all the imprints should vanish as the yogi reaches the highest state. Patañjali says in *Kaivalya Pāda* (IV.7), the actions of the yogi are neither white nor black or grey. Obviously there are no fruits of non-white and non-black actions. This is where *kuṇḍalini śakti* merges with the soul - the union of the *prakṛti* and *puruṣa* or *śakti* and *śiva.*

- Thank you, sir. This is a very important and clear clarification. -

So, the whole *yoga sādhanā* answers about *cakra.* To open the *sahasra daḷa (sahasrāra cakra)*, you need *aṣṭadaḷa yoga.* We do various *āsana* to awaken the physical energy and filter it by backbends, forward bends, inversions. For instance, we do inversions in order to bring psychological and glandular control. By doing *Sālamba Śīrṣāsana, Sālamba Sarvāṅgāsana, Halāsana, Setu Bandha Sarvāṅgāsana,* we experience the quietness of brain. The disturbed, perturbed and out going mind, scattered mind, is stabilised when we do *prāṇāyāma.*

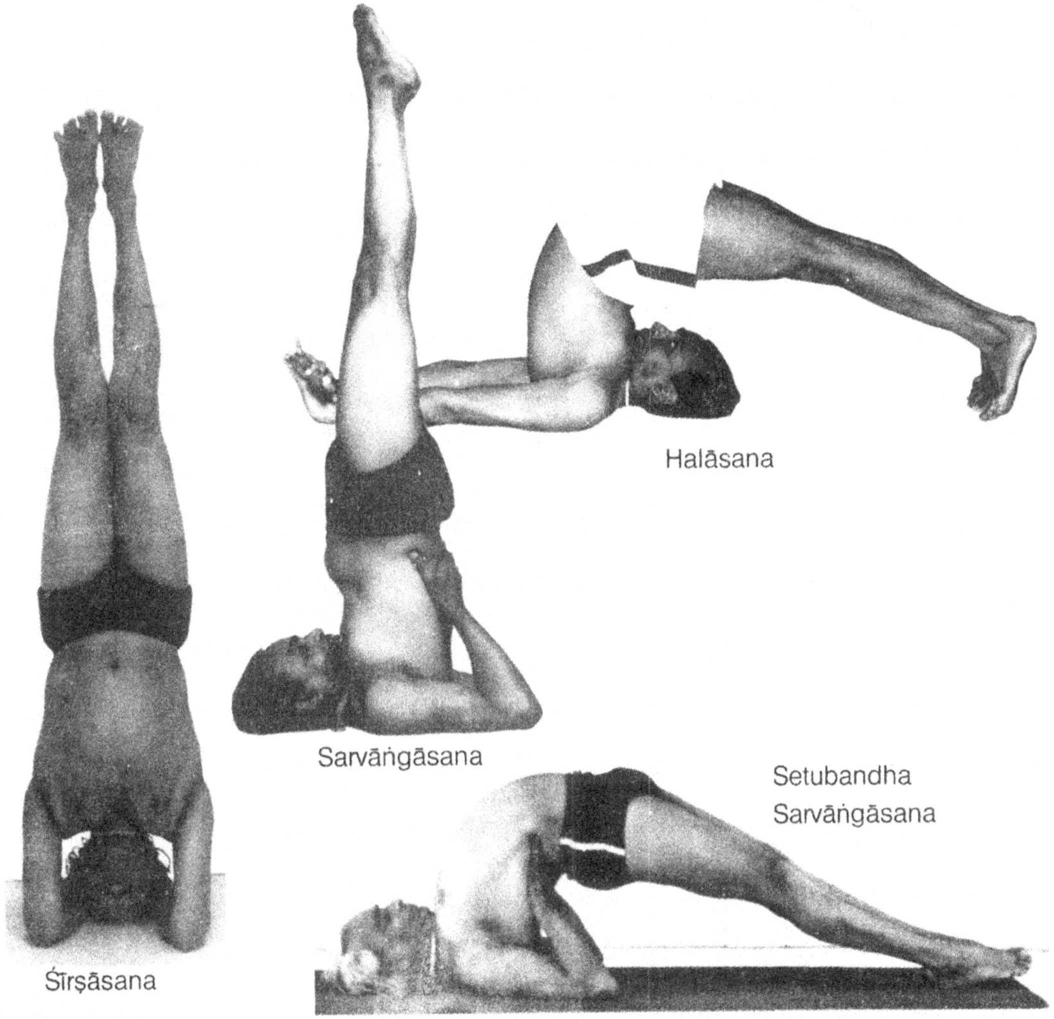

Plate n. 35 – *Sālamba Śīrṣāsana, Sālamba Sarvāṅgāsana, Halāsana* and *Setu Bandha Sarvāṅgāsana*

Upaniṣads say that *prāṇāyāma* is *parama tapas* – the greatest *tapas. Pūraka* is the **G**enerator of energy, *kuṁbhaka* is the **O**rganiser of energy and *recaka* is the **D**estroyer of unwanted or destructive energy that has to be thrown out. So **GOD** is *prāṇāyāma* and *prāṇāyāma* is God.

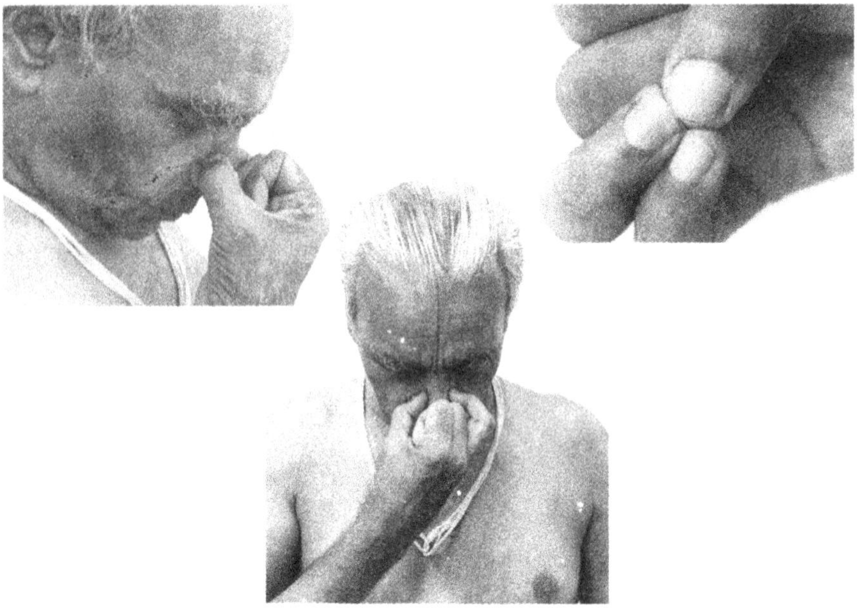

Plate n. 36 – Correct placement of the fingers for digital *prāṇāyāma*

Similarly, cosmic energy is known as *viśva-caitanya-śakti*. The *śakti* is in the gross atmospheric air, when we do the digital *prāṇāyāma*, the beauty is in the placement of the fingers so that the *prāṇa nāḍī* takes in the refined energy which is known as *prāṇa*. For example, the *Haṭhayoga Pradipīka* (II.64)[1], mentions the usage of digitals for *prāṇāyāma* such as *Sūrya Bhedana* and *Nāḍī Śodhana*.[2] This drawn-in energy is stored in *kumbhaka*, which then is absorbed into the *cakra* for storage. So the *cakra* are the store house of this refined energy which remains as divine energy.

---

[1] *Yathodaraṁ bhavetpūrṇamanilena tathā laghu* /
Dhārayennāsikāṁ madhyātarjanībhyāṁ vinādṛdhaṁ // (*H.Y.P.*, 2.64)
JYOTSNĀ OF BRAHMĀNANDA
madhyātarjanibhyāṁ madhyamā tarjanibhyāṁ vinā anguṣṭhānāmikākaniṣṭikābhirnāsikāṁ dṛḍhaṁ dhārayet / *Anguṣṭhena dakṣiṇanāsāpuṭaṁ nirudhyā anāmikā kaniṣṭhikābhyāṁ vāmanāsāputaṁ nirudhya nāsikāṁ dṛḍham gṛhṇīyadityarthaḥ* // Meaning: Without the index and middle fingers, place the right thumb on the right side of the nose and ring and little fingers on the left side of the nose – is the meaning of the stanza.

[2] The reference for "non-use" of the index and middle fingers has created confusion and misguided many in the placement of the fingers and thumb on the nostrils.

I would like to mention how the digits have to be placed here; factually, the tips of the fingers and thumb have to be placed not only evenly but also parallel to each other; carefully, skilfully and with advertence, for *Nāḍī Śodhana prāṇāyāma*. This parallelity of placing the fingers, with the ring and little finger for right pressure comes only when the index and middle finger are both flexed and fixed at the mound of the thumb.

As there are seven *cakra*, there are *sapta prajñā* as well. The *prajñā* evolves in seven provinces – *saptaprānta bhūmi* (See *Y.S.*, II.27). You have to connect the *saptaprānta bhūmi* through *aṣṭāṅga yoga* practice. These are namely, *śarīrajñāna, prāṇajñāna, manojñāna, vijñānajñāna, ānubhavikajñāna, rasātmakajñāna* and *ātmajñāna*. It is a journey from physical body to the spiritual body. These seven phases of *jñāna* trigger the *cakra* and the union of *śarīrajñāna* with *ātmajñāna* is the *kuṇḍalinī* power.

So why I don't use this word *'kuṇḍalinī'*, s-o cheaply, is , because of its divine nature. Patañjali recognises it as *prakṛti śakti* and *ātman* as *puruṣa śakti*. As Ishvarakrishna says in *Sāṁkhya Kārika*, when *ātman* sees this *kuṇḍalinī*, she is like any married woman who does not come in front of any man except her husband. In other words she belongs only to her husband as a respectful woman. "He desists, because he has seen her; she does so, because she has been seen. In their (mere) union there is no motive for creation." (*Sāṁkhya Kārika*, 66). Patañjali expresses the same, *kṛtārthaṁ prati naṣṭam api anaṣṭaṁ tadanya sādhāraṇatvāt* (*Y.S.*, II.22), meaning, the relationship with nature ceases for emancipated beings, its purpose having been fulfilled, but its processes continue to affect others.

I don't like to address *kuṇḍalinī* that cheaply. I show my respect to *prakṛti śakti*. As a *yoga sādhaka*, I respect this *śakti*. So I do not speak of the Power of this Devi. I respectfully pay my reverences to this *śakti* and nothing beyond.

– Thank you, Sir. –

Q.- Soon we are going to enter into the twenty-first century. Lots of people are planning and talking about 21st century. Now, how to do yoga for the 21st century? Is it a continuum or do you have some vision?

I have no vision because first of all I don't know if I shall live up to the 21st century.

- When I look at you, I can't imagine you are 80 years old. -

That I don't know. You know, life is like an eternal river, which flows from the mountains to the sea. Life has no beginning, life has no end. But when God gives us an individual life, we need to discipline it in order to use that life for betterment of one's living. Yoga is as old as *Hiraṇyagarbha* who is the creator. Though it is millennium's old it is still an exhilarating art.

I must say that it is the grace of my *guru*, who told me to carry this yoga wherever I can. I took it by creating the interest and made it popular. Obviously, any science cannot develop unless it becomes popular. So my early idea was that since yoga was unknown, I was thinking of how to spread the message so that people begin to practise it. I know, if the majority of the people practise yoga, then to survey its effect, utility and the changes that take place in the practitioners is possible. If two-three people do and get benefited, it cannot be proved as science. If hundreds and thousands of people do, and if they are tested for research in yoga, it will have a far greater impact than it does now.

Science on body and mind has advanced and there are new treatments for new diseases also. But a surprising thing is that those who are sure of the symptoms of the disease and their knowledge of curing the disease are afflicted with the same diseases. As the mirror reflects, the yogic practice fortunately reflects the health as well as ill-health of each individual. Health has various dimensions. Like physical, moral, mental, intellectual, conscious, conscientious and divine.

Heyaṁ duḥkham anāgatam (II.16), of Patañjali's *Yoga Sūtra,* is for gross intellectual people. Disease, suffering, afflictions don't come to the surface to be known soon. Some diseases don't show the symptoms immediately and may affect one a little later; like cancer and AIDS, where the incubation period is long.

Patañjali uses the same frame theoretically – *sopakrama* and *nirupakrama*[1]; some may be immediate, some may take time. Today's language for that is incubation. What does incubation mean? Patañjali uses *sopakrama* and *nirupakrama.* The effect of the *karma* may be soon or later. Therefore, for jaundice the incubation period is six weeks, and for AIDS twelve years or so.

Patañjali also had said the same. He also speaks of treatment. He says that these afflictions could be in one of the four stages. These stages are dormant, attenuated, interrupted or fully active. This he puts theoretically that afflictions could be sometimes fully active *(udāra),* so also dormant *(prasupta),* dull and attenuated *(tanu),* or it could be interrupted *(vicchinna)*[2]. I took this *sūtra* on therapeutic level, and then I started working on diseases. If the disease was very active *(udāra),* I had to work from the periphery. If it was dormant *(prasupta),* I had to go into the internal body. In chronic diseases I had to lessen its intensity *(tanukaraṇa)* and see that the attack of the disease was postponed *(vicchinna).* Similarly, I thought of *sopakrama* and *nirpakrama* and whether I could check it in the incubation period thus leading towards *heyaṁ duḥkham anāgatam*[3]. Why allow time for the disease to come later? Let me touch the roots, let me penetrate and touch the inner body.

---

[1] *Sopakramaṁ nirupakramaṁ ca karma tatsaṁyamāt aparāntajñānam ariṣṭebhyaḥ vā* (*Y.S.,* III.23). The effects of action are immediate or delayed. By *saṁyama* on his actions, a yogi will gain foreknowledge of their final fruits. He will know the exact time of his death by omens.

[2] *Avidyā kṣetram uttareṣāṁ prasupta tanu vicchinna udārāṇām* (*Y.S.,* II.4). Lack of true knowledge is the source of all pains and sorrows whether dormant, attenuated, interrupted or fully active.

[3] The pains which are yet to come can be and are to be avoided (*Y.S.,* II.16).

As you have got an inner mind and an outer mind, you have got inner body and outer body. Physical intelligence is only on the peripheral or structural body. That physical intelligence affects and reacts on the organs of the physiological body - *prāṇamaya kośa.* This is what we call chemistry, which produces a lot of essences *(rasa)* in the body. In Sanskrit chemistry is named as *rasāyana śāstra.*

The physiological body, which is fed by the actions of the structural body, acts as the arch and span of the bridge between the physical body and the psychological body. If there is no middle body, there is no direct connection between physical body and the psycho-mental body. So the physiological body is the bridge which connects these two, and the psychological body and the intellectual body are connected to our mind. *The ākāśa,* the *ānandamaya kośa,* is bridged by consciousness – *vijñāna* and *prajñā.* They are all bridges and we have to cross over these bridges. When there is a break there is a disease. But if we cross over we are healthily moving from the gross to the subtle and to the subtlest of health.

As you questioned me, I would say that yoga is a continuum. However, health is very essential. What we observe is that the new style of life, new problems, new diseases and new medicines are increasing the problem. Patañjali too talks about disease. He says that disease is a first major obstacle that stands in the way of health and yoga. If the body gets affected, breath gets affected; if breath gets affected, the mind gets affected. He has already declared, *heyaṁ duḥkham anāgatam* (II.16), the pains which are yet to come can be and are to be avoided. Now, we have to make use of it. He is indicating preventive measures through this *sūtra,* but he also warns that it is a full subjective responsibility. Everyone should adhere to single-minded effort in order to prevent[1]. He is indirectly pointing at the life-style that is needed. He reiterates this advice in case any latent, hidden impression of disease remains, reintroduce yoga into the system[2]. Break in practice, break of faith in yoga will lead towards decay, so continue yoga.

The health-consciousness has come. All the health schemes are ready. Millions of dollars are spent on research work on medicine to cure and prevent the diseases. But all these are objective approaches towards health. Nobody is touching the root-cause of unhappiness, sorrow and diseases. Nobody thinks of preventing the root-cause. We have everything yet have nothing, because we have lost human value. Life of mankind is not only for enjoyment. Man is an intelligent being but carrying the imprints of animals. The doctors are known for giving health as a yoga practitioner too does, but there is a difference. The difference between a

---

[1] *Tatpratiṣedhārtham ekatattva abhyāsaḥ* (*Y.S.,* I.32). Adherence to single-minded effort prevents these impediments.

[2] *Hānam eṣāṁ kleśavat uktam* (*Y.S.,* IV.28). In the same way as the *sādhaka* strives to be free from afflictions, the yogi must handle these latent impressions judiciously to extinguish them.

medical practitioner and a yogic practitioner is that for any yogic practitioner defect is known at once through his own practice. But a medical practitioner has to check his own health. A heart specialist dies with heart problems because he is callous and does not look after his own health. Though doctors are responsible for giving health, they have no way to find out the way to come out from their ill health. They do not listen to their inner voice. Yoga teachers are the ones who have dialogue with their bodies. Therefore, in the 21st century, what we need is the subjective health, which can come only through yoga. Objective health comes through medicine, but it is like a bandage hiding the wound inside. Hence, in the 21st century, where people have become more intelligent and more understanding, they have to go for subjective health, which is vibrant.

Health is like a live wire. If the red-hot wire is covered with ash, you may think it is cool and you may touch the ashes, which may burn you. Only through yoga does one guage health. Health that is gained through yoga acts as a burning instrument to know if something goes wrong. So I am sure in the 21st century, if we take yoga not on the physical or physiological levels but as I explained, with alignment of intelligence and consciousness, then we can see a better world in the 21st century, where many people have to say good-bye to medicine and have to say good-day to yoga.

Q.- You spoke about doctors, and you spoke about yogis, and now yoga teachers, yoga teachers being able to see ahead. But many yoga masters, some of them having lived a monastic life, have died with sicknesses. Unlike you; you are so busy, you are a family man, with six children and all that. How is it possible for you to be so healthy at this age? And how is it that those people failed?

My friend, you know the most important thing in my life is my regular practice of *āsana,* which I started at my young age for gaining my health. But you all know that I had suffered from tuberculosis, typhoid, and many other problems. My *guru* taught me how to get back life, where I could live and not be a parasite, so I took to yoga. I continued practising *āsana,* even when I was not knowing any of them properly. Then he asked me to go and teach in Pune, and that's all.

Because he had ordered me, I took it as a challenge and I accepted, though not knowing much on the subject.

You know that I am not educated, I am a failed matriculate. Obviously there was no chance for me to get any job. So my capital was only those few *āsana* that I learnt from my *guru.* I thought, let me see if I can work and make a living out of this subject. He taught me for two years, as I was in Mysore between 1934 and 1936. His teaching was irregular. One day he would suddenly call and heap everything on me and then starve me from knowledge for days. Though I had this irregular teaching my practices were regular. This regular practice tutored me with such knowledge that I will be the last man to ever stop. I am not one of them who say that they have reached the level where the *āsana sādhanā* is not required. If their practice is gone, then according to *Gītā* they are *yogabhraṣṭa*. Due to negligence, yoga masters died from sicknesses.

Though my *guru* taught me *āsana* for health reasons, my ethical approach and mental zeal was such that I did not practise those for the sake of health but to find out the hidden values. No doubt, I gained health and could earn my bread. But some inner force, inner drive, made me go beyond health. I did the same *āsana* but the practice was not the same. Even today I did only six *āsana* for more than two hours without wasting time in between. My *Śavāsana* is a separate practice apart from *āsana* and *prāṇāyāma*. I don't even move my mind from one place to another. My consciousness remains confined to my place – the core.

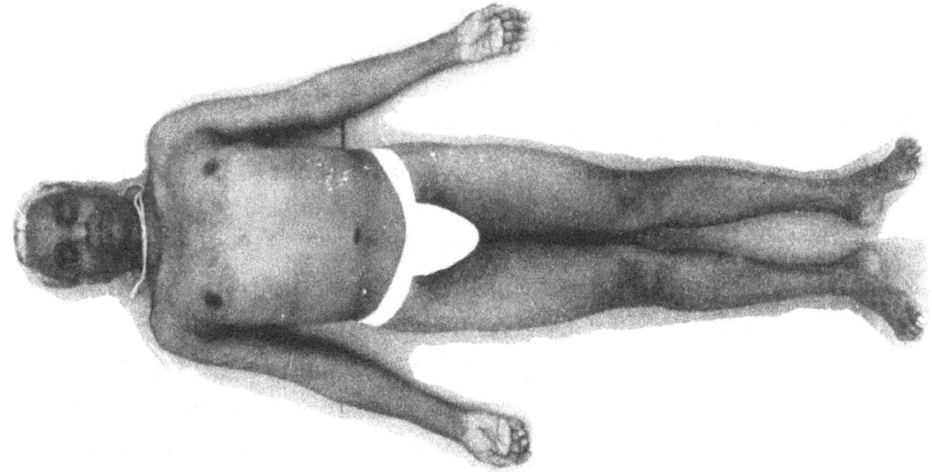

Plate n. 37 - *Śavāsana*

So, the question is not whether I have advanced spiritually. I do not need any certificate from others. It is not for others to know or judge whether I have seen *ātmā* or not. But *āsana* is the one that has built me, which has showed me the route towards my Self and God. I will not flinch from this route. That is why I am still practising, and naturally I am healthy. Health is a by-product, but an essential one. I am now a free man in word, thought and deed. Remember Patañjali's word *vyādhi* at the beginning of the text and how he ends with *puruṣārtha śūnyānāṁ.*[1] In an unhealthy person it is impossible to happen where he is devoid of the fourfold aims. It is then an incomplete work. How can the *guṇa* be involuted, when one is polluted? So let us not go on this ego-trip. Let us accept our limitations and stick to practice. *Sādhanā* is more important than *sākṣātkāra* or *mukti.* The *bhaktan* says, "Let me always be a *bhaktan* and not a *muktan."*

But then there is age. You know, my *guru* came here to Pune for my 60th birthday. He at that time insisted that I should stop *āsana* practice, because I had turned 60. I respected his words. After three months. I became completely dull and stupid, both physically and mentally. I lost those healthy sensations which I had. I soon overlooked his advice and went back to my instinctive elements. Today, even the tips of my fingers are alert. There is no difference between this inner tip and that of the outer tip of my palms or feet.

Believe me, I respected him and experienced the pitfall in *sādhanā.*

He gave me a *japa mālā* for *dhyāna.*

I asked: "Did you have any ill effect from continuing practice?" He did not reply. I stopped my practice as a sign of respect to him. My body became like a log of wood.

Mild *āsana* had no effect on me. I determined to gain back control again and today I stay in *Kapotāsana* for 15 minutes.[2]

Today I do not practise for physical strength but for mental tolerance and forbearance, and certainly not for exhibitionism.

When I used to visit Madras, *Gurujī* would ask me, "Are you practising?" I used to say, "I have not left it." Then he said, "You must be a very courageous man." "Are you doing *Naṭarajāsana?"*, he asked. I said, "I am doing everything." But then, in 1979, I met with an accident and I lost everything. Though I am fighting to get back, I say I am slowly coming back. Again there was another accident and again faced a set-back. I am still trying to the best of my capabilities. The knee complains; arm complains. They say, "We are ageing". Still I am continuing. Now I am far far better. After my knee injury, I had lost *Vīrāsana, Padmāsana...* I got them back after 10 to 12 years of patience with efforts. Now I am trying even *Kandāsana.* We, human beings, are proud to express progress on the intellectual level. I say there is an intelligence in the body as well. It is true intelligence. Because that intelligence knows how to do it, it guides me in my practice. Age frightens anybody. My age also frightens me, saying that it cannot take it. I did not cajole nor gave a military order to do. By sheer will power, I calmly endured pain but I did not provoke the pain. When I was young the body was very active but the mind was not willing. Today the mind is willing, but the body is not willing.

[1] *Puruṣārtha śūnyānāṁ guṇānāṁ pratiprasavaḥ kaivalyaṁ svarūpapratiṣṭhā vā citiśaktiḥ iti* (*Y.S.*, IV.34). *Kaivalya,* liberation, comes when the yogi has fulfilled the *puruṣārtha,* the fourfold aims of life, and has transcended the *guṇa.* Aims and *guṇa* return to their source, and conciousness is established in its own natural purity.

[2] See Plate n. 44.

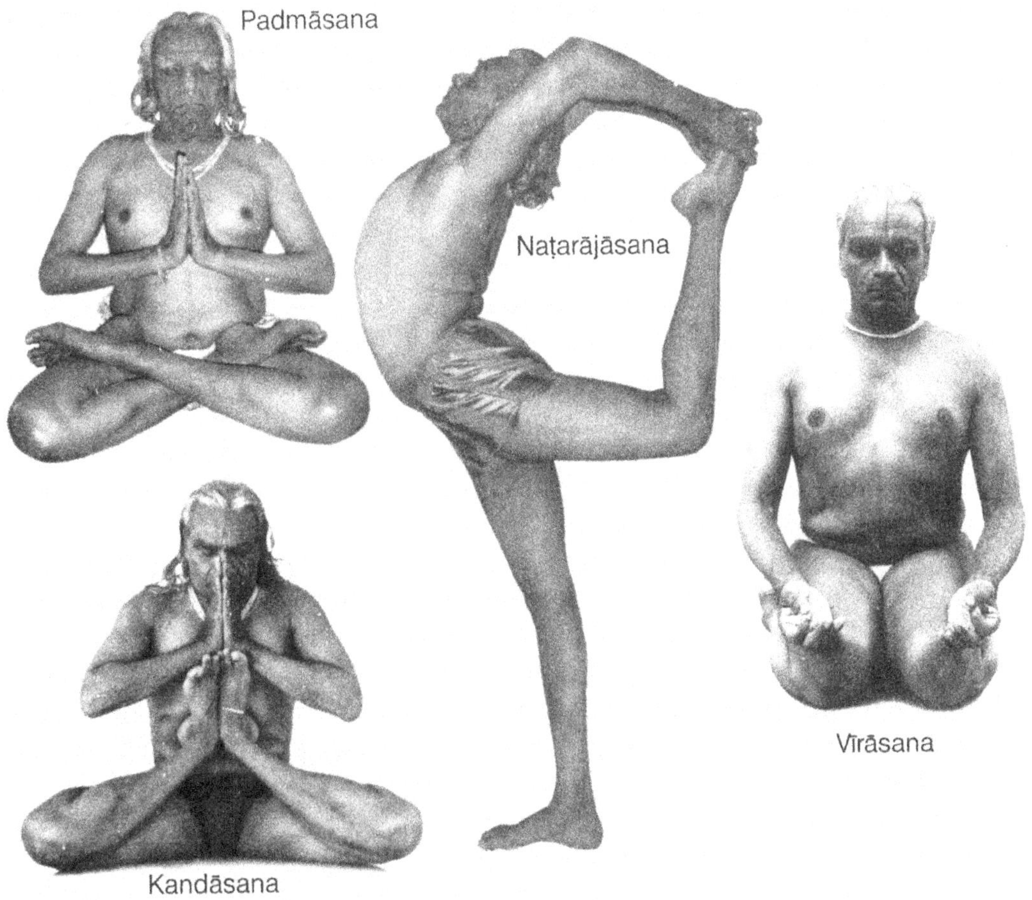

Plate n. 38 – *Natarajāsana, Vīrāsana, Padmāsana, Kandāsana*

Like this, the fight is going on, but I have not left practice. Excuses are easy ways for escape. At eighty I can say that I need no practice. I could cover it also by saying that I have reached a higher level of consciousness. But I don't want to hide my weaknesses. I do *prāṇāyāma* for one hour each day, I practise *āsana* for four to five hours and teach also in some classes. I am definitely in medical classes. Sometimes, I give guidance in the classes, as I want youngsters to shine soon as good teachers. People say that there will be a big void between me and my young teachers. I think, I can close this void by guiding them with correct directions.

In old age fear comes and it is the worst enemy. Facing this fear, one should continue so that it keeps one away from fear.

I do *Vṛkṣāsana.* My legs are far more stable than youngsters'. Why I am saying this is because if I give room for carelessness at this age, I lose the feel of touch of the intelligence in the body sooner than I can think of.

Many so-called yogis cannot stand and cannot walk, and tell a lie that they are advanced in their spiritual plane. It is a pure lie to say that they are on the spiritual line. Honestly, they want all the comforts except hard work, but yoga demands hard work with intellectual attention and awareness. If my body and mind give way, then I tell the truth, that I have lost the grace of yoga.

- *Thank you.* -

God bless you.

(END first day)

* * *

Day Two: 22 February 1997
(in the Main Hall, R.I.M.Y.I., Pune)

Q.- Uncle, yesterday you cleared a lot of doubts about yoga. Today I would like to take up the next area, which is the application of yoga.

How is it that something like yoga which is supposed to be one of the six *darśanas* has come to be now, one of the most accepted systems of health care applicable to practically every day type of work we have today. How did this happen?

Sometimes, when the industrialists start factories with the aim of value for national production, they find some by-products by chance which they never thought of emanating in their trials, and their usefulness turns out as their main profitable product. Though yoga's means and aims are highly philosophical, I think the same thing is happening in this subject also. It brings on its journey *śauca,* which means health in modern terminology, and *santoṣa,* happiness, and on account of that, this has gained momentum in the 20th century because its by-product, health, has attracted people.

The majority of people appear to be healthy but in the true sense are not really healthy. Stress, strain and speed of modern life have brought competition between man and man, which is pressurising life a great deal. The pressures are not only on a psychological plane but also on the neurological flame. This pattern of life is introducing a negative stress on today's life. This negative stress is bringing about deterioration in one's body and mind. On account of this, disturbances on the physio-psychological body are blocking the neurological flow of energy into the system in imbalancing the psyche of man further. This invited problem has made man to search ways and means to gain back neuro-psychological health and to forget his sufferings.

Here yoga plays a great role in replacing the negative stress by positive stress to overcome those currents which sap one's life. Therefore I cannot comment on the title of your book, *Awakening of the Body*. But actually what is required is not awakening of the body, but awakening the intelligence of the body, which should be utmost in your thoughts. The intelligence of the body is no doubt a factual intelligence. For example, a man may say, "I can do *Padmāsana*," but this statement is only from his mental frame. The intelligence of the knee has to convey to the intelligence of the brain its weaknesses and difficulties in performing *Padmāsana*.[1] Here, the intelligence of the brain that prides that it can do *Padmāsana*, gets restricted due to stiffness or pain in the knees. While trying *Padmāsana*, if one realises the pains or injuries of the knees, but does not know how to deal with them under adverse circumstances, he finds an escape path in abandoning to try means to get to *Padmāsana;* but goes for medication or for an operation. Is this the answer? He won't mind if he loses the knees. Is this the sign of health?

My point is different. I think the other way round. How am I to handle the factual intelligence which is hidden, dormant in the body of the knees and tap it diligently to get freedom from pains, so that one day I eventually perform *Padmāsana?* This is called awakening of the body's dormant, hidden intelligence wherein the sensory nerves and the motor nerves communicate with each other to find ways for a workout to get *Padmāsana*. The joints might have gone dry or cartilages or ligaments might have been injured. Under these circumstances, it is yoga that has means and ways to overcome these hindrances. Instead of thinking of alternative medication or surgery, one has to find out alternate methods in *āsana* itself to find relief.

The practice of *āsana* triggers and rekindles that dormant intelligence and makes it to surface. People who have taken to yoga get the feeling that there is sense of health in their knees or around the area of the knees such as hips and ankles and handle those areas to release the load on the knees. I have given relief to lots of people with knee injuries. That spread by word of mouth and caused yoga to become popular. This way it is a science in its own right.

What Patañjali says on the first two aspects of *niyama*, namely *śauca* and *santoṣa*, the United Nations are now taking seriously in their thinking for world's peace and joy for the 21st century. Patañjali has said it thousands of years ago.

Śauca means cleanliness and this means health, and health is *śauca*. Cleanliness conveys keeping the entire system of the human body to function properly and harmoniously. How and why it has to function is an epic study in itself. Here, I think in the practice of *āsana* one begins to understand how and why. Fortunately, yoga begins from the cognisable body and in

---

1. See plate n. 4.

course of time takes to cognise the mind as well as the interior and inner most sheaths of the body. This is what Patañjali means when he speaks of *śauca,* which is in today's terminology – holistic health.

Santoṣa means contentment, mental happiness. When one gains physical health, naturally the next stage is happiness *(santoṣa).* As a good number of people have taken to the practice of *āsana* and *prāṇāyāma,* they have derived both health and happiness. If I am emphasising particularly *āsana* and *prāṇāyāma,* it is for the reason that these can be explained, shown, demonstrated, as they are cognisable to all. What is taking place in presentation can be seen exactly. So, *āsana* gives direct perceptible knowledge, and when they are put into practice, one can factually conceive those perceptions as intelligence and consciousness feel the illuminative light emanating from the body.

Though Patañjali gives eight aspects of yoga, the first two *(yama* and *niyama)* are only indicated on a theoretical level. The other three, namely *āsana, prāṇāyāma* and *pratyāhāra,* are both theoretical and practical. These three enlighten one from the gross sheaths towards the subtle sheaths. That is why importance has come to *āsana* and *prāṇāyāma* because they can be seen, explained and experienced. The other three, namely *dhāraṇā, dhyāna* and *samādhi,* are the wealth of yoga, which are only experienceable. That is why the middle part of yoga, i.e. *āsana* and *prāṇāyāma,* being an evolutionary part of human growth, has been appreciated by many and it has taken a major role.

Unless and until this major role of body and mind is experienced, one cannot go to the subtlest part of *dhāraṇā, dhyāna* and *samādhi.* When the *sādhaka* reaches this subtle level, then *darśana* begins. Hence, the ways to understand what *darśana* means begins when one reaches a certain state of maturity in *āsana* and *prāṇāyāma. Darśana* means a mirror. If the mirror is clean, it reflects; if dusty, the reflection is distorted. Second meaning of *darśana* is looking, seeing the mind by the mind, experience, vision, sight, view any doctrine. This means the body, mind, intelligence and consciousness have to be clean and clear like a clean mirror for the Self to reflect without deflections or refractions. *Āsana* removes the dust and impurities that cover the mind, intelligence and consciousness. This I say is divine health, as the vision of the Self is sighted. On account of this healthy feeling through *āsana* and *prāṇāyāma,* yoga not only has become very popular, but I boldly say that *āsana* has become a root practice for one to move towards its philosophy as *darśana.*

All know that body is perishable. But see what Kālidāsa says, *"Śarīramādyam khalu dharmasādhanam".* Body is essentially needed to follow religious and righteous duty. Is not nescience *(avidyā)* the cause of unhealthy body and perverted thoughts? Caraka says, *"Dharmārthakāma mokṣāṇām ārogyam mūlam uttamam".* For the four aims of life *(dharma, artha, kāma, mokṣa),* the health of the body and mind is essential. We need stamina, enduring capacity, forbearance to accept stress and find ways to overcome them. *Āsana* and *prāṇāyāma* build *prakṛti śakti* to generate *puruṣa jñāna*.

When *prakṛti śakti* activates *puruṣa jñāna*, then it is a perfect health and energises one. It is for us as yoga teachers to make people understand how to channel that energy which flows from health to utilise it for emancipation. This is the interior aspect of yoga as *darśana*, which you asked, and all of us have to work for it, so that the body reflects on the core with right re-reflection without refraction.

Today people speak of *dhyāna* like fast food. Without *jñāna* there is no *dhyāna*. And this *jñāna* comes with long uninterrupted *sādhanā* of *āsana*, *prāṇāyāma* and *pratyāhāra*. The wisdom of our *ṛṣi* in yoga was elevation and bliss *(abhyudaya)* and final beatitude *(śreyas)*.

Patañjali has not said that yoga is meant for peace. Even in sleep one remains peaceful, yet why are we suffering? Nobody asks that question. Therefore, yoga is for culturing your nerves, culturing your fibres, culturing each and every cell so that the body says, "I am clean and I don't want to pollute my clean environment." This is the gamut of yoga *darśana*.

Q.- Uncle, you have worked with a lot of sick people, you have discussed with a lot of medical people, I'm talking about the Western system of medicine called allopathy. You have taught a lot of medical people. According to you what is the failure of Western medicine?

Health cannot be purchased by drugs or by modern medicine. We have to admit that medicine and specially allopathy has advanced to a great extent. The doctors have done wonderful work on the human machine. They lost the link, as they are content in telling people that a static life is good health. Is just existence enough? Their discoveries are prolonging the life span. But health is not prolonging saying, "I am getting on". Health is positive and dynamic. As health is dynamic, body too must remain dynamic and also the mind and intelligence. Life is recognised for its dynamism. So this type of dynamic health is not presented by modern science at all. *Yogāsana* and *prāṇāyāma* lay the foundation for the study of positive health. I have taught people and as far as my experience goes *āsana* and *prāṇāyāma* makes one do the day's work without any strain and at the same time helps them to feel fresh the next day as if a new life has begun. A disease free life is the first stage of health. Then to make a disease free person to be healthy in mind, intelligence and conscience are the further stages of health.

The body is like a bow. You should know how to hold the bow in order to aim the arrow. You should know that if you point the bow in any direction you cannot use the arrow. You require firmness, stability, resistance, attention, and the power in this bow of the body. This is built up by the arrows of *āsana* and then the same *āsana* are used as arrows to hit the target that is the *Ātman*. Unfortunately today the target of yoga has stuck with handling diseases.

Diseases can be divided into various categories. Gross ill health is physical illness. Physical illness in turn puts pressures on the mind. Modern medicine cannot remove this pressure which affects the mind. The practice of yoga not only removes the pressure that comes from the body's illness but releases tensions on the mind and consciousness.

The *ṛṣi* and yogi did not forget the importance of health of the body. For instance, the *Varāha Upaniṣad* uses the word; *ratna pūrita dhātu*. The word *ratna* means a gem, jewel, a precious stone; according to our *Upaniṣadic* terminologies *rakta* (blood), one of the *saptadhātu*, should be just like a gem. Now, why is the blood, which is liquid, compared to a solid gem? The blood is not watery. Its contents are not all that liquid. The contents and the percentage of these contents, what you call R.B.C., W.B.C., haemoglobin, plasma, platelets, and so on have to be there. If any of these particles and chemicals of blood is in want, then health is affected. The food we take becomes chyle in no time, then its first immediate transformation is blood. Therefore, the food must be pure and nourishing. If that blood should be like a gem, you should know how much effort one has to put for that to become a gem. From this angle I say that *āsana* plays a very major role in cleansing the blood. In *āsana* and *prāṇāyāma* practice, the consciousness acts as a needle, while the eye of the needle is the intelligence. The fibres of our body are the thread. When you have to insert the thread into the eye of the needle, if the fibre of the thread is loose, you cannot insert, so you sharpen it by making it wet, and then the fine fibre is passed through the eye of the needle. This loose thread that is made to pass through the eye of the needle is the mind. Then the mind fades out, but the thread is sewed by the needle to remain in contact with the eye and the needle, i.e., intelligence and consciousness.

The fibres of our body as thread are used by the needle (consciousness) to stitch as a fine muslin cloth. The *āsana* teach us this art of stitching so that the consciousness is made to interweave as a single muslin cloth the entire physical body to become a psycho-intellectual body. This is what *āsana* does. I won't say that western medicine has failed in its job. I can only say that it does not know of this special function of yoga.

According to Patañjali the intelligence progresses in two stages, *savitarkā* and *savicārā*. *Savitarkā* and *savicārā* (analysis and synthesis), are functions that belong to the seat of the brain. The sewing teaches us to analyse and synthesise the *āsana* practice inside the body. Even if it is a toe, you should know whether it is sewn properly or not, and if the intelligence too has reached that level or not. The pointed end of the needle being consciousness, it has to take the intelligence along with it for it to follow the body. If the consciousness moves with the movement of body, then it is subjective health. This makes the consciousness to be in close contact with each and every pore of our body. And when the whole needle (consciousness), the eye of the needle (intelligence) and the thread (fibres) are brought together, it is *saṁyama.* We know that *dhāraṇā, dhyāna* and *samādhi* is *saṁyama*; so we say, *trayam ekatra saṁyamaḥ*[1]. Have we talked of *āsana, prāṇāyāma* and *pratyāhāra* as a *saṁyama?* Firstly, the external organs, namely, body, mind and intelligence should be made to get integrated. *Āsana* works on body, *prāṇāyāma* on energy and *pratyāhāra* on the intelligence to sharpen so that they get integrated in order to apply *(viniyogaḥ)* for next three aspects of yoga. The first triangle is of body, mind and intelligence. The second is *dhāraṇā, dhyāna* and *samādhi. Dhāraṇā* is a sensitive intelligence which takes you towards the consciousness, and consciousness builds you to understand what is the soul and non-soul – *ātman* and *anātman.* To separate *atman* from *anātman* comes through conscience – *viveka.* Connecting these two triangles of yoga brings that light of wisdom, which flows like a river in the body. The status of this wisdom is *sarvathā vivekakhyāti.* Know that it will not be a sudden leap. But if the stage of *sarvathā vivekakhyāti* has to come, the status of intelligence has to reach the height of spotless, stainless state, which is *nirbīja samādhi* – the ULTIMATE END. What else does one need but to embrace yoga? Patañjali says in the second chapter *vivekakhyāti,* and ends the fourth chapter raising it to the height of Everest[2]. The whole journey of yoga is from *vivekakhyāti* to *sarvathā vivekakhyāti.*

The evolution towards *saṁyama* by integration of the trio body-mind-intelligence through the *saṁyama* of *āsana-prāṇāyāma-pratyāhāra* the yogi moves towards the higher *saṁyama* of *dhāraṇā-dhyāna-samādhi*

Through *yogāgni* (fire of yoga) one has to light *jñānāgni* (fire of knowledge). These two fires have to enter and move in the entire body, nay, the entire existence – *ātmāgni* – of human being and keep one from the body to the core completely aware and healthy. That's where the modern science has failed and yoga has not. And that's why yoga is still being practised, the refuge for people to get back their lost health. In short, health means awareness and awareness means health.

Q.- Differences exist in health care systems but all have certain principles, for example there is the question of pathology, organisms in allopathy. *Āyurveda* speaks about *vāta, pitta* and *kapha.* Acupuncture talks about energy meridians. Are there certain principles in yoga?

---

[1] These three together – *dhāraṇā, dhyāna* and *samādhi* – constitute integration or *saṁyama* (*Y.S.,* III.4).

[2] *Yogāṅgānuṣṭhānāt aśuddhikṣaye jñānadīptiḥ āvivekakhyāteḥ* (*Y.S.,* II.28). By dedicated practice of the various aspects of yoga impurities are destroyed: the crown of wisdom radiates in glory.

Prasaṁkhyāne api akusīdasya sarvathā vivekakhyāteḥ dharmameghaḥ samādhiḥ (*Y.S.,* IV.29). The yogi who has no interest even in this highest state of evolution, and maintains supreme attentive, discriminative awareness, attains *dharmamegha samādhi:* he contemplates the fragrance of virtue and justice.

Yes, there are different health care systems but very few know the various facets of health. There is ethical health, physical health, mental health, emotional health, intellectual health, health in consciousness, health in their conscience. All put together is divine health.

Well, we are closer to *āyurveda*, yet we differ. If *āyurveda* speaks on *vāta, pitta* and *kapha*, yoga takes five elements as the base. As far as the health care is concerned, it is the five elements; in these five, the three elements, *āp, tejas* and *vāyu* play the role of health. But when it comes to philosophy, it is *triguṇa*[1].

Here also, Patanjāli speaks in one way of the integration of *sattva, rajas* and *tamas*, which means *sāmyāvasthā*. In one way it is the union of the three *guṇa*. Hence it can be termed as *guṇa-saṁyoga*. It is another type of *saṁyoga* in *yogasādhanā*.

See, first of all you should know that we are made up of *pañcabhūta; pṛthvī, āp, tejas, vāyu* and *ākāśa*. *Gandha, rasa, rūpa, sparśa* and *śabda* are the infrastructures of these five elements. These two, *pañcabhūta* and *pañcatanmātra*, have to co-ordinate very closely for clean health.

Pṛthvī, the element of earth is the foundation. So our body is predominantly the element of earth, the heavy part of the *pañcabhūta*. *Ākāśa* is the lightest element, ether. *Pṛthvī* indicates the firm foundation whereas *ākāśa* indicates space. If *pṛthvī* is the base of body, then *ākāśa* is

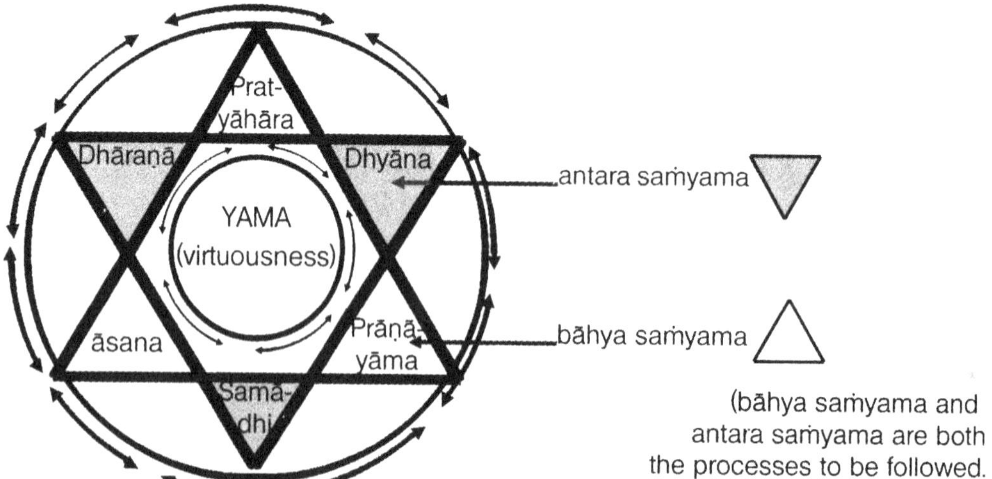

Plate n. 39 – The *Yantra* (triangles) of yoga

[1] See *Aṣṭadaḷa Yogamālā*, II.41, p. 282, *"Practice of* prāṇāyāma". About *āyurveda*, see vol. III, section III, pp. 141-168.

the space of the body. *Ākāśa* has no boundary, so the core inside has no boundary. It is *cidākāśa*. *Āp*, water element, *tej*, fire element, and *vāyu*, air element, work within the field of earth and ether. Imagine a factory. The structural building of the factory is earth having a place for the factory to function along with all the sections. Now the factory will have all raw material – again earth, to manufacture the product. This production is possible with the help of water, fire and air. These elements may be in the form of electricity, foundry-fire, magnetic earth or any other form, but basically all these elements exist in it in different forms. These days in any business we see whether production can be distributed. This is called marketing. Similarly, with raw materials of *pṛthvī*, the product is manufactured with the help of *āp*, *tejas* and *vāyu*, and finally distributed in the global market, that is space, ether. Well! This is just an example to study how they work in our body. The earth element – the body – is used with *saptadhātu* – chyle *(rasa)*, blood *(rakta)*, flesh *(māṁsa)*, fat *(meda)*, bone *(asthi)*, marrow *(majjā)* and semen *(śukra)* – as the raw materials which are blended and moulded through *āsana* and *prāṇāyāma* for producing the energy by the elements of *āp*, *tejas* and *vāyu* for distribution in the space of the body, i.e., *ākāśa*.

The characteristics of the five elements are solidity, fluidity, heat, mobility and volume. The properties of these five elements are smell, taste, sight, touch and sound. Again these are all hidden energies. *Āyurveda* speaks about *tridoṣa* – *vāta*, *pitta* and *śleṣma*. We as yoga practitioners say *vāyu tattva*, *tejas tattva* and *āp tattva* are the cause for ill health. When the *tridoṣa* are vitiated, the health is shaken. For us if the balance of five elements which exists in each cell of the body in certain ratios gets disturbed, the disease establishes itself. However, yogis have connected these *tridoṣa* to the three *guṇa*, *sattva*, *rajas* and *tamas*. Normally the *doṣa* are connected with body and *guṇa* with mind. But these three have interconnections. They act, react and interact with each other. They have close relations, one affecting the other. The *triguṇa* and *tridoṣa* are helped by *āsana* and *prāṇāyāma* to bring balance through the three *bhūta* (water, fire and air) within the frame of earth and ether, and the chemicals that blend are used for distribution.

The two – *pṛthvī* and *ākāśa* – do not directly participate in action. The functioning happens by the three elements – *āp*, *tejas* and *vāyu*. The practice of *āsana* and *prāṇāyāma* creates the firmness in the earth element and makes the ether to contract and expand as per need. *Annamaya kośa* is a vessel or container and *prāṇamaya kośa* is the content. The first one is the capsule which is filled with energy.

That is why *prāṇamaya kośa* is called *āp śarīra*, *manomaya kośa* as *tejas śarīra* and the *vijñānamaya kośa* as *vāyu śarīra*. The *annamaya kośa (pṛthvī)* acts as a producer while *ānandamaya kośa (ākāśa)* acts as a distributor. If there is no buyer, the production is a waste. So, who is the seller and who is the buyer? The body, senses of perception, organs of action, mind, intelligence, I-consciousness, consciousness and conscience are the purchasers, and the storehouse of energy being the core, he sells and distributes.

Take any type of medicine, allopathic, *āyurvedic* or homeopathic or any other. When they are used, they trigger the elements in the body to work faster or slow down as per need. They advise to continue medicines for as long as is required to maintain balance in these elements. They may not be knowing that the elements trigger, but that is their prescription. This is the truth.

Suppose we do *āsana* and *prāṇāyāma*. They play a tremendous role in building up the health of the body, the health of the mind and the health of the intelligence. But it requires tremendous will power, and that is why people go for drugs and medicines. If they have will power there is no need because all these things are there inside us as a defensive force to balance these elements. The practice of *āsana* and *prāṇāyāma* definitely brings harmony between these three elements. For example, when one gets nausea, one does certain *āsana* according to the prescription of the teacher and the nausea disappears. When one is constipated, one does inverted *āsana* and the constipation disappears. When one is dull, certain *āsana* practice removes the dullness. So whatever āyurveda guides for the control of the *vāta*, *pitta* and *śleṣma*, yoga does through the three elements of *āp, tej* and *vāyu*. Please know that *vāta* belongs to the element of *vāyu* (air), *pitta* for *tej* (fire), and *śleṣma* for *āp* (water). If the elements are controlled the *doṣa* are controlled.

Hence *āsana* can play a very major role. But due to want of will power, people prefer medicine. But can medicine be a permanent cure? I say no because of the *upaniṣadic* word, *ratna pūrita dhātu*. One of the seven *dhātu* is *rakta;* we call blood. The *rakta* should be filled with the gems of quality, which means a bio-chemical change. Today the gems in blood means haemoglobin and 'T' cells. These are the *ratna pūrita dhātu*. Words may be different but the contents are almost identical. Those ancient words that were taught centuries ago *(ratna pūrita dhātu)*, stand true even in today's modern science. AIDS sufferers, after doing yoga in Pune, when tested, found that their 'T' cell counts had improved. This 'T' cell count in blood is the *'ratna pūrita dhātu'* of our *Upaniṣads*.

If we can understand the old science and connect to the new science, probably we'll bring both the understanding of medicine as well as yoga closer together. But unfortunately a big gap is there in between.

I think now the real time has come to speak on subjective health. The medical science treats health objectively. It is now for us to connect the subjective experience in health of yoga with the objective views on health with modern medicine.

I spoke previously about *savitarka* and *savicāra*. We all know Patañjali is the author of *Āyurveda*. See how beautifully he connects the *savitarka, savicāra, ānanda* and *asmitā* of the brain with the intelligence of the heart. Patañjali advises that pure *asmitā* of the head *(sabīja samādhi)* has to be treated by the intelligence of the heart with *upekṣā* – indifference. Here, he leads one to *nirbīja samādhi* by *maitrī, karuṇā, muditā* and *upekṣā*. If one studies, *savitarka* and *savicāra* are the opposite branches of *maitrī* and *karuṇā*. Then the branch *ānanda* of the head and the branch *muditā* of the heart come close to each other. This way Patañjali shows how they should come close together in order to balance the intelligence of the heart with the intellect of the head and the intelligence of the body. The seat of the individual self is the head and the seat of the Universal Self is the heart. The union of the individual self – the head *(jīvātmā)* with the Universal Self – the heart *(paramātmā)* is yoga. When the intelligence of the head and the intelligence of the heart are made to function in the field of *āsana* and *prāṇāyāma*, that dormant energy, which is hidden and unused is brought to shine out. Then the triangular action of *vāta, pitta* and *śleṣma* of the body get the right treatment to develop their maximal potency and to work in concord.

So not only in the 21st century, but in the coming centuries, yoga will have its value, because it is the only science which balances the elements of the body, the intellect of the head and the intelligence of the heart.

Q.- Doctors have some specific approaches to specific problems. For example someone goes with a heart problem, they take an ECG. Is there anything like that in yoga?

It is interesting to note that today, after so many years, modern science is gradually accepting indirectly the principles of *yama*, that smoking is bad for health. But if we speak on the principles of *yama*, people say, "Oh you are teaching ethical principles, which is nonsense!" Now, science has come closer to yoga saying that the smoking affects the lungs. As to the principles of *yama*, smoking is cruel for the lungs. Molesting or harassing sexually, is it *brahmacarya?* Stealing the products of intelligence and patenting them, is it *asteya?* Can false and hearsay accusations be considered *satya?* The greed which kills others, is it *aparigraha?*

I am pointing out all these because the principles of *yama* are meant to trigger the *dharmendriya*. The sense of conscience, *dharmendriya* is the conscience, which pricks when first the feeling of guilt touches and hurts. *Yama* is the medicine for a clean conscience. Each thought, each action, each motive, each intention has to be rubbed on the touchstone of *yama*.

There is a beauty in our ancient system of understanding the values of life. They are, as you know, *dharma, artha, kāma* and *mokṣa*. They cover in short duty, wealth, pleasure and emancipation. *Dharma* and *mokṣa* are the spiritual aspects, *artha* and *kāma* are the worldly aspects. Have we ever thought of why the sages have put *artha* and *kāma* between *dharma* and *mokṣa?*

The mind moves like a brook without banks with no discipline[1]. *Artha* and *kāma* are placed in between *dharma* and *mokṣa* in a sequential order. You know of *rīti* and *nīti*, which we commonly use.

In sociology *rīti* means norms. These social norms are based on the culture of the land. *Rīti* is the behaviour and character of individuals. It shows the ways of adjusting to society's norms so that no harm befalls the community. *Rīti* is a *dharma* where thinking, custom, conduct and purpose are channelled by the sense of duty..

What is *nīti?* It is an individual code of behaviour. The society needs the firm foundation on *nīti* and *rīti*, which means ethics and morality. While dealing with society, *rīti* is essential otherwise we are considered below the level of animals. *Nīti* uplifts each individual to the higher level of consciousness. Both *rīti* and *nīti* are interdependent on each other. *Nīti* leads what we aim on these four *puruṣārtha*. Our aims and objectives have to be positive and direction too should be right. For example, giving health to people is positive thinking, while destructive thoughts like cruelty, dishonesty, covetousness, are negative. Human beings can only think of morals, and not other creatures. In this sense, *rīti* is *dharma* and *nīti* is morals. The principles of *yama* and the principles of *niyama* come under *nīti* and *rīti*.

Artha means wealth and *kāma* means pleasure. These two have to be in between *rīti* and *nīti*. This is what yogis have taught us. The yogis were leading a married life because they were living between *dharma* and *mokṣa*, or *rīti* and *nīti*. They were using *artha* and *kāma* within the discipline of *dharma* and *mokṣa*. If *artha* and *kāma* are meant for the accomplishment of disciplined worldly life, *dharma* and *mokṣa* are meant for the accomplishment of spiritual life. If we discipline ourselves in *artha* and *kāma* and do not use them for pleasures *(bhoga)*, then our thoughts get moulded towards emancipation *(apavarga)*.

Bhoga is enjoyment of pleasure and *apavarga* is freedom from pleasures. *Rāga*, attachment or clinging, is the root cause of bondage. *Virakti* or non-attachment leads towards freedom. In order to follow *dharma*, you need *artha*. Wealth is needed to live with contentment. *Kāma* means not only worldly enjoyments but covers *siddhi* also. One has to be non-attached to *siddhi*, otherwise one is tempted towards attachment *(rāga)*. If one gets caught in the *rāga*, *mokṣa* will be too far for him. So one needs to direct these forces of *artha* and *kāma* towards higher aspects of life, namely emancipation. If one directs one's powers of wealth carefully without greediness, then emancipation is nearer. So, freedom from *rāga* means coming closer to *mokṣa*.

Today's science has said that almost all diseases sprout from the liver. The liver, the heart and kidneys are the three major organs in our body. According to *āyurveda*, when the liver

---

[1] See page 210 of this article

is overstrained the kidneys take on the work. When the kidneys and liver are overstrained the heart takes the work in order to rest the liver and for the kidneys to recover. The heart rests when the kidneys recover and kidneys rest when the liver is activated. This is how the body wisdom works. This is how the nature alone steps in and does this job. If one becomes weak, the other works for it. *Āsana* and *prāṇāyāma*, being a natural method of healing, work on liver, kidneys and heart consciously and at the same time rest them also. If the liver is dull, we have to think whether the head of the liver or the right side or the left side or the bottom or the middle is affected. Accordingly the *āsana* are to be adjusted for each segment to activate. As there are so many *āsana*, one has to give a thought of how and where so and so *āsana* penetrate different parts of the liver. In the same way, similar approaches have to be there for the kidneys, the heart or on any other organ or area.

For instance take our practice of *Viparīta Daṇḍāsana*, *Kapotāsana* or *Vṛśchikāsana*. The medical field say they are contortions. They do not see anything beyond this. If they are true scientists, without branding them as contortions, it is their job to find out what happens to the ventricles of the heart in *Viparīta Daṇḍāsana*, what happens in *Kapotāsana* or *Vṛśchikāsana*. The heart has got two banks, the front and the back. The open-heart surgery is done from the top portion of the heart but a yogic operation is attentive intellectual treatment that is done from the back of the heart. Like surgery, in yogic treatment the needle of the consciousness is made to pierce through the arteries as natural surgery. We have to use that discretion to find out

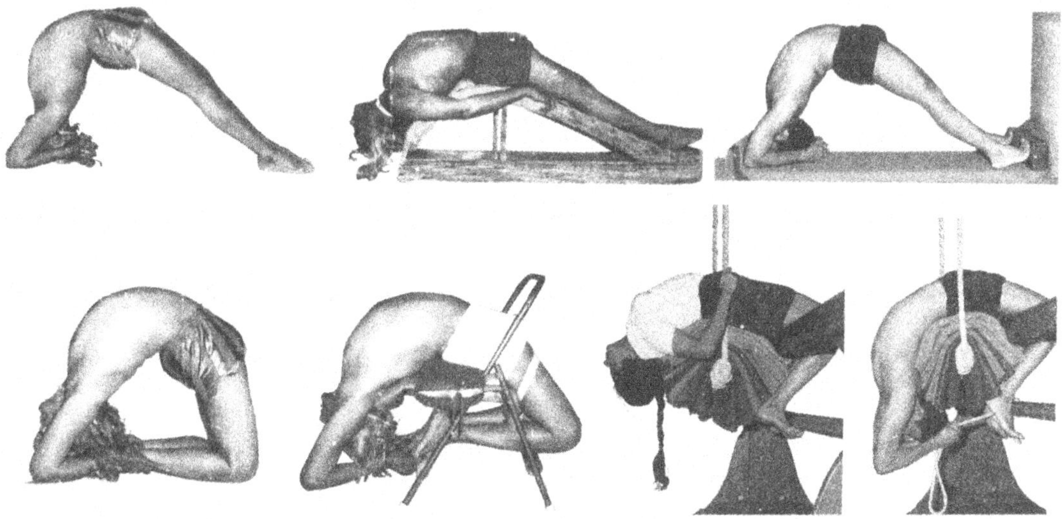

Plate n. 40(a) – *Āsana* Independent and supported *(Viparīta Daṇḍāsana & Kapotāsana)*

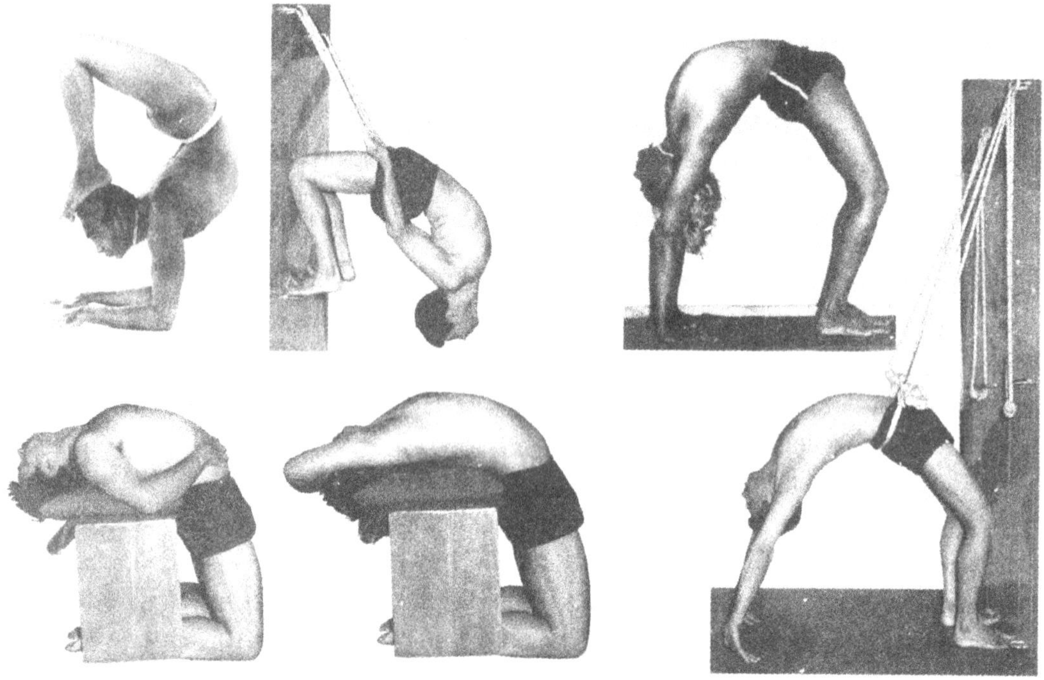

Plate n. 40(b) – *Āsana* independent and supported (*Vṛśchikāsana, Urdhva Danurāsana and Ustrāsana*

whether the consciousness is piercing the inner parts of the heart. Here, the *vijñānamaya kośa* does research subjectively in these *āsana* like *Kapotāsana, Vṛśchikāsana* and *Viparīta Daṇḍāsana* to trace whether the intelligence and consciousness do pierce to remove the narrowness in the arteries. As the patients cannot work independently, props are used to work on those areas with comfort without creating a fear complex in the patients. I feel that scientists without applying their scientific mind are calling these movements contortions and are failing in their duty to see the greatness of other sciences.

I am neither a scientist nor a medical man. But God has blessed me with an intuitive vision through which I have been gifted to study my body as well as others'. The scientists have studied the body objectively by external means. Each *āsana* helped me to understand the living body. The practice of these *āsana* gave me clues to study and work on various parts of the organic body and understand how to reconstruct and rejuvenate through expansion, extension and relaxation.

The yogis found out ways and means to work on the liver and the kidneys by not straining the heart so that it is kept healthy, free from cardiac diseases. Today, due to mental and intellectual stress, nobody works on organs like liver, kidneys, pancreas and intestines to remain healthy. As these major organs are neglected, heart attacks have increased.

At least one good thing in *āsana* and *prāṇāyāma* is that they help in curing diseases, and if it fails to cure, at least it minimises and creates power to endure.

Without structural adjustment, 'body awakening' is impossible. As long as the structural or anatomical body is not done with active attention and balance, body intelligence cannot be cultivated. It is the same with *prāṇamaya kośa*. If the *prāṇamaya kośa* or organic system is not attended to and aligned properly, the vital organs cannot remain healthy. Therefore, *āsana* and *prāṇāyāma* help in coordinating the skeletal body with the organic body and vice versa. The balance to attain is hard. But this is real health.

Therefore, it is important for a yoga practitioner to maintain his own practice using his body mechanism as a laboratory to come to a right conclusion to treat ailing persons. Doctors refer to the authoritative books, whereas we have to refer to our own body with judicious practice of the *āsana* with observation and adaptation. We need to keep our eyes wide open to watch the patient's body, its structure, its presentation when he or she is doing the *āsana* or *prāṇāyāma*. We have to give our eyes to look at his expression on face, the texture and colour of the skin, and ears to watch the sound of breath, vibration of nerves and recurring aches and pains in each *āsana* as they communicate the physical tolerance and emotional endurance.

So, I would say that the practice of yoga can indicate what the disease could be. If modern science has progressed to measure each defect, yoga can use its own parameters seeing the body and mind and their interaction to know the condition of a patient. Any ailment expresses itself on one's face; from the facial expression in certain *āsana* the teacher can spot the problems. Yet there is no harm in checking the patient's conditions by electronic means, which may help the teacher of yoga to go in for treatment according to scientific diagnosis.

Q.- Uncle, one more point, which is also something again as the western system of medicine. I would like to ask you, when you as a yoga master look at a person, is this observation condition-based or does it also take into account the individual?

I will not say that this observation is condition-based. It is rather experience-based. Secondly, we have to take into account the individual. In fact, this is indicated in *Yoga Sūtra* by Patañjali.

You know I will give you two examples. First see Patañjali's way of tracing the disease symptom-wise: *duḥkha daurmanasya aṅgamejayatva śvāsapraśvāsāḥ vikṣepa sahabhuvaḥ* (I.31). Sorrow, despair, unsteadiness of the body and irregular breathing accompany the distraction of *citta*.

Though the word *sahabhuvaḥ* is used to be in concurrence with the other distracting factors, actually if you ask me, these are the symptoms of diseases. We have to revere this *sūtra* as it is closely connected to our life. *Duḥkha, daurmanasya, aṅgamejayatva* and *śvāsapraśvāsa* express the effect on the mind, particularly on the nervous system, tremor or shakiness or pain of the body, hollow and shallow breathing, fickle mindedness. All these Patañjali says are nothing but psychosomatic conditions. They are the symptoms of *vyādhi, styāna, saṁśaya, pramāda, ālasya, avirati, bhrāntidarśana, alabdhabhūmikatva* and *anavasthitatva*[1].

When you see the person, you see what type of *duḥkha* he has, what type of *daurmanasya* he has, what type of reaction there is on the body, quality of breath, to get the sense of how he reacts to the treatment and what type of treatment convinces the patient while guiding in the *āsana*. But before commencing the treatment give a thought on groups of *āsana* and work out the needs of the patient before introducing those *āsana* so that he finds relief and gets convinced of cure. No doubt, we have to treat individually, but one who has confidence and capabilities can take more patients, which often builds a healthy atmosphere by working together. Yet slight adjustments in *āsana* and *prāṇāyāma* have to be done as per the needs. Suppose one has got a liver problem, first I have to find out where and which part of the liver is affected, whether the top or the middle or the bottom or the side. Accordingly say, take for example *Dwi Pāda Viparīta Daṇḍāsana*,[2] I modify the *āsana* to work on the exact area that is affected, without going for other *āsana*. Similarly, the teachers have to learn to adjust the *āsana* that works for healthy functioning of the liver whether they are forward, backward, lateral or twistings but to get the right effect from the action. I hope the teachers know these subtle delicate adjustments. Scientifically the foundation of each *āsana* is very accurate, but slight adaptation for the patients to derive maximum benefit is needed.

- *For the individual.* -

For that individual or for 'that' patient where the problems exist. Though the prescription of the *āsana* does not change, in the beginning one should know how to adjust and adapt a particular *āsana* according to the patient's need. Suppose someone has a prostate problem, affecting the urinary system, then one has to think in which way the *āsana* has to be taken so that the patient too feels that the adapted *āsana* is showing some effect. The teacher has to work on the *āsana* consulting the patient to get his re-actions so that the consciousness is

---

[1] *Vyādhi styāna saṁśaya pramāda ālasya avirati bhrāntidarśana alabdhabhūmikatva anavasthitatvāni cittavikṣepaḥ te antarāyāḥ* (*Y.S.*, I.30). These obstacles are disease, inertia, doubt, heedlessness, laziness, indiscipline of the senses, erroneous views, lack of perseverance, and backsliding.

[2] See plates n. 41 & 42.

brought to involve him in sensation and verify whether the adjustment activated the part or not. The teacher may be active and intelligent, but he has to get the feedback from the patient whether the affected part is responding or not. This way, not only the teacher learns and gets confidence to handle the case by knowing the effect of each *āsana* but become good in the healing art through yoga whereby he builds up faith in his patients also. While introducing the *āsana* to a patient, there could be a certain pain, which a skilful teacher can change into an pain that the patient welcomes. They say "It's good, though it is painful." This means that those *āsana* are congenial in giving healthy sensitivity and act as effective cure.

In the early days yoga was not practised as therapy, though it has the healing qualities. In today's mental weather, yoga has gained popularity as therapy and hence, the attention has increased more on its therapeutic values.

The main subject is 'Awakening of the Body'. If the yoga teachers know how to intelligise the dormant intelligence of the body, then they are sure to help in curing various ailments. I've tried on cardiac patients, as well as those with open-heart surgeries, and I have also helped those who were advised for an immediate operation and are alive and kicking without undergoing surgery.

The majority of cardiac attacks are due to a guilty conscience. Desire, anger, greed, infatuation, pride and malice add further to mental stress. People's minds and dexterity act as slow poison, which one may not realise. For example, it may be at a job planning for a higher job by hook or crook, by pulling down their own colleagues. Is this not a guilty conscience? No doubt, I feel blockage takes place due to mental stress, consuming wrong food, oily substances and so forth.

I will give you one example. I had a cardiac patient. The open-heart surgery was done about three years ago. He was coming to the class. Though I had not taught him, I knew that he was a God-fearing person. When I came to know that he had a heart attack, I thought, "How could a God-fearing person get a heart attack at this young age?" I couldn't believe that this man had an open-heart surgery. I asked his wife, who is also a yoga student, whether her husband had any bad habits. She confidently said, "Nothing, nil!" I said, "I cannot take your words. So please ask him whether he is hiding something". The lady persisted asking her husband, yet the answer was, "No, I had no bad habits at all." When he came to the class, I asked in front of his wife, "Tell me the truth, don't hide, because by hiding, you will pay with your life. Were you smoking?" He said, "Yes." His wife said, "I have not seen him smoking in my life, though I was married 25 years ago, not once!" And he was a chain smoker in the office and he was having cardamom and clove in his mouth on his way home, to hide the nicotine smell.

- Smart -

Yes! As he confessed his weakness, he asked me, "How did you know all these things?" This is intuitive knowledge, which came to me through my *āsana* practice.

As I was teaching him, he saw great improvement. The insensitivity from the left side began to disappear and life came back to him. But the problem began when I introduced *Sarvāṅgāsana* after several months. Believe me or not, the moment I took him to *Sarvāṅgāsana* he started gasping for breaths. According to Patañjali, the symptom of laboured breathing came into my mind. In half a minute's time, he became pale. I wondered how it could happen, when I've taken almost a year to introduce *Sarvāṅgāsana*. I could not believe it. He was doing backbends, which are definitely more strenuous compared to *Sarvāṅgāsana*. Fortunately on that day there were physicians and surgeons in the class, practising. I told them to look what had happened. They could see something wrong, and advised me not to make him do *Sarvāṅgāsana*. I asked the patient's permission whether he was willing to try again. I tried several ways changing the methods. I couldn't trace the cause of his laboured breathing only in this *āsana*. Lastly I took *Sarvāṅgāsana* by taking his legs backwards to extend and expand his diaphragm and his immediate reaction was, "relief". But about breathing he said it was the same. I carefully looked at his diaphragm in the *āsana* and called the doctors to see that the diaphragm is not in its position. They were surprised to see the defect and asked me how did I find out that the diaphragm is not in its place. In backbends or in *Śīrṣāsana*, he was never panting, because in these *āsana* there was no compression on the diaphragm. In *Sarvāṅgāsana*, due to the load and pressure on the diaphragm, he began panting. I told him that something had gone wrong at the operation theatre. He at once said, "*Gurujī*, I had entirely forgotten about it. The operation was done two years ago, and you have brought the memory back. A few days after the operation I was told to take normal food. I took my normal food and began vomiting. This happened repeatedly. So, I was admitted again for a check up. They put me on saline for a few days and then asked me to try food in small quantities. Yet the same problem recurred. Then sonography and M.R.I. were done. They realised that they had stitched the diaphragm at a higher level". *Sarvāṅgāsana* guided me that something has gone wrong in his diaphragm and reminded him, which he had forgotten. The doctors had told him that nothing could be done at this stage but to learn to live with it.

Today the same person does fifteen minutes of *Sarvāṅgāsana*, the diaphragm has moved to its original place. Tell me, can the medical people alter this? When yoga can alter such changes, is it not a miracle of yoga? The diaphragm that was stitched close to the heart has been moved to the position where it should be. Now, he enjoys *Sarvāṅgāsana* and feels the extension up to corners of the chest wall where he was not feeling the movement before.

People call yoga quackery? Is it quackery? Their ethics is that a doctor should support another doctor. But in yoga we are alone responsible, and hence we have to be doubly cautious, even though the case may be very difficult to handle. We have to see that he maintains the condition for some time and when some change occurs, one can proceed to minimise the problem and go ahead for cure, keeping this in mind and see it does not relapse.

Regarding another heart case. Dr. Vakil of Mumbai who got the first prize for discovering *redolpha*, was a cardiologist. He was treating his mother for a cardiac infarct, and she was not allowed to climb steps even at home. She got upset by these restrictions and came to Pune for a few days to try yoga. Dr. Vakil's wife was learning yoga from me. Within one month I made her climb up and down. The doctor came to see her and was surprised to see her climbing steps with comfort. Then she wanted to go to Mahabaleshwar and I told her to go but to continue her practices. You will be happy to know that after yoga, she lived for ten to twelve years more. By the grace of God, yoga has made suffering people recover and live happily.

The required practice of *āsana* for different ailments does not change, only they have to be adapted to the demands of the situations. Mild *āsana* are introduced to start with, then as the body tones, varieties of *āsana* are introduced to interpenetrate for total eradication, while in medicine prescriptions are changed too often if the patient complains of no change.

If by chance you refer to the earlier issues of *Yoga and Health* magazines, they mention that Mr. Iyengar's key is the challenge he accepts in various diseases. I did start working on diseases as the demands were more and financially cheap also. I will not allow the disease to aggravate but work to succeed to bring credit to yoga. The right method always has a wonderful effect. With this in mind, I worked and people benefited. I know that yoga being a natural science, its results might be slow, perhaps giving pain in the beginning, but later sure to improve. Probably now yoga has been accepted as a therapy and it is for the younger generation to work to maintain the prestige of yoga.

Q.- Yesterday in our private talk you brought out a very interesting point. I think it's important for us to share it with others, the idea of *sabīja* and *nirbīja*.

Ah! Everybody speaks about *sabīja samādhi* and *nirbīja samādhi* – seeded and seedless *samādhi*. While reading the *Yoga Sūtra* one has to keep in mind the contents that are expressed, whether they fit in to the other aspects of yoga from *yama* to *samādhi*. Sometimes Patañjali may have used a particular idea or concept in one *sūtra*. It is for us to think whether it is applicable to other petals of yoga. For example you read the effects of *yama* from *niyama* and the effects of *niyama* on *yama*. If you follow *śauca*, *santoṣa*, then *ahiṁsā*, *satya*, get involved.

Similarly, *tapas* has an effect on *asteya, svādhyāya* on *brahmacarya* and *Īśvara praṇidhāna* on *aparigraha.* Actually, *niyama* acts as a foundation, base, pillar, support for *yama.* The principles of *yama* indirectly indicate what the human mind runs after. By practising *niyama,* the *sādhaka* naturally follows *yama.* If one does not follow *niyama,* then one is far far away from following the *yama.* Either way *yama* and *niyama* are inter-supportive for cultural development. The *bīja* (seed) of *yama* is in *niyama* and the seed of *niyama* is in *yama.*

Patañjali speaks of *citta-prasādanam* (*Y.S.,* I.33), wherein he advises a favourable, serene mind to pleasures and pains, virtues and vices, and compare this with the effects of *āsana* where he frees himself from dualities (*Y.S.,* II.48). Both express almost identical effects. When he explains in the successive six *sūtra,* (from *Y.S.,* I.33), he shows various ways of support for a favourable disposition of the consciousness. Even, he goes to the extent by *sūtra, yathābhimata dhyānāt vā,* (*Y.S.,* I.39)[1], asking the *sādhaka* to choose an object according to one's taste. In this *sūtra,* he interestingly takes one closer to the core of being which is dearest to all. This is the *ātman.* It means that you can have the soul as *ālambana* or support. While coming to the actual subject of *aṣṭāṅga* yoga, he speaks of alternative means or supports in detail to reach that *citta-prasādana* state of which he speaks in I.33.

In the context of *samādhi,* he has very clearly mentioned about *sabīja* and *nirbīja.* In the *Vibhūti Pāda,* he speaks about *dhāraṇā, dhyāna* and *samādhi.* Now these three are the foundation for *saṁyama. Saṁyama* cannot happen unless these three aspects get together; and unless the *saṁyama* happens the deliberate acquisition of *siddhi* is impossible. *Saṁyama* becomes foundation for deliberate *siddhi.* Though he defines *dhyāna* in *Vibhūti Pāda,* he uses *dhyāna* in *Sādhana Pāda* as support to stop the fluctuations of consciousness created by gross and subtle afflictions[2].

Patañjali defines *dhyāna* as *tatra pratyaya ekatānatā dhyānam* (*Y.S.,* III.2). This word *ekatānatā* indicates continuous uninterrupted flow of attentive awareness. Does this qualitative attribute *ekatānatā* apply to *āsana* or not? Is this uninterrupted attentive awareness an *ālambana* or not? When Patañjali talks about *ālambana* or support on so many places, can we not work out in line with his thoughts in the *āsana* and *prāṇāyāma* for the benefit of its followers?

The vessels hold water. If the floor is uneven, the water spills out. Similarly, even the ground must be even for the pot to rest firmly, so that the contents remain without disturbance.[3] This analogy holds true for the body, the mind and the soul.

---

[1] The consciousness becomes disposed and serene by meditating on any desired object conducive to its steadiness.

[2] *Dhyānaheyāḥ tadvṛttayaḥ* (*Y.S.,* II.11). The fluctuations of consciousness created by gross and subtle afflictions are to be silenced through meditation.

[3] A typical water vessel in India is not flat at the base, it is rounded.

The body is the floor, the jar is the mind, and the content in it is the soul. So when we do the *āsana* we have to stabilise all these aspects. Naturally the body becomes the support *(sabīja)* for the content – the soul. Similarly the body is the support for *āsana.* Otherwise the mind spills out and disturbs the core.

After explaining *ālambana,* let me take you back to *āsana. Āsana* is *sabīja* as well as it can be *nirbīja.* If you recollect the illustrations in *Light on Yoga,* you see all *āsana* are done without any supports except the floor. Today, the mentality of people has changed to such an extent that they don't want to face any physical strain. Awakening of the body to them is totally nil. No doubt they have intelligence. But there is a tremendous space or void between their bodies and their intelligence. In our practice of *āsana,* we close the gap and hence there is no void. There is unity: we work to unite the body, the mind and the soul. Being prone to comforts, they want health with ease, as they like easy money.

Therefore, I have to find means, *artha. Artha* means not only wealth, but also purposefulness, aims and utility. These means are the various designs of gadgets as support *(bīja).* With the help of *Yoga Sūtra* I.39, I applied my mind to various gadgets and tempted the students that they can do all the *āsana* as they are in *Light on Yoga* without strain and congenial to one's heart and head.

Now I call a student of mine to do so that I can show you *Dwi Pāda Viparīta Daṇḍāsana* on a chair and present how one can concentrate on parts of the body to get a simple uninterrupted stretch.

I make him do the *āsana.* Now I adjust his thoracic dorsal spine on the frontal edge of the seat so that the shoulder blades touch the front edge of the chair and that it cuts the shoulder blades firmly by asking him to press the feet on the wall parallel to the chair or on a box to support his heels. This adjustment stimulates the heart.

For liver, spleen, bladder and pancreas, I take the same *āsana* but move his legs below the chair keeping them on the bricks where I make him feel the auto-massage taking place in this position.

Then I move his feet down to the floor for the knees to get not only straight, but also to join and grip together. This not only works on the knees but also on the sacro-iliac area. This way, one *āsana* can be used as a remedy for various problems through careful adjustments.

Take AIDS. First I have to think what *āsana* have power to dry the genital organ. AIDS patients feel not only wetness but also heaviness in the organ. As it remains wet, I have to work finding ways to dry the wetness first. As beginners cannot do independently the *āsana,* we teach them by using bolsters and pillows for the head. Then to trigger alertness in the body, we use various supports and make them do many *āsana.* This treatment is by *sabīja āsana.* The

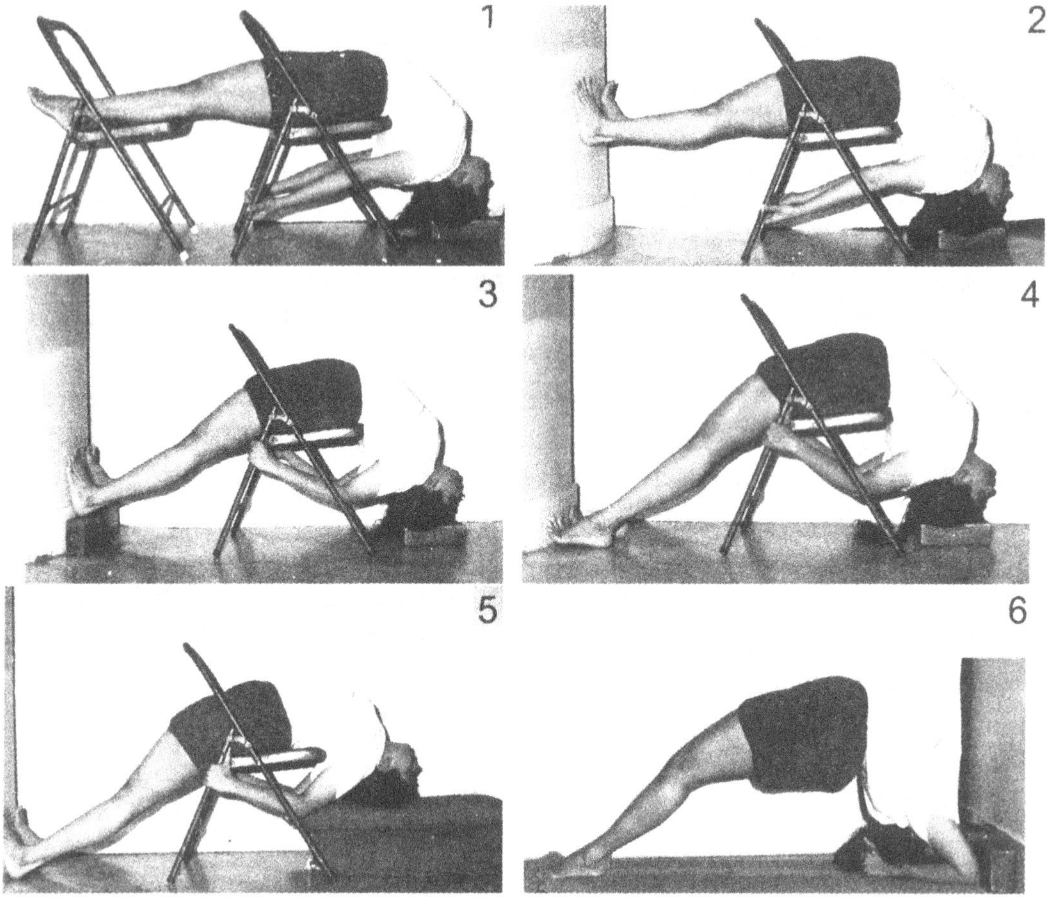

Plate n. 41 – *Dwi Pāda Viparīta Daṇḍāsana* with supports – 1. on a chair with feet on box, 2. parallel to the floor, 3. on two bricks, 4. feet down, 5. head support, 6. elbows to the wall.

props act like a bed but keep one relaxed with no strain. When one begins to do independently one has to recollect the quiet feelings that are experienced in *sabīja āsana* and introduce them in *nirbīja āsana.*

When we do the same *āsana* independently we hold the body for a long time, (especially when the body is not trained enough), where the brain becomes active and hard, which makes one feel as if one is straining the other systems of the body. So, instead of working on the organs, the brain is strained without any effect on organs This is why we use the props as support especially in therapy, so that the organs are made to work and not the brain.

Is it not a science when we develop gadgets like this? Please understand what medical people do to help a patient walk, we do the same in the yogic line.

Now, in the same *Dwi Pāda Viparīta Daṇḍāsana,* though one works independently, he takes the elbow support against the wall to get stability in the *āsana.* Because his elbows are fixed to the wall, he gets the grip to do the *āsana* well and at the same time he develops the strength and endurance. This is how I build up from support *(sabīja)* to go towards *nirbīja āsana.*

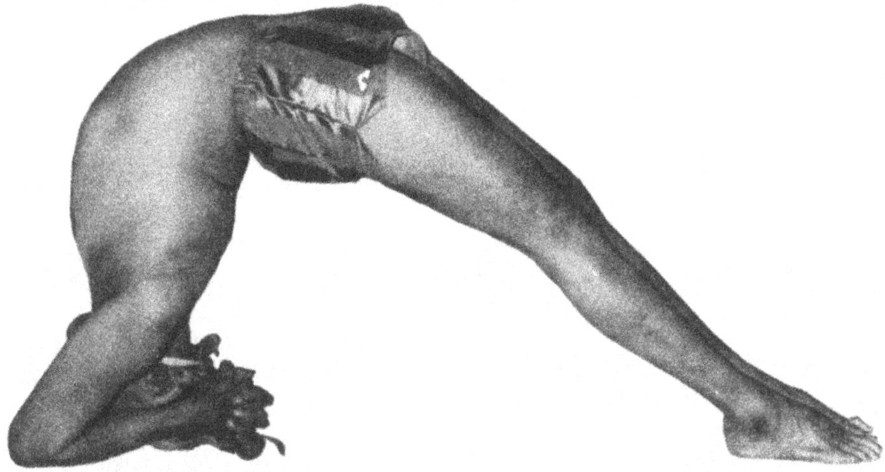

Plate n. 42 – *Dwi Pāda Viparīta Daṇḍāsana*

For one who has not done yoga at all, whose physical awareness is not yet lit-up, we teach the same *āsana* with cross bolsters. This is how we begin to teach. From here we build up ideas to take him further and further in the *āsana.* Here, my attention is to open the lungs automatically by re-adjusting the diaphragm for horizontal expansion so that at a later stage, he breathes deeper, and then *prāṇāyāma* is introduced. This building in lungs is still *sabīja.*

After all these trails, he will be made to do the *āsana* independently. There is absolute stability and no shakiness. When the *āsana* comes this way, it is *nirbīja āsana.* You see how the muscles are toned by grades to react healthily so that one remains quiet in brain and active in body. This is *sthiratā* (steadiness) and *sukhatā* as well. I think this *sukhatā* has no tinge of laxity. Whereas with the supports one acts and relaxes now and then. By props, when they get rest, they are happy. When one has to do independently, they face hardships. At the end, when mastered, it turns into *nirbīja āsana.*

Nirbīja āsana are done only when one is free from bodily pains and intelligence and consciousness move naturally and freely without hindrances in the limbs of the body.

– Does that mean that they should be able to stay stable for a length of time? –

Yes, when the body gets toned, its intelligence is awakened, to hold the *āsana* with ease and comfort.

You see, these gadgets and props are built up by me because of the patients. It is their need that worked on my intelligence as an *ālambana* to find out means to achieve maximum befits with a minimum effort. Hence, I consider them as proxy teachers, which makes me to think and learn.

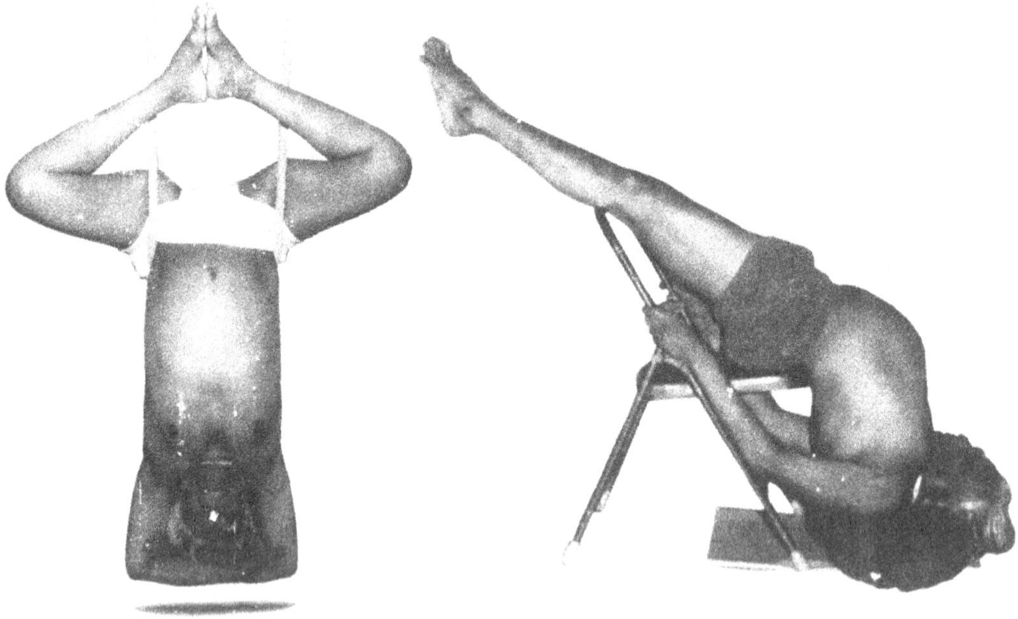

Plate n. 43 – *Śīrṣāsana and Sarvāṅgāsana* on props.

- You must have done it all yourself. -

Naturally, I cannot make others guinea pigs to experiment to earn credit for myself. I did everything on my own. As we use the hand on the back in *Sarvāṅgāsana* as *sālamba*, I make people do the same *āsana* on a chair.

We all know that *sabīja samādhi* has various grades[1]. Similarly, *sabīja āsana* also has grades. Our *guru* taught us *Sālamba Sarvāṅgāsana* with hand support as well as *Nirālamba Sarvāṅgāsana* without support of hands. Why *sālamba?* Because one does better. Support acts as a safe vault for the mind.

Take *Kapotāsana* with support. You see no strain and no efforts, whereas if the *āsana* is done independently, there is struggle. Also a lot of preparations in bending backwards are needed to do *Kapotāsana* independently.

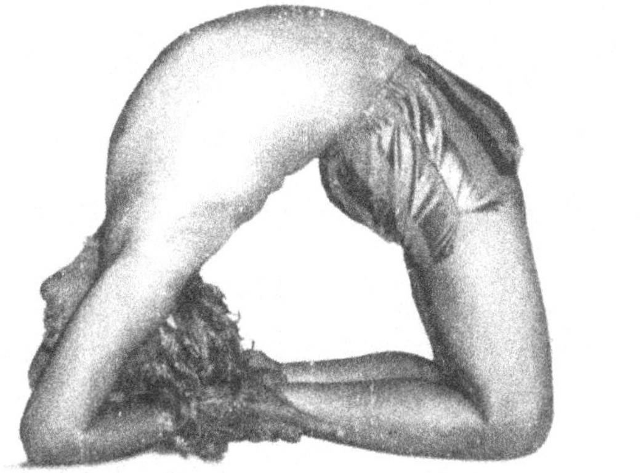

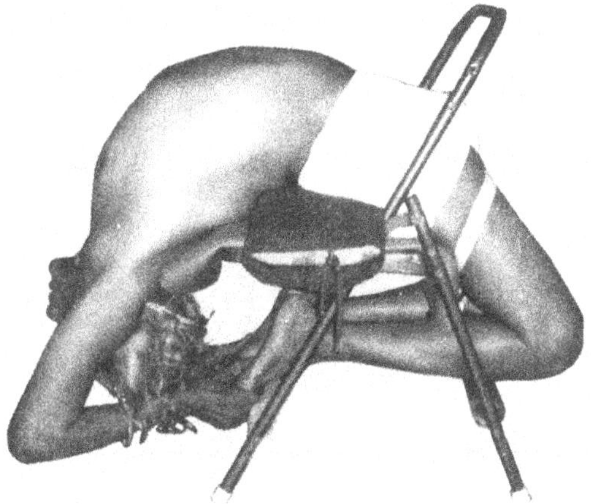

Plate n. 44 – *Kapotāsana* using support and independent

Watch now *Halāsana*, *Halāsana* on the box, the way we treat the patients. The brain is relaxed here. Because the weight of the thigh muscles are rested on the stool, therefore no tension is felt on the diaphragm and one breathes easily. In this state the brain relaxes and witnesses the action.

When the child is in the womb, the head of the foetus is downwards. This *āsana* almost imitates the shape of the head in the womb. In this, the position of the head makes the brain to remain at a subterranean level, as if one is in hibernation. The patient cannot perform wrong, because this bench will tell him which part of the right leg and left leg are touching the bench for him to adjust himself. I said this as "monitoring". If one does a wrong *āsana* independently,

---

[1] *Tatra śabda artha jñāna vikalpaiḥ saṅkīrṇā savitarkā samāpattiḥ* (*Y.S.*, I.42). At this stage, called *savitarkā samāpatti*, the word, meaning and content are blended, and become special knowledge.

Smṛtipariśuddhau svarūpaśūnya iva arthamātranirbhāsā nirvitarkā (*Y.S.*, I.43). In *nirvitarkā samāpatti*, the difference between memory and intellectual illumination is disclosed; memory is cleansed and consciousness shines without reflection.

Etayaiva savicārā nirvicārā ca sūkṣmaviṣayā vyākhyātā (*Y.S.*, I.44). The contemplation of subtle aspects is similarly explained as deliberate *(savicāra samāpatti)* or non-deliberate *(nirvicāra samāpatti)*.

Sūkṣmaviṣayatvaṁ ca aliṅga paryavasānam (*Y.S.*, I.45). The subtlest level of nature *(prakṛti)* is consciousness. When consciousness dissolves in nature, it loses all marks and becomes pure.

the brain is not in a position to rectify the wrong, whereas with the props support the brain tells the practitioner that this leg is resting well, and that the other leg is not. When one works independently, energy flows like a brook: the stronger side pulls, the weaker side remains silent. If the body *(ghaṭa)* goes wrong, the content moves wrongly.

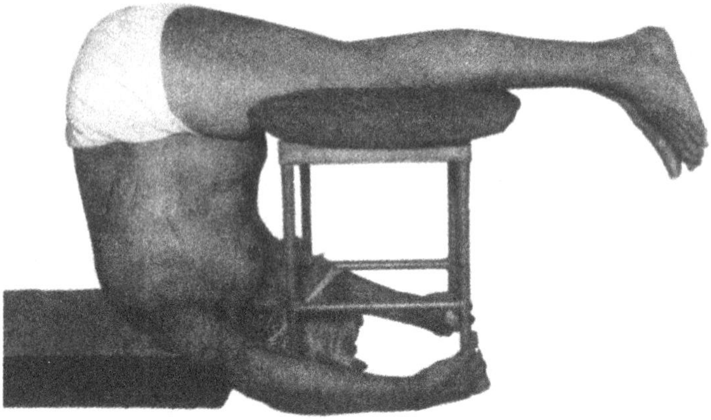

Plate n. 45 – *Halāsana* using support

See *Vṛśchikāsana* on the rope, *Ūrdhva Dhanurāsana* on the rope. That's how we teach the beginners to create confidence. Without creating confidence, it is not worth forcing people to practise independently. In my days, we were afraid of our masters. Probably that experience you must not have had. Today the students control the teachers.

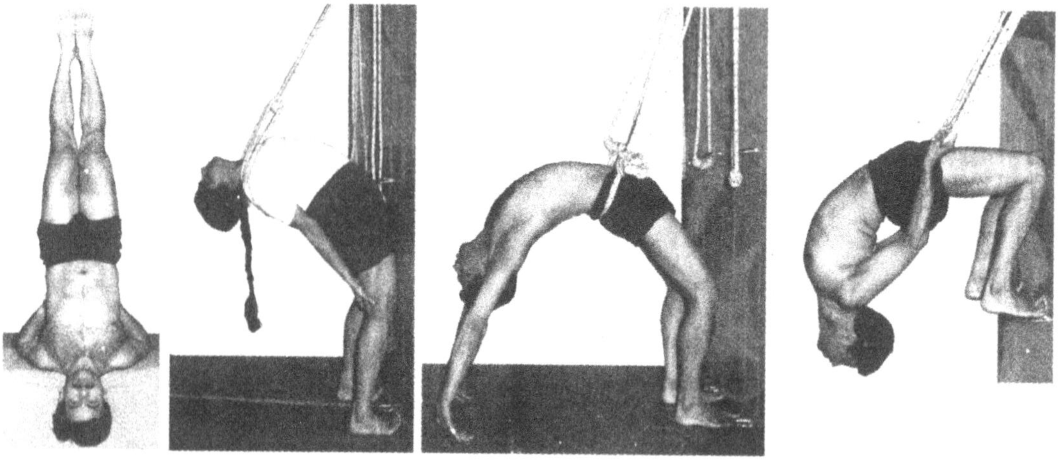

Plate n. 46 – *Sarvaṇgāsana* without strain, neck curvature, *Ūrdhva Dhanurāsana* and *Vṛṣikāsana* using ropes

Let me show you for cervical spondylosis. See the noose around the neck. The noose around the throat leads to death. But in this way one comes out from *mṛta* (death) and proceeds to *amṛta* (nectar). The dead neck becomes alive. The spondylosis cases remain on traction in the hospitals for weeks. Here, I treat them like this and it takes minutes and not weeks.

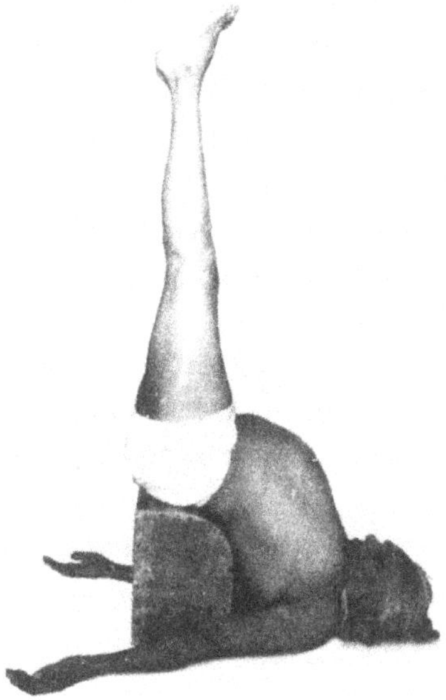

Plate n. 47 – *Viparīta Karaṇī* supported

For thyroid problems, we teach *Sarvāṅgāsana* without putting any strain on the neck and throat. The doctors advise not to do *Sarvāṅgāsana* for thyroid problems, but we work without creating fear complexes. As science is meant to give hope, I find out means to help them but I never confuse the patients. In this method of doing, the chin goes down, the chest is kept open with no strain on the thyroids. This is how we start and then slowly raise the back of the head as they show improvement. Later, when they feel ease in the throat, we take them to the classical *Sarvāṅgāsana*. The way we take the *āsana* helps to lessen the swollen thyroids and breathe easily. I take *Viparīta Karaṇī* both in head balance and neck balance; see how the props are used to do these two. In these there is no neck pain and no headache. Even for cold and cough, we make them do these *āsana*. So, the yogic science has given a methodology where one can practise without fear. But today's modern science creates more fear than confidence.

For us the gadgets are like today's intensive care unit. In olden days there were only general wards and rare special wards, but not intensive care units. Science has advanced and the new electronic equipments are used for monitoring which send messages to the doctors wherever they are. These yogic gadgets, props and blankets do monitor the *āsana* so that the doer cannot do or go wrong. The props and gadgets rejuvenate the system but never exert. Here extension, expansion and circumduction take place without creating load on the brain or the nerves, whereas if one tries independently, exhaustion is felt before one experiences relief.

Yogis have the subjective experience and modern science has objective views of body functions. If we can present modern views with the oriental subjective experiences, a new movement of understanding on the living body may shine forth in the 21st century. Then I am sure yoga will shine with more glory.

This is what science of yoga has given us, but somehow or other we have lost it. By the grace of God and by the grace of my *guru* I started finding means for people to hold on to it like a leech and I am seeing them sticking to it. From here, I hope the present generation builds further means to generate interest for the coming generation.

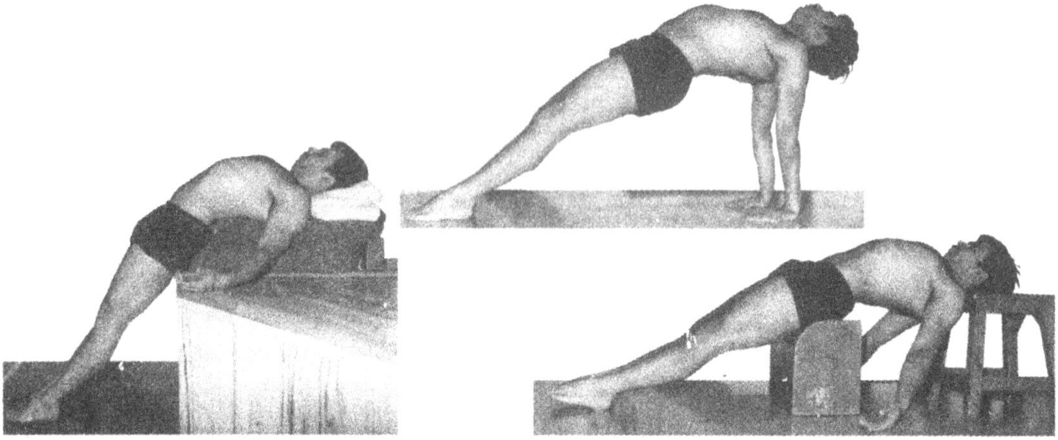

Plate n. 48 – *Purvottānāsana* with support for head, passive, less support, active

Q.- Uncle, last question. As a yoga teacher, if we have to help somebody, who is in trouble, what is required? Is it the intelligence? Is it practice?

Both. First practice, then intelligence.

First of all, you have to have experiential knowledge through experimental practice. For this you need an inquiring mind. In medicine there are guinea pig tests. In yoga the teacher has to do the guinea pig test on himself. While doing, he has to learn the art of observing the adjustments taking place not only on the anatomical body but on the organic body on their own, whether they are right or wrong and to rework on them. He has to learn how to interact with himself and his system and find out by re-adjustments that he introduces and traces reactions that take place in the system. This way, there has to be a self-studying process in practice. By this process the teacher develops and sharpens in his intelligence and cultivates smartness in re-adjustments. When somebody approaches with a problem, he has to give his ears to listen thoroughly to the problems of that person. Then, as a teacher, he has to think and do some homework with his experiences, the ways to deal with it. This is a kind of *pratipakṣa bhāvanam* (countering with the knowledge of discrimination) (*Y.S.,* II.33).

We think that Patañjali has spoken of *pratipakṣa bhāvanā* in the context of *yama* and *niyama*, which is a wrong thinking. In fact the teacher has to feed his *sādhaka* the process of using the thinking power. In *pratipakṣa bhāvanā* Patañjali gives the key on this subject of thinking, which can be applied in the process of learning *āsana*, *prāṇāyāma*, *pratyāhāra*, *dhāraṇā* and *dhyāna*.

Now, coming to your question, if somebody comes with a problem, we need to put ourselves into that situation in order to identify the problem subjectively, which helps the teacher and the taught under each one's emotions. It is not to be misunderstood as a kind of emotional attachment. But it is a kind of "see through" process. According to modern science, it is sonography, where we as teachers need to feel patient's physical and mental vibrations through reciprocations.

Well! I question myself, "Suppose I have this same type of problem as the patient has, how do I face it? How do I practise?" This way, the teacher has to work and develop that sensitivity and intelligence by trying on himself, imitating those problems in himself, and how those problematic tensions lessen. If the teacher feels even one percent change, then he should know that it will have twenty to thirty percent effect on patients. This way he has to learn to minimise or eradicate the doubts of the patients' problems and tensions.

Due to my many years of uninterrupted practice, my body's intellectual sensitivity has reached that level that not only do I understand the problems but touch the afflicted part and adjust myself so that no mistake takes place in handling the patient. By advising the patient to do on his own, he may commit mistakes on account of want of knowledge and understanding. Without experiencing himself, as a teacher if he cannot carefully observe in the patients he cannot create that awareness.

To understand where he may go wrong or commit mistakes, I imitate his non-illuminative intelligence and perform the *āsana* which I try on my own and note in my heart the mistakes that commonly occur in the *āsana* when a beginner does on his own. Then, as a toned person I work on him with the intermediate stages of those *āsana* before I take him to the final position. This way, I give a required guidance step by step by suggesting necessary ways so that he gains confidence and relief at the same time.

This is the practical way of dissection that I observe, first on my own, then on the patients. Regarding teachers, I advise them to read books that are available to understand the symptoms and causes of various diseases. Modern science has presented very well the causes and symptoms of innumerable diseases. Unfortunately yogic science has not presented the symptoms of various diseases, but has expressed the various effects of yogic practices. Fortunately, Patañjali, with the pen name Caraka, has given in detail in his treatise on *āyurveda*, the *Caraka Samhitā*, the causes and the symptoms of diseases.

The author of yoga and *āyurveda* is the same person. Though both are *mokṣa śāstra*, dealing with spiritual emancipation, one starts from *citta* (consciousness) and the other *śarīra* (body). *Āyurveda* begins with the body and ends with the soul, while yoga begins with the mind, goes towards body and then takes one to reach the soul. But there are lots of identities between these two *śāstra*. One views on health and the other on the ways to acquire health. One treats with medicaments and the other by the usage of mere will power to tap the hidden defensive energy. After taking medicine, whether it is *āyurveda* or modern, the doctor advises means of exercises to the patients. Caraka goes further in suggesting that, if the medicament fails, to take to yoga. This shows that the author was aware of the value of yoga subjectively to recommend this to those who do not find benefit from *āyurveda*. Both the sciences, yoga and *āyurveda*, know that the health in the structural and organic body, keeps the mind healthy and how the pettiness of the mind disappears when one is healthy, and how the thinking process is transformed.

Since accuracy and perfection in *āsana* are required, the teacher should have a good knowledge of the structural body. No doubt, by educating the body through *āsana*, one learns a great deal about the functions of the body. As the architect and structural engineer co-ordinate together to put up the building, the teacher too has to live in each *āsana* connecting the intelligence of the intellect with the intelligence of the body. This co-ordinated study gives a feeling to a teacher of what is a correct *āsana*. From here, the teacher should learn to internalise the mind in his *āsana sādhanā* to penetrate the inner cave of the body. Having grasped through books about the symptoms of various diseases, the teacher has to think which *āsana* would work on those symptoms, which is an essential part in treating the patients. In case the knowledge is limited, the approach gets limited; if the experience is vast, then the avenues for treatment would be vast. If a patient has a headache, he only says, "I have a headache", but will not be knowing the cause of it. It may be due to indigestion, tension, want of sleep, neurological disturbance or hereditary. The teacher has to find out clues by talking to the patient and select series of *āsana* according to his felt experiences. He needs to experience each *āsana* subjectively to feel which *āsana* creates heaviness, lightness, relaxation, tension, hardness and ease. Through experimentation, he has to get right experiential feeling and knowledge. This way of studying the symptoms and putting into practice guides the teacher in the ways of approach to work on diseases.

Probably the yogis traced millions of *āsana* for hundreds of muscles and joints which move and flex in hundreds of ways in various degrees in forward, backward, right lateral and left lateral movements, besides adduction, abduction and circumduction. Practice with study gives ideas to a teacher with innumerable alternative *āsana* to work on various diseases. For adduction, abduction and circumduction actions the yogis use terms like *dakshiṇa*, *vāma*, *utthita*, *supta*, *pārśva, parivṛtta, viparīta, adhoḥ, ūrdhva, pūrva, paschima, uttāna*[1] and so on. If one gives a thought to these terms, then it is possible to understand the terminologies of occidental and oriental sciences. The yogis might have thought of how to prevent disease and provide a cure when it is already there. The yogis, by using trunks of the trees, rocks and stones in their practices for extension and relaxation, were experiencing *manolaya* (quietness in mind). The props which you see do the same.

Each *āsana* has a name. They have literal meanings and those have to be studied by students as well as teachers. They convey the parts of the human system which help one to adapt the *āsana* in deriving maximum benefits. In the beginning prescribed *āsana* do help and as one improves in body attention, sensitivity develops in indicating that the body can take the complex *āsana* to activate the core of each organ.

So what is required is sensitive practice with the power of observation to catch even the minutest transformation that flashes in the practice of each *āsana*. This requires total sensitive intelligence, dedication and devotion.

Lord Krishna emphasises in *Bhagavad Gīta*, that the yogi needs *vyavasāyātmikā buddhi*[2], which means experienced wisdom. The practitioner should have a single flow of attention, without oscillation. His mind should not be on achievements or on fame. He has to practise with the sense of absorption and with an open mind. This makes the mind to look within, to move within, and to be within. He has to savour the flavour and the essence of true knowledge *(rasātmaka jñāna)* through his experienced knowledge. This flavour surfaces when one repeatedly filters and re-filters the same experience to bring out the *"vyavasāyātmikā buddhirekeḥ kurūnandana"* of Lord Krishna.

With this flavoured knowledge, when the teacher treats a patient, he has to trigger the intelligence and consciousness to feel exactly the reactions taking place in each and every *āsana*. For this, the teacher has to be well conversant in techniques and should be armed to know how to mould his techniques to fit in to the responses of the patient according to his emotional and intellectual capacities.

We all know that medicines are prescribed for patients and they are asked to come after three or four days for a re-check. This treatment is purely on scientific technical grounds, with no communication of man to man or heart to heart; while in yogic treatment, emotional contact plays a major role.

---

[1] *Dakshiṇa* – right; *vāma* – left; *utthita* – extended; *supta* – supine; *pārśva* – sideways; *parivṛtta* – rotated; *viparīta* – inversion; *adhoḥ* – downward; *ūrdhva* – upward; *pūrva* – front; *paschima* – back; *uttāna* – intensely extended.

[2] *Bhagavad Gīta*, II.41.

Yoga follows *śodhana kriyā* and *śamana kriyā* as in *āyurveda*. *Śodhana* is filtering the cellular system. *Āsana* does that very well. Then, there is *śamana kriyā*, a pacifying process. *Śavāsana* and *prāṇāyāma* play a major role in *śamana kriyā*. So *śodhana* and *śamana* go hand in hand. When cells are intelligised, the soothing and pacifying process begins. As the patient cannot bear discomfort or pain, the props are used which helps in pacifying the system. When we treat the patients, the intelligence alone cannot help, but emotional approach is also needed. Heart to heart communication helps half way in the healing art. Even if one takes ten people at a time, the teacher has to be in contact with all. With years of experience behind me, I have tasted the fragrance of each *āsana* to such an extent that I see faster and help my teachers how to see so that they learn without boring the patient or in wasting time in handling many at the same time.

According to Patañjali *vitarka* and *vicāra* are needed on the intellectual side. These two aspects do not sprout from emotion. First I have to know how to use my experiences and my 'feel' of *āsana* technically, as techniques help the patient. At the same time, the felt feelings and sensitivities are converted into techniques. Then I watch the patient's reaction and how the *āsana* expresses in his body. Each *āsana* has its own body expression which can be noticed on their faces. As I see their faces changing and the heart expressing delight, I know that so and so *āsana* is congenial to them. If some rejection is visible by facial and emotional expressions, I at once change the methods to strengthen their mind and create confidence by re-adjusting that *āsana*. I think yoga teachers have to work first with the given techniques and watch the student's re-action. If necessary, they have to change the techniques at once to give a soothing sensation.

Recently we had about ten to fifteen cases of high blood pressure in the classes at one time. There was an American doctor here, Dr. Ray Long. He had come to learn yoga, to see how yoga helps on blood pressure. Along with him I took nearly three medical classes. I used to work with the high blood pressure cases and he would take the reading of their blood pressure. Before he could take the readings, I used to tell him that such and such patient's pressure had risen. He took the readings and was surprised to see that the pressure was on the higher side. Then I used to readjust the patients in the same *āsana* for Dr. Ray Long to test, telling him that the pressure had dropped. Then he was surprised by my readings without any instrument. He told me, "If we treat high blood pressure patients, we have to wait for three days to get the report from the patient, whereas here in all the cases the B.P. comes down the very same day, in a matter of one hour".

I would say that if yoga is accepted in general by the society, then health care centres are not needed. In the West yoga has become so popular because they search for natural remedies and yoga gave them what they were looking for.

Today, we have to educate people first on the philosophy of the body, then the philosophy of the mind, and later we have to take them to the philosophy of the soul. Deliberately, I am using the word philosophy. It is easy to say, "Go beyond the body and mind." But one cannot go unless one has the wisdom of the body. The wisdom of the body and mind has to be gained. I know that body is perishable, but I do not want it to perish by our carelessness. As Patañjali says, when the *adhyātmaprasāda* has to take place, the *ātman* is engulfed by *prakṛti*. *Ātmā* is covered or shadowed by *prakṛti*. The thoughts *(vṛtti)* cover it. We need to uncover it. Then there is no search, the search comes to an end. Even that *ātmabhāva bhāvanā* comes to an end[1]. This is the state of real wholistic health. This *sūtra* on *ātmabhāva bhāvanānivṛttiḥ*, covers also *śarīrabhāva bhāvanānivṛttiḥ*, *manobhāva bhāvanānivṛttiḥ*, *buddhībhāva bhāvanānivṛttiḥ*, *ahaṁkārabhāva bhāvanānivṛttiḥ*. When one observes these step by step, then the division disappears, the *dvandva* disappears, the dualities of body and mind, mind and soul disappear.

The confluence of three sacred rivers – Ganga, Yamunā and Saraswati – is called *Triveṇi sangam*. Similarly, the *Triveṇi sangam* is within us. Yoga begins first on uniting gross self (the body) to the subtle self – mind, intelligence and consciousness. When these gross and subtle selves join the *ātman*, the Self, or *Puruṣa*, it becomes *Triveṇi sangam*. Practice of *āsana* and *prāṇāyāma* consecrates the cells of the physical body (Ganga) and the aspects of mental body (Yamunā) to get wedded to the Self (Saraswati).

I have taken much of your time in explaining the depths of yoga's wealth. If one diligently practises in blending the intellectual and emotional sheaths, I am sure the essence of yoga pours out in making one not only a good teacher but a noble teacher of yoga.

– Thank you, Uncle. –

[1] *Viśeṣadarśinaḥ ātmabhāva bhāvanānivṛttiḥ* (*Y.S.*, IV.25). For one who realises the distinction between *citta* and *ātma*, the sense of separation between the two disappears.

THE INWARD PATH FOR A BETTER WORLD*

On December 1998, the Iyengar Yoga Festival was held in the city of Pune, India, to commemorate the eightieth birthday of Yogachārya Shri B.K.S. Iyengar.

Once this event concluded Gurujī had the generosity of meeting us and giving this interview, in which he exposed his impressions about the development of Iyengar yoga in Spain, and explained again general views of yoga and some more particular concerning his teaching at the Convention.

Q.- *Gurujī*, it has been a privilege to have your presence and inspiration during your last two visits to Spain. They were unforgettable moments, imprinted in our hearts. Please, could you tell us your impressions on the development of your system in our country?

I am proud of this development as well as the emotional oneness which I felt in Spain. It has touched me more, because in other places people speak with a calculated intellectual head but you people are more emotional and speak from the heart, which is clean.

Therefore, I am confident that the senior pupils like you, getting together should build up a good foundation, not only for the health of the body, but also for the peace of mind in the whole community. However, this expression has now become very common, so it is better to say that you build up intellectual stability and clarity. Intellectual indecision leads to instability. This definitely disturbs one and so it needs the attention for mutual understanding with one another.

---

* Interview by Vicky Alamos, Xavi Alongina and Jose Maria Vigar, at the library of the Ramāmaṇi Iyengar Memorial Yoga Institute, on 16th December 1998. Published by *Yoga Jwāla,* the magazine of the Spanish Iyengar Yoga Association, n. 1, 2000.

Yoga is the science of the heart. You people appear to have good *saṁskāra* and I think it is a great thing to see. With these good impressions *(saṁskāra),* if you all work together and exchange, you will surely build up a society where your expression of joy and peace could be seen by others.

Q.- The Spanish Iyengar Yoga Association is newly made with the other Iyengar Yoga Associations in the world. Could you advise us in the inception of this path?

The ideal of global awareness has taught us many things apart from business. We are like brothers and sisters. Hence, we have to live together naturally. We all belong to the family of this planet – the Mother Earth. I know that it took a long time in Spain to form an Association and am glad that it is going on well. Spanish people have the right temperament; as such it is well established with the practice of yoga, it definitely adds to your culture since you all have already this quality. An Association is meant to further this friendly approach and unity between teachers and students.

Q.- What was your reaction when you knew that Spain was, together with the United Kingdom, the second country in the number of participants, to attend the functions for your birthday?

It clearly shows the eagerness and enthusiasm which are there in you all to get the best, as quickly as possible, from yoga.

I was touched by the way you all work in groups and I know that it takes time for the Association to grow in maturity; but I think, as spiritual discipline has no barriers, no demarcation, slowly a congenial factor could be built up, so that all feel oneness in each other. One may reach soon the goal and the other may reach late. As you all practise with love and affection, I consider this as a sign indicating that you are close to your hearts.

- Thank you, Gurujī, *for your appreciation. Let me come to the next question.*

Q.- When you teach you insist on the importance of *yama* and *niyama* in our practice. Could you explain the relevance of these two universal principles for the maturity of the practitioner?

When we think of *yama* and *niyama*, we should first of all understand the ethics of the body: the ethics of the nerves, of the mind, of the intelligence, of the cellular system, of the circulation, and the ethics of the neurons of the brain and so forth. All these factors are involved in ethics. If proper attention to correct discipline is not attended to, then it becomes heedless practice, which is the opposite of *yama* and *niyama*. Discipline is ethics *(nīti)*, but some unfortunately mistake ethics as an ideological forced discipline. While you are doing the *āsana*, when you apply your wisdom, it is *yama (nīti)*[1], and what to do comes under *niyama*. Other word for *niyama* is *rīti*[2]. It is a mode or method of performance. So if one understands what not to do and what to do, then you understand the principles of *yama* and *niyama*.

As I said in the Convention, in the practice of *āsana* each individual should become an interior decorator. Without the mind, without the intelligence, can we decorate the inner body? So these disciplinary principles of *yama* and *niyama* must be followed in the practice of *āsana* to make the seer rest in each and every place of the body without any impediments or obstacles. Regarding *āsana* practice, I am speaking of Patañjali's *ahiṁsā* and *satya*, in a practical way.

While doing the *āsana* we have to find out: Which part is aggressive? Which part is non-aggressive? Which part is in the right direction and which part is not? If one does not do the *āsana* as it should be presented, then does this practice come under truth? Is not truth a discreet judgement of each motion and action? You all have seen the scale of justice. The central part is the one that presents prudent sound judgement. We have two legs, two arms, two sides of the trunk, two eyes, two ears, and so forth. All these are to be evenly weighed so that the needle at the centre does not tilt and that needle for us is consciousness. This is what I mean by discreet judgement as truth.

If you take *yama*, one uses these ethics towards social life, while one uses *niyama* as individual ethics. Normally one observes these two to live in the world: but in the practice of *āsana* it is a beauty to know that *yama* and *niyama* are subjectively observed in each muscle, tendon, joint, capillaries and so forth.

Suppose you are asked to do *Tāḍāsana*, if one knee is extended and the other knee backwards, where is *satya*? If one leg does well, do you think you are right in your perception? Is it not your sense of duty to search where the right sensation is coming from one part of the leg while the same sensation is not coming on the other leg? This discretion comes only when you think with deliberation while doing the *āsana*. Without the implementation of *yama* and *niyama* they cannot be done. In fact, *yama* and *niyama* are all implicit in the practice of *āsana* but one does not watch. Similarly, the other aspects of yoga namely; *prāṇāyāma, pratyāhāra, dhāraṇā* and *dhyāna*, are also implicit in the *āsana*.

---

1 *Nīti*, or science of human norms, values and behaviour, is another synonymous term for *yama*. It means guidance and hence involves ethics (what not to do).

2 *Rīti* means method or mode, or what to do. Again a synonymous term for *niyama*.

Q.- How should the life of a practitioner be once his limited daily practice is finished?

In olden days practice of yoga was different from today. In those days the kings were looking after the yogis, so they had no economical and financial problems. Everything was supplied by the rulers. Now we have to earn our livelihood and at the same time practise yoga. This is the difference today. The times have changed. It is very difficult to survive without an economic base.

Today, yoga works economically for us because the intelligence of the body, of the mind and of the heart are utilised in such a way that there is no wastage at all. The energy and intelligence are focused towards the interior world (world within the body) instead of on the external worldly pleasures, where energy is wasted in indulgence of the pleasures.

As we have to earn our living, it may take a longer time to reach the zenith. So we have to balance between living in the external world and living in the internal world. As we go for jobs to survive, we do not nag or complain about it. Even if a survey is taken of people before they started practising and after practice, it can be proved that they finish their jobs faster than non-yoga practitioners. Due to yogic practices you deal with people with modesty, honesty, quickness and firmness. One does not notice this, but in the practitioners there is clarity in thinking. So they do the job fast. Hence, there is satisfaction both in the employer and the employee. One can see in those who are not yoga minded, they nag about their office work. I don't think any of my yoga students do that, and this is equipoise in them. The quality of the work that they do improves to a great extent.

- So, this is also a way of practice. -

Yes, It is a way of practice: "How to adopt and adapt according to the situation". Remember the scale of justice. Then you experience the beauty of yoga.

Q.- The next question, *Guruji*, is: how to avoid the contentment that could become a kind of drain for the practice?

You are right. There has to be a balance between contentment and discontentment. When you say: "I am contented", stagnation sets in. You may say that you are contented, but internally you may be hankering for achievements. Is not brooding and hankering an obstacle in the rules of *yama* and *niyama?*

The internal brooding cannot be seen from the outside. You may say that you are a contented person, but you know what is inside you. However, *santoṣa*, the contentment exposed in the *Yoga Sūtra*, is different. One should be content with what one achieves today but one should not be ambitious for further achievement in practice. Knowledge has a beginning but it has no end; so the moment you go on practising, the subtlety will set in; naturally there comes the inquisitiveness to bring that imprint back in your body, mind and self. And that is the new positive experiences, which set in without ambition and should be developed and cultured to proceed further.

If you remain contented, then you do not proceed further, then your knowledge gets stagnated and becomes stale. Your *sādhanā* has to be like a river. The water of the river does not remain stagnant. If it is stagnant, it is no more a river. The flow of the river cannot be demarcated as having a beginning, a middle or an end. It originates at one point and reach the ocean at the other point. Similarly your *sādhanā* should be like that. Knowledge originates from the core as a seeker and leads you towards emancipation as seer like the river joining the ocean, which is its culmination. Use contentment as a stepping-stone in order to continue the *sādhanā*. Do not do *sādhanā* with a dissatisfied and negative mind, but with cheerfulness. See that contentment does not put a full stop to your *sādhanā*. A practitioner of yoga should be contented with what he has achieved. Since there is plenty to know to reach the final goal – emancipation the discontentment has to be there. I call this as the divine discontentment. Have contentment in worldly achievements but have discontentment until you reach the final goal in the spiritual kingdom.

Q.- In this Convention, *Prashant* has explained to us the three aspects which distinguish Iyengar Yoga from other systems: technicalities, sequencing and timing. The next day, during the class, you added the fourth aspect: the sequencing of the technicalities in each *āsana*. Would you please elaborate this for the sake of the readers of *Yoga Jwālā*?

No thought of sequencing the *āsana* was considered before. One would pick up any *āsana* according to one's taste. However, I brought the awareness of sequencing during practice. Now, the sequencing has become a known fact at least for my pupils. When the patients approach their yoga teachers for their problems, these teachers ask me. Obviously, I have to give sequences of *āsana*, because we have to study how the toning has to take place so that there is no untoward effect in their systems. For the sake of the patients, I have to learn the sequences of *āsana* altogether in a different way. But it does not end here. We need to have the sequence of movement in the performance of the *āsana*. We have to create a sequence that recovers health gradually, like a sapling which grows into a tree. Often the plant is trimmed for healthy growth. Is it not? Similarly, we have to trim the sequence for an *āsana* so that the energy may not flow in the wrong directions aggravating the problems. This is the sequence in technique. So while doing the *āsana* one has to see that the sapling of the *āsana* grows gradually into a healthy tree of *āsana*.

We have hundreds of muscles, hundreds of joints, circulatory system, nervous system, mental system (mind, intelligence, memory, etc.), what you call psychological and intellectual application and so on. We have also to sequence these ingredients of nature while doing the *āsana*. The technicalities explained in *āsana* and *prāṇāyāma* are not merely the techniques but are meant to unfold oneself from within to balance all these various systems of the body. We need to bring attention, memory, intellect and perception in the process of performing the *āsana* to derive the best maximum effect. The utilisation of this apparatus, namely the body and its systems, as well as the mind and its systems, has to be such that the apparatus is used in a sequential order. They have to be used in a balanced order also. Finally, the intelligence has to surface everywhere so that no imbalance in body, nerves, mind and intelligence occurs. If one is in slumber, one pinches to find out whether one is wakeful, sensitive and fully aware. In a similar manner we have to see whether the intellect is pinching, pricking, touching and surfacing accurately everywhere in the body while doing the *āsana*. Is that awareness balanced or not? Then you'll realise that in some parts we are aware, in some parts we are not. That is why the other day I explained to the entire class only the sequential adjustment in each *āsana* by sequencing the skin, the capillaries, the tendons, joints and muscles of each and every part of the body. I am sure many of us must have followed and understood the very approach at all levels of body and self. This comes under *brahmacarya* as the seer is made to move in each cell of the body.

One advantage in this Convention was, whether for the raw beginners, beginners, or advanced students, I presented from scratch, giving various definitions of each and every division of the body, how to make the mind to reach there with the intellect and how to balance the intelligence and the mind evenly, so that when they are practising there is no difference between body and mind. That is what I taught this time. If you all interpret this in your practices, then I think it will not be difficult for any to reach the zenith in the field of yoga.

When this sequencing is learnt, there is no difference between the seer – *dṛṣṭā* – and the seeker, because the seeker is the seer, the seer is the seeker. When the seer does not see, he remains a seeker. The moment the seer sees, then the seeker transforms into a seer.

I thought that I should give this experience, otherwise you may take it that only the sequencing of *āsana* is important and you may lose the importance of this conscious inward sequencing also. That is why I added the fourth one, where you approach *prakṛti* – the seen – sequentially. If the seer has to come in contact with the seen, one has to bring the seen to the level of the seer[1], therefore the seer needs to reach the seen at each and every level. Under the bright light everything becomes clear. Similarly under the light of the seer, the seen becomes clear. For this reason the sequencing or unveiling process is important. One has to approach one's *prakṛti* sequentially.

All the students should know that the fourth sequencing includes the subjective sequencing of the mind, the 'I' and the intelligence with the consciousness. These three subtle ingredients of consciousness move, reach and send the message to the soul – the seer: "Sir, I feel that I have touched here, there and everywhere in the body. In case you feel that I have not touched, guide me, what I have to do?" This self-enquiry, self-appealing itself is the sequencing of the seen for the sake of the seer in the *āsana*.

– *Thanks for the details,* Gurujī. *Now it is clear. Let me move to the next question.* –

Q.- *Sthira sukham āsanam* is usually translated as: "sitting comfortably in a posture" but you offer us the spiritual aspect of the *āsana* practice when you interpret this *sūtra* as: "I am the *āsana*, *āsana* am I", from your knowledge and experience. Could you please explain it further?

This "I am the *āsana* and *āsana* I am" is experienced in every *āsana,* but how can I make you to experience it? It has to be in your qualitative experiential practice. You have to bring that state of activity in your intelligence and consciousness, but it is impossible for anyone to imprint this feeling on you. So one has to work attentively within the sequence I have just mentioned. You have to observe and get absorbed. In this way, I am sure these questions would be answered by your own self rather than listening to me *(Gurujī smiles)* and then suddenly says: "Here I got the clue". *(Gurujī takes a book and puts it vertically on the table.)*

See: this is the front page, this is the back page. Imagine that the back page is the back of the calf muscle, and the front page is the front of the calf muscle, is not the front page parallel to the back page? Similarly, you have to observe the length and touch of the back muscle and feel the even contact with the skin. Then adjust the length of the front muscle with the bone to

---

[1] *Sattva puruṣayoḥ śuddhi sāmye kaivalyam iti* (*Y.S.,* III.56). When the purity of intelligence equals the purity of the soul, the yogi has reached *kaivalya,* perfection in yoga.

be evenly in its contact. This is how the study should be done. Now take the width of the calf. Does your intelligence flow on the inner side of the calf or on the outer side? If intelligence touches both the parts, then it is a perfect positioning of the intelligence of the calf with the intelligence of the seer. Then you are in *āsana* and *āsana* you are. This is *sthira sukham āsanam.* It means like this you have to adjust each and every part of the body parallel to each other and the Seer has comfortably settled in each cell and in each part of the body. *(Gurujī smiles.)*

Q.- During this Convention we have been told not to do pneumatic *prāṇāyāma,* but to practise it as exposed by Patañjali in the *sūtra* II.51: *"bāhya ābhyantara viṣaya ākṣepī caturthaḥ",* in which he explains the fourth type of *prāṇāyāma*: the non-deliberate and effortless *prāṇāyāma.* Should we understand this learning process in the same way you have just exposed for the *āsana*?

Yes, this conveys the same meaning.

Patañjali says, in the *sūtra* II.49[1], that the normal breath being unrhythmic, you have to make it rhythmic and that after succeeding in it, you have to hold the breath – *kuṁbhaka.* He says in the next *sūtra,* II.50[2], that after holding the breath, you have to know which part of your body – *deśa* – the seer is touching, which part of the body he is not touching. After that he mentions timing – *kāla.* He speaks of timing, but not on chronological time such as four counts (inhalation), eight counts (retention) and sixteen counts (exhalation). When you count, are you doing *prāṇāyāma* or are you counting? Nowadays *prāṇāyāma* has become a mechanical process. Patañjali has not mentioned counting. On careful study I understood that the grip of the torso must not be by you but by the core of the being – seer *(ātman).*

In *kuṁbhaka* the seer surfaces in the body. One has to watch how long the seer is firmly in contact with the peripheral body. Though the seer has receded or turned his back from the torso in *kuṁbhaka* many practitioners stick to the counting in numbers. This cannot be *prāṇāyāma,* because the seer has receded and ego has surfaced. So you have to act to bring the receded seer to surface and that is "time" – *kāla.* You have to learn by reading Patañjali over and over to understand the depth of *prāṇāyāma.* How long is the seer in contact with the

---

1 *Tasmin sati śvāsa praśvāsayoḥ gativicchedaḥ prāṇāyāmaḥ* (*Y.S.,* II.49). *Prāṇāyāma* is the regulation of the incoming and outgoing flow of breath with retention. It is to be practised only after perfection in *āsana* is attained.

2 *Bāhya ābhyantara stambha vṛttiḥ deśa kāla saṁkhyābhiḥ paridṛṣṭaḥ dīrgha sūkṣmaḥ* (*Y.S.,* II.50). *Prāṇāyāma* has three movements: prolonged and fine inhalation, exhalation and retention; all regulated with precision according to duration and place.

physical body? That is the *kāla*. The moment this contact vanishes, then that time does not count, as it becomes just a forceful *kuṁbhaka* or pneumatic *prāṇāyāma* as I told you.

Saṁkhyā. *Saṁkhyā* means number; counting the number of cycles time as well as standing for precision. As Patañjali has used *kāla* (time), before. I am sure *saṁkhyā* stands for precise in movement of breath as well as placement of chest and spine.

Then he guides one to do *dīrgha*, i.e., long, smooth, deep inhalation and exhalation. When this long, smooth breath is made subtle, it becomes *sūkṣma*. Here stability and subtle touch of the seer in *kuṁbhaka* are also involved.

In one *sūtra* he has given five methodologies for *prāṇāyāma*. If one studies step by step one understands how complicated and refined his approach is. In the *sūtra* II.51[1], he says the beauty of *prāṇāyāma* is in doing without volition. As I said: "I am the *āsana*, *āsana* I am", here: "the breath I am, I am the breath". If *prāṇāyāma* is practised the way Paṭañjali guides with careful attention and implementation, then it is not pneumatic. Pneumatic problems come when you hold the breath with *'aham'* or by the force of the brain and muscles. Then the neurones of the brain get affected. This is pneumatic *prāṇāyāma*. Forceful inhalation and exhalation exert the cells of the brain, nerves and sometimes blood vessels may rupture, which may end up with various problems. I hope you understand now what the pneumatic *prāṇāyāma* is.

Prāṇāyāma is the hub of a spiritual *sādhanā*. Therefore, you cannot do egoistically, but by surrendering the intelligence to the seer.

Evolution of the seer towards its frontiers is inhalation and involution of the body, senses, mind, intelligence and consciousness towards the seer is exhalation. In *kuṁbhaka* there is neither evolution nor involution. As long as the seer maintains without disturbing the elements between inhalation and exhalation, it is spiritual *kuṁbhaka*. In *antara kuṁbhaka* the seer is evoluted and in *bāhya kuṁbhaka* the elements of nature get involuted.

What is evolution? *(Gurujī shows it to us doing a forceful retention after inhalation.)* Many do with jerks and physical force like the way I showed you. Then some just count or grip the brain, not knowing the body is loose. But this is not evolution as both body and intelligence get disturbed. *(Then he shows without force.)* Exhalation being the process of involution, one sinks the body as well as the seer. Watch my exhalation. I keep space between the inner intelligence and the inner spindles of the body and the skin.

There has to be a thorough understanding and communion from the skin to the core during inhalation. The seer should fully occupy the body with equipoise both in longitude and latitude of the torso. One has to learn to see whether energy, intelligence and seer are accurately

---

[1] *Bāhya ābhyantara viṣaya ākṣepī caturthaḥ* (*Y.S.*, II.51). The fourth type of *prāṇāyāma* transcends the external and internal *prāṇāyāma*, and appears effortless and non-deliberate.

balanced from the perineum up to the top trunk. You feel the lightness and exhilaration. In pneumatic *prāṇāyāma*, you won't feel lightness, but heaviness in the brain and rigidity in the body.

If you follow Patañjali carefully, then there is no danger in *prāṇāyāma*. You asked earlier about the sequencing of *āsana*, where the sequencing of motion and action are to be involved in body, mind, intelligence and consciousness. Now see the beautiful sequencing of *prāṇāyāma* by Patañjali: There is *bāhya vṛtti* – exhalation, *ābhyantara vṛtti* – inhalation, *stambha vṛtti* – *kuṁbhaka*, *deśa* – place, *kāla* – timing, *saṁkhyā* – precision, *dīrgha* – long, *sukṣma* – subtle. "Learn first which part the seer is touching, which part the seer is not touching". Is the seer in contact with the entire trunk *(deśa)* during exhalation, inhalation and retention. This has to be observed and attended to.

Then he comes to *kāla*, timing. Study how long the seer is in commune with the physical, psychological and intellectual bodies. You know, we have the skeletal body *(annamaya kośa)*, organic body *(prāṇamaya kośa)*, mental body *(manomaya kośa)*, intellectual body *(vijñānamaya kośa)*, body of consciousness *(cittamaya kośa)*, and the body of joy and bliss *(ānandamaya kośa)*. How long will it take to touch all these sheaths? That is what he means by duration, and not the chronological duration. Then he comes to *saṁkhyā* – the precise and subtle adjustment. We have to see whether we are maintaining the subtle touch in our *pūraka*, *recaka* and *kuṁbhaka*. If all these sequences are not rhythmically maintained, then it is not a *prāṇāyāma*.

He speaks further of *dīrgha* and *sūkṣma*. First he advises to learn prolongation of all the three factors of *prāṇāyāma* and after learning prolongation of them, he wants us to proceed towards subtlety. Even when one holds the breath, he says, timing is unimportant but the feel of the presence of the seer is important.

The highest type of *prāṇāyāma* is the one which is done from the seer. When it comes from the seer, it is beyond deliberation.

Q.- In this Convention we have practised *āsana* followed by *prāṇāyāma* or *prāṇāyāma* and then *āsana*. Could you please explain under which circumstances can we practise this way?

I said to Geeta and Prashant, alternately to take *prāṇāyāma* first and at the end, because I wanted the students to know how *prāṇāyāma* affects before and after *āsana*.

In the morning before *āsana* class you could do better because there is no strain on the lungs, and when I took the *āsana* class first the fibres of your spindles were stretched and strained, so you could not do *prāṇāyāma*. So when people say: after practising *āsana* do *prāṇāyāma*, know that this is also a mistake. It may suit the beginners, because they do not stretch their lungs like the more toned practitioners. I wanted to guide teachers who have assembled here to experience which type of *prāṇāyāma*, before *āsana* or after *āsana* is helpful.

You must all have noticed that the rhythm does not come after *āsana* practice. You feel the cells of your lungs are taut.

Why did I take *prāṇāyāma* on the last two days without making you to sit? Because the fibres which were already extended in the *āsana* could be strained further if I had asked you to sit. Therefore, I did not allow the spindles of the body to become hard and prick the fibres. Hence, I made you to do *prāṇāyāma* in *Śavāsana*.

All the things I did in the early days I wanted you to study and experience those different changes before and after *āsana*. I wanted each teacher to know practically the good and the bad of everything in yogic practices. I hope you got the knowledge and understanding of when to teach *prāṇāyāma*, to whom, at what time and which one.

Q.- There have been participants with different levels of practice in this Convention; we have practised different types of *prāṇāyāma*. Could you please explain your methodology?

I kept in mind the overall presentation as many were of different levels of practitioners and I had to teach *prāṇāyāma* accordingly. For example, take *Ujjāyī prāṇāyāma*. This even a raw beginner could not do due to restriction in lungs. *Ujjāyī* hardens the cells of the lungs. *Viloma prāṇāyāma* does the opposite as interrupted breaths give interval for the cells of the lungs to recover. *Antara kuṁbhaka* pressurises the cells of the lungs, hence I began the class with exhalation in *Viloma prāṇāyāma*.

This is how one has to study and learn. That is why I taught you all on attention with exhalation. I tried to educate you all to learn how to introduce *prāṇāyāma* to start with. The strain that you feel in *Ujjāyī* you do not feel in *Viloma prāṇāyāma*.

I have shown you ways so that you know how to train various parts of the torso before attempting *kuṁbhaka*. Here *Viloma prāṇāyāma* is taught as a first step to acclimatise in toning the lungs. This way one builds sustaining power in the lungs for other types of *prāṇāyāma*. Afterwards one has to experiment which *prāṇāyāma* fits according to the physical and mental conditions. Hence, I do not fix the programme saying today you do *Ujjāyī* or *Viloma*. Suppose you cannot do *Ujjāyī*, switch to *Viloma*, then tomorrow think of *Ujjāyī*. Regimentation should not be there either in *prāṇāyāma* or in *āsana*. Remember *maitrī* – friendliness. There should be a co-ordination and friendliness between the spindles of the body and the spindles of the mind.

Q.- You speak very frequently of the intelligence. In the western world it is often mistaken with the mind. Would you please explain the differences between both of them?

Mind is a gatherer and intelligence is the discriminative power. Mind cannot discriminate; mind sends the message to its master, the intelligence. That is why our Indian philosophers divided the five sheaths of the body: *annamaya*, *prāṇamaya*, *manomaya*, *vijñānamaya* and *ānandamaya*. These five belong to the five elements, namely *pṛthvī*, *āp*, *tejas*, *vāyu*, and *ākāśa*[1].

Therefore, when we are doing the *āsana* and *prāṇāyāma* the most important thing is that we have to feel these five elements co-ordinating and co-operating with each other, tracing the five sheaths. Suppose you take a deep inhalation with a forced movement of ascending order of the rib cage, then *pṛthvī* only works and there is no contact of *āp*, *tejas* or *vāyu*, and that is why the Indian people at once say that *manas*, the mind, is a gatherer, sending messages, and leave the discriminative power to the intelligence.

Haṭhayoga Pradīpikā (IV.69-77) speaks of four states of practices for four types of practitioners. First is *ārambhāvasthā*, where a beginner does on the outer layer of the body, which is known as peripheral, physical yoga. The next is *ghaṭāvasthā*. Here, the practitioner goes from the peripheral body a little deep towards the inner body. Then comes *paricayāvasthā*. Here the mind acquaints with the sensation of the body. This is *maitrī*. Now the mind says to the body: "Let me introduce my master, my boss, the intelligence *(buddhi)*, to you". The moment the mind introduces the various parts of the body to the intelligence, then the mind disappears. Then the scene of intelligence corrects the wants of the body as the body in its own language asks, "Please, guide me through the spindles of the motor nerves and sensory nerves how they should work". Hence, the intelligence is called *vijñānamaya kośa*, known as *buddhi*, wisdom, faculty of intellectual intelligence.

Between motor nerves and sensory nerves there has to be synthesis. If these two work synthetically, then the mind disappears. For example you, Xavi and I were old friends and you introduced me to José María. Once you introduced me to José María, you go away from the picture, as the connection now is between me and José María. Here, Xavi is the mind, who disappears when once he introduced to me as intelligence to José María as body. This is known as *paricayāvasthā*.

Paricaya means introduction. The mind introduces the body, the senses, the organs to the subtle sense, which is intelligence and we call it *sūkṣmendriya*. We don't include *manas* – the mind – in *sūkṣmendriya* as *annamaya*, *prāṇamaya* and *manomaya kośa* are gross bodies *(sthulendriya)*, and *vijñānamaya* and *ānandamaya kośa* – intelligence, consciousness and self

[1] See *Aṣṭadaļa Yogamālā*, II.41, *Practice of prāṇāyāma*, p. 282.

- are subtle body *(sūkṣmendriya)*. The body along with its organs, senses and mind give us gross sensations and gross knowledge, whereas the intelligence, consciousness and self give us subtle sensations and subtle knowledge. So from gross senses you have to go towards the subtle senses. These have to be guided by the subtle senses to subdue the gross senses. Today we only use the three external ones, neglecting the other two.

That is why, while sequencing the *āsana*, I want you all to bring the subtle senses, the intelligence, consciousness and self to surface in each and every *āsana* sequentially.

We have got *manomaya kośa*, mind *(manas)* as fire, and *vijñānamaya kośa*, intelligence *(jñāna)* as air. If one has to be active, fire is needed; otherwise, he remains inactive. Fire ignites the intelligence to move, as it belongs to the element of air. Without air the fire gets extinguished, and when united it fuses a new energy.

The final state is *niṣpattyāvasthā* or the state of culmination or maturity where the dualities disappear and the yogi realises a unified state of consciousness.

Q.- The *Yoga Sūtras* are difficult to understand for us since they do not belong to our tradition; however they are referred to very often during our practice. Would you please advise us on the methodology we must follow to understand and make them implicit in the practice?

It is true. *Yoga Sūtra* have four chapters namely *Samādhi Pāda, Sādhana Pāda, Vibhūti Pāda* and *Kaivalya Pāda*, in which Patañjali speaks of the views, ways and effects and finality of yoga respectively. You have to keep on reading and re-reading these *sūtra*. Then as a study you have to categorise the *Yoga Sūtra*. Wherever the word *citta* comes, take these *sūtra* on one side, wherever the mind comes, take these *sūtra*. In this manner, if you can categorise the *sūtra*, then the imprints will be good. Similarly, see how many *sūtra* Patañjali allots for *yama, niyama, āsana*, and so on. This way you learn quick to understand the *sūtra*.

Just now, you asked me about the mind and the intelligence. Now, how many times does Patañjali refer to the mind? He refers to the mind in five *sūtra*. Among those five *sūtra*, he only tells how the mind improves qualitatively in two. In the two other places he explains the two phases of mind; namely, *daurmanasya* (despair) and *saumanasya* (cheerfulness). Mind can get depressed and can be uplifted. Then the fifth time he refers to the speed of the mind, which can be as fast as the seer when totally ripe.

He gives us two *sūtra* where the mind can be improved qualitatively through the practice of yoga. The first one comes in *Samādhi Pāda*. *Viṣayavatī vā pravṛttiḥ utpannā manasaḥ sthiti nibandhanī* (*Y.S.*, I.35). It means that if the mind has picked up a certain object of its interest, one has to make it work on it, so that the mind becomes stable. Here he does not speak of restraint but to go with the object totally to maintain the steadiness of the mind. You have to allow the mind to flow with that object. It does not mean to go with sensually alluring object, but to that object which can conduce the mind to get stability. Now, the mind which has to pick up the object has to get cleansed, so Patañjali refers to two phases of it – *daurmanasya* and *saumanasya*[1]. The impediment in our progress on the yogic path is the dejection and disparity of mind. The sorrowful and distressed mind needs treatment so that it gets elevated, uplifted and cheerful. The *śauca* as a *niyama* has to be followed and practised for the distressed mind to become cheerful to practise yoga with the freshness of mind.

Suppose I am doing the *āsana*, my mind has to go with that *āsana* in and out completely, then I am a real practitioner of yoga, because I made the seer to look and stay everywhere. The mind has to remain ever fresh to do the *āsana*, to correct the *āsana*, to adjust and readjust and maintain alertness. For this, *āsana* has to be done with *saumanasya* and not *daurmanasya*.

Before going to the state of *sthiti nibandhani* or stabilising the mind, he says to uplift the mind from the state of *daurmanasya* to *saumanasya* through *niyama* and make it fit for concentration through *prāṇāyāma*. When the mind has become a fit instrument for *dhāraṇā* – concentration, then make it stable by picking up an object of its taste in order to have the graceful diffusion of consciousness. And finally, in the third chapter, he speaks of the speed of mind – *manojavitvaṁ*[2]. *Manojavam* means the speed of mind. When the mind is purified to the level of the seer, the mind can match the speed of the seer to be with him. The fluctuating mind also has speed but its speed is to go away from the seer whereas the pure mind goes with the seer since such a mind knows its destination.

This elaboration can give you some idea about how the evolution of mind takes place, how mind has to be educated, cultured, refined and utilised.

So if you learn to look at the *sūtra* this way, then you get a background. I have done it, but it might take some time for you to bring this to practical application. Wherever *citta* comes, I have set in one list, wherever mind comes I have set in another; what are the impediments in the first chapter, second chapter, third chapter, fourth chapter, wherever they come; collect and

---

1 *Duḥkha daurmanasya aṅgamejayatva śvāsapraśvāsāḥ vikṣepa sahabhuvaḥ* (*Y.S.*, I.31). Sorrow, despair, unsteadiness of the body and irregular breathing further distract the *citta*.

Sattvaśuddhi saumanasya aikāgrya indriyajaya ātmadarśana yogyatvāni ca (*Y.S.*, I.41). When the body is cleansed, the mind purified and the senses controlled, joyful awareness needed to realise the inner self, also comes.

Dhāraṇāsu ca yogyatā manasaḥ (*Y.S.*, II.53). After *prāṇāyāma*, the mind becomes a ripe instrument for *dhāraṇa* (concentration).

2 *Tataḥ manojavitvaṁ vikaraṇabhāvaḥ pradhānajayaḥ ca* (*Y.S.*, III.49). By mastery over the mind, the yogi's speed of body, senses and mind matches that of the soul, independent of the primary causes of nature. Unaided by consciousness, he subdues the first principle of nature *(mahat)*.

make a ready reckoner. This way of categorisation will be good to learn. Then you have to find out the near similarities in the *sūtra* which connect to your practices, and so forth. For instance, though you get details of *prāṇāyāma* in *Sādhana Pāda*, Patañjali speaks of it also in *Samādhi* and *Vibhūti Pāda*. You have to see how he touches the subject, then its application becomes easier for you. I think this would be of great help to you all to learn the essence of Patañjali's *Yoga Sūtra*.

YOGA – HEAD TO TOE*

Part ONE – MENUHIN AND IYENGAR

Q.- How should we describe you on our programme?

Just a human being with two legs and two arms. *(Laughter.)*

Q.- When you were young, people thought you were going to grow up to be very weak and weedy, didn't they?

Yes, because I was born at a time when the world was attacked by the Spanish influenza, so I was probably having the flu in my mother's womb itself and that affected me a great deal. Although several millions of deaths all over the world were there, God made me survive, but minus health and strength.

– But you had a very big head for your body, didn't you? –

Yes.

Q.- Why was that?

When I was a child I could not even lift up my head, so I had a problem. I never thought I would have health and strength in my life. I don't know why the head was big though the body was small.

---

* Interview by Mark Tully for BBC Radio 4, in Pune, 7th & 8th April 1999.

Q.- How did this weak young child who was not at all confident that he would ever be healthy in his life choose to go in for yoga?

From birth to the age of thirteen, after influenza, I developed malaria, after malaria I was laid up for twenty-one days with typhoid fever. Then the doctors examined me and found I had tuberculosis of the lungs also. That frightened me a little that I may be a drag in life. So I thought better to commit suicide rather than continue living a dependent life. Fortunately my sister was married to a yoga master who said, "Why don't you do some *yogāsana*, you may gain health?" This tempted me to try yoga.

My brother-in-law learnt yoga in Nepal. He was a great scholar and he passed successfully all the *darśana* - *Nyāya, Vaiśeṣika, Sāṁkhya, Yoga, Pūrva Mīmāṁsā* and *Uttara Mīmāṁsā* (now known as *Vedānta*) in a short time. Then his teacher advised my *guruji* go to Muktinārāyaṇa Kṣetra, near Nepal, to know the practical aspects of yoga, under this great *guru*.

- And that's where he learnt his yoga? -

Yes! His *guru* was *Shri* Ramamohana Brahmacāri.

- Your guruji sounds to have been a very very strict person. He used to make you walk miles just to leave your books and then come back again after school... -

Yes, he was a very very strict disciplinarian, and I couldn't go against his wishes. I had to walk eight miles up and down each day. Though the *yogaśālā* (the Institute of yoga) was only about ten minutes walk from the school, he wanted me to go home, just keep my schoolbooks and come back to *yogaśālā*. This was really a great strain on my fragile health. This overburdened my body's strength which affected my education. Even though I was practising yoga, I couldn't gain health even after months of practice.

Q.- When did your health then start to improve?

Only after coming to Pune as a yoga teacher to teach yoga from 1937 to 1940 I began to gain health and understood what health could be because I began gaining physical strength. Until then I had no good health or physical strength.

- And that was through yoga that you started to understand this. -

Well, I think it is true that I began understanding both health and yoga. Please know that I never did anything except yoga. In those days there were no available medicines and if there were any, I could not afford them, so I had no other way than yoga. Secondly, I had the job of teaching. People called me to teach yoga in schools of Pune for six months. This offer came as a God given gift. My *guru* being very strict, I thought it would be a good opportunity to be a free lancer rather than to be under the thumb of my *guru*. The moment my *guru* asked me to go and teach, I was very happy to move away from his clutches.

- But you have a picture of your guru *here in the Institute, so you obviously still respect him a great deal. -*

If he had not put the seed of yoga, probably the world would not have known me, and hence I am grateful to my *guru* for sowing the seed of yoga in me. Through him I developed this yoga sapling to grow into a healthy tree, and later it went on growing as an orchard one after the other.

- This was your destiny, in a way. -

It seems so.

- You believe in destiny, obviously. -

Well, if there were no destiny, probably I would have been working as a clerk or something in life. When I started yoga I could not even bend my back because I was in bed for years, I was like a log of wood. This illness was probably a destiny for me to find a means. Destiny brought me to yoga, and the very destiny played with me to teach yoga in Pune and various other places of the world.

Destiny not only brought name to yoga, but fame to my *guru* and me.

Q.- Was your *guru* a deeply spiritual man as well?

Well, see, it is very difficult for me to explain his spiritual level when I myself did not know what 'spiritual' means. As there is a comparative study in intellectualism, one can say he was more intellectually up-beat than others. But in spirituality it is very difficult to say whether one is highly qualified unless the other has drunk the nectar of spiritual life himself. At that tender age, for me he was a great scholar and a *pundita* and had the *mantrajaya*.

- Means... -

He had the power of the *mantra*. For example, he takes the ash, says a *mantra* and gives that ash to the patient as medicine, the patient would come back the next day and say, "I'm better". That is his *mantrajaya*. Having seen such instances myself, I say that he must have had some spiritual power and without that spiritual background such things cannot happen.

Q.- And did his success go to his head at all, was he arrogant at all about it...

Being an intellectual, he was intoxicated to some extent. As far as I knew him, there was arrogance in him. When he grew old, I could see him mellow a great deal. When he was in Mysore, he was proud, both in brawn and brain.

I can only speak of him as long as I was living with him in Mysore for two years. I do say at that time he was an intoxicated intellectual and proud of his knowledge.

Q.- And is arrogance one thing that yoga tries to reduce?

Frankly speaking yoga should sublimate arrogance. Unfortunately some people, who do not find equals to humble their intellectual pride, arrogance might rule him. If there were such intellectual persons equal to him, probably, humbleness would have come to him on its own. He was like an intellectual monarch, naturally that kept him as the king of the scholars.

Q.- How did you develop your distinct way of doing yoga?

When I was called to Pune to teach yoga in schools and colleges I had to develop a distinct way in order to attract them towards yoga. Probably I am the pioneer to bring yoga into schools and colleges in 1937 and I am the pioneer to teach yoga in mixed classes where men and women, boys and girls were working together.

- Did girls learn yoga before? -

As far as I know, I had not seen.

– So you introduced it to women as well... –

Yes, in '37 I introduced yoga to women. When I was invited to teach in Pune, not only was I in poor health, but has no teaching background. As a teacher I was not knowing the subject to work with confidence. Chance came when I was not really knowing anything. When I came to Dharwar with *Gurujī*, I was asked to teach yoga for women. This was the only background I had when I was sent to Pune by my *Gurujī*. From then onwards I started teaching in girls' schools. In this sense, I introduced yoga to girls and also started a separate class for women in the ladies club of the Deccan Gymkhānā Club called Vanitā Viśrām.

Q.- What about other contemporary yoga teachers, did they think that this was heresy, that you were doing completely the wrong thing...?

No, no, no! Nobody said that I was doing the wrong thing. Only they attacked for teaching on a mass scale. The so-called yogis of the day were of the opinion that yoga is taught one to one and a lady teacher should teach ladies and not a man. Secondly, as I had a shattered health, and began to work on physical fitness in schools and colleges, that made them think that the teachings are on the physical level and not at a yogic level. Later I became conscious of alignment. I was keen on bringing the alignment of the body with the co-ordination of the mind so that the body and intelligence co-function. But as far as I know nobody said what I was doing and imparting was wrong.

Q.- What is really different about Iyengar yoga compared with other yogas?

Today the technique has improved to such an extent that we call it high tech. I thought that when we do each of the *āsana*, we should have zero pressure. I have to adjust my muscles, I have to adjust my joints so that the pressure is not too much on one side or too less on the other side. That's known as zero pressure. The moment I learnt to bring zero pressure, the mind used to become very light and in that lightness I could feel distinctly the functioning as well as the non-functioning of the inner body. From this I learned that there is something in this presentation which keeps the mind as an alert instrument not to be as an actor only but an observer also.

Q.- That's interesting, an instrument of observation, not as an actor, how do you stop the mind working as an actor?

Well, I thought of body and mind as twins and learnt to keep them apart. This way I learnt when the body should be as an actor and the mind as a witness, and when the mind to be an actor and the body as a witness. That is how I learnt to use the body on mind and mind on body. You see that the intelligence has two avenues, one avenue towards the head and the other one towards the heart. This way, it has two avenues. When I'm acting I totally get involved, and therefore, I have to change my brain to become a witness when the mind acts and I reverse the mind to witness when the brain dictates. By this way I began working to acquire perfection in *āsana*, by maintaining the frame firmly and at the same time keeping my brain calm. That's how I started interpenetrating and interweaving to move the mind and brain deeper and deeper from the outer body towards my inner body.

- Now you've talked about the extreme accuracy of your āsana *or positions and the need for perfect balance. Really, some people have criticised you for saying that in a sense your yoga is too harsh... -*

Yoga is a disciplined subject, it cannot be done casually or with harshness. By casual attempt one can gain a casual understanding and harshness leads to crudeness and roughness. But discipline appears to many as harshness. Similarly in my case the word 'aggressiveness' has been used. One can use words with different meanings. I'm an intensive practitioner, I'm an intensive and sensitive teacher. Many might call my intense approach harsh or aggressive. Words may be different. But I teach with the feel of my heart. The way I go into the subject, not only inspires my dull and lazy students to be active but also electrifies their intelligence in understanding the subject.

- But you are certainly not, as I understand it, trying in a way to torture the body in the way the people who do physical training.... -

No, no! It is not the torture of the body. You see, we have only the body as an instrument. If you ask Mr. Menuhin, he may say he's an artist when there is a violin in his hands. If there's no violin, he cannot express his artistic musical qualities. For me my body is like a piano or a violin or whatever you may call it. So I have to tune each and every part of it. The nerves in our body are like the strings, the brain is the intellectual part which is similar to the sound production from the instrument. The nose is the bridge of any instrument through which the breath is adjusted at every stage of the *āsana*. The spinal vertebrae are the knobs of the instrument, so I have to tune the knobs of the spine to such an extent that the nervous system, which starts from the spine, do not over-extend or under-extend. If there is under-extension the sound does not come, if it is too tight the string snaps. So, one has to keep the exact pressure so that the tuning of the body takes place in such a way that one can listen to the inner vibration of the sound of the body. As far as I am concerned, I hear the sound, the vibration, and adjust to get equilibrium in body, mind and self while in *āsana, prāṇāyāma* and *dhyāna*.

Q.- One experiment which I believed you conducted once was to get some army cadets, young boys, and divide them in two, one lot did the army PT which is very western really, and the other did yoga. What was the result of that?

You see, it was in 1955, the National Defence Academy invited me to teach the cadets. With all the efforts of the staff members, some could not come to the standard that was needed in the army.

Major General Habibullah was the commander at the time. He was suffering from dysentery, which he developed while fighting in Burma, now Myanmar. He came to me for treatment and got rid of his dysentery. The moment he found results, he asked me whether I could teach some cadets. "We have some cadets who are not at all on the required standard to be in the academy", he said.

– They're substandard? –

Maybe the way he approached me conveyed this idea. He requested me whether I could build them up to be on a par with other cadets. General Habibullah had seen my demonstration and had experienced my way of teaching. Seeing that I was active, dynamic and alert, he asked me to devote two days a week for those cadets to see what progress they make. This is how a six months' course started.

The officers were asked to have a check on these students. I did a good job in six months and built up their physical and mental calibre to such an extent that their physical power as well as their memory power increased, which made the Authorities to retain yoga in the Academy subject to the available funds. This went on for years. As it was not a compulsory subject, sometimes the Authorities said that they had no funds and dropped me and sometimes they would call me or my staff members back to teach again. This is how it was going on until 1995.

During this period I had the honour of giving a demonstration in the presence of Khrushchev and Bulganin who visited India in 1957. Bulganin sent word while I was performing to show what all I know. This impressed them and both came to me and congratulated me.

In fact, at that time, I was teaching the commander-in-chief of India, Gen. Srinagesh, along with Major General Habibullah.

Q.- Has yoga spread to Russia?

Yes, in 1989 the Health Ministry of the Government of Russia invited me as a State guest to convey and demonstrate as an alternative medicine. Officials were so much impressed that I was asked to train many who showed interest to learn. Now there is an Iyengar Yoga Association in Russia and there are about a dozen yoga institutes in Russia, at various places. Even my books are now available in Russian language.

- You talked about healing somebody with dysentery. -

Yes, yes.

- Now that sounds on the surface of it an odd thing for yoga to do, I can understand healing someone with ankles like mine, broken ankles or something, but... -

No, yoga is not a physical exercise, it's an organic exercise. When one has to do the *āsana,* one has to work not only on the anatomical body, but also on the organic vital body. Then one has to reflect, re-study, re-observe and re-adjust the physical as well as the physiological bodies. As one does the *āsana,* there are lots of things involved. One has to learn certain things, un-learn and re-learn certain things. This way, the process goes on.

As yoga functions on the organic body, the effect is bound to be on the organic body. It certainly plays a better role on the organic body as well as on the mental body more than on the muscular and skeletal body.

Q.- But it also plays a role on the muscular body as well, doesn't it?

Well, I said earlier that the musculo-skeletal body is the foundation. Obviously without activating the musculo-skeletal body, the organ i.e., body, cannot be healthily strengthened.

In medical science there are extension, flexion, abduction, adduction, circumduction of the muscles, and so on. Actually, I use these movements while doing *āsana,* specifically the organic body. The science doesn't speak about the abduction, adduction, circumduction of the liver, the spleen, the pancreas or the intestines, the lungs. In *āsana* we have got all these various organic actions to function where we get these abduction, adduction, circumduction movements to reach that highest level of health in the organic human system. And that's why *āsana* play a great role.

Q.- Have doctors objected to your treating people and said that you don't know how to do it, you're not medically qualified, and that sort of thing?

Fortunately, no one objected to my approach. I have addressed and demonstrated in many medical conferences and the patients who came to me were recommended by medical practitioners. Even today doctors recommend and send their patients to me. If you ask the patients in the therapeutic classes, you will come to know that most of them are recommended by the doctors. Often when the doctors fail, they say, "Try this man".

I only work to prove that yoga has a curative and preventive value. By the by, I have many highly qualified doctors as students and patients who come for their remedies.

A few years ago surgeons and physicians from the Army hospital came several times to watch me treating patients of various illnesses. After carefully observing the changes in the patients, they told me that what they appreciated in me was the confidence I create in the patients. These words of theirs are enough for me to say that yoga had won their hearts.

Q.- You are left to step in, in the most difficult cases of all, when the doctor has not been able to do anything.

Yes, because of the confidence the medical fraternity has on me and my yoga practice. It is they who send patients to me and when the patients go back and tell their doctors, they feel happy with their patients. I have created confidence in the medical field, that yoga has a good effect without ill-effect.

Q.- And when you do this remedial yoga, which we saw yesterday, is it something which worries you, that you might lead people to have great expectations and perhaps not achieve those expectations in full?

Definitely their expectations are high. But it is for me to create confidence in them, that yoga would benefit them. No doubt God has given the healing power. My job is to perform and if they recover very fast, I say wonderful. If they don't recover, I say, I have an opportunity to study and learn from their shortcomings. By chance if other patients come to me with the same problem, as I have had previous experience, I proceed with new applications to treat them. One thing, I am happy to see is that I've not injured anyone and I've not sent anyone away disappointed. Either they benefit or are made to endure without mental pressure.

- Never? -

Never. I've taught a lot of people, not one can say I've disappointed.

- You've healed so many people... -

Though I say with an emphatic, "Yes.", you see, after all we are all human beings, therefore limitations will be there. Yet, while experimenting on myself, if I have achieved so much, that itself is research. How has medical science made progress? Did they not do experiments? The same thing I have done on my own body, which I used as a laboratory for me. In my whole career the patients that I have handled, if written in book form, I think it would definitely surprise the medical world.

Q.- Some people criticise your yoga for being too much to do with the body, organs, mind, not enough to do with the spiritual.

My dear friend, body, for me, is a gross self, mind is a small self and the real Self is the finest of the Self. People do not realise, but our own philosophy has given a beautiful example. Can the water be held without a vessel? If the floor is uneven, can the vessel stand on the floor? So the body is the container and the content is the Self. If the container is placed accurately, the content remains undisturbed inside. I say the neo-yogis do not understand the difference between the container and the contained. If there is proper communication between the container and the contained, there is no jerk or vibration in the content. If the vessel is placed crookedly, the water level will be disturbed inside. Otherwise, not. As I said earlier, Menuhin was an artist on a violin, Clifford Curzon was a piano artist, so also was Malkuzinski and Jacqueline Dupré on the cello. For me, the body is my instrument where I had to explore the inside hidden content to surface through the practice of *āsana* and *prāṇāyāma*.

Q.- But do you then go on to teach them how to cope with the self, or...

Well, how they come to me I have to teach them. In the beginning I may use the disjointed and disconnected body. The ankle does not listen to the knee, the knee does not listen to the hip, and the hip does not listen to the spine. So first I co-ordinate them. Then I go to each area to find out whether the mind has engulfed those in that position. When I teach you and you do *Tāḍāsana*, I say you have to get the same feeling that I have, i.e., bottom feet touching the floor evenly, maintaining steadiness in body, and mind remaining as straight as a palm tree. This is applied to all *āsana*. Even if you do an advanced *āsana* like *Naṭarājāsana*, you have to feel that the mind is exactly even to that of the frame of the *āsana*. We've got about 700 muscles, 300 joints, so each and every part, the inner, the outer and the middle part have to be balanced in *Naṭarājāsana* accurately like *Tāḍāsana*[1], or any other *āsana*, and that is, for me, spiritual practice.

In olden days, people were calling 'divinity' for today's 'perfection'. When the word perfection is used, it means, "You have to be precise, you have to be flawless". It means you have to be divine. *(Laughter.)* Words may change, but the feelings cannot change. Is it not? *(More laughter.)*

Q.- But my understanding of it is that the final true yogi is the one who attains something through *sādhanā* called *samādhī*, and that *samādhī* is when, in a way, he loses his self completely.

Yes... *Sādhanā* is the foundation for *samādhī*. As I said the extent one's practices are faultless, he loses his identity of the small self but live with the sight of the Self.

– ...and get united with the divine. –

---

[1] See *Aṣṭadala Yogamālā*, vol 2, plate n. 15.

With the divine, yes. As man is made up of two components, nature and soul, there are two powers in our body, the power of the nature and the power of divinity. The aim of yoga is to blend these two, the power of nature and the power of divinity together..

Q.- Have you yourself achieved *samādhi?*

Myself... if I say yes, I'm an arrogant person. If I say no, you say I'm raw in yoga. As I said before, it is very difficult to express the experiences. When I do *āsana*, I'm completely an introvert. When I'm practising I forget myself but live in the Self. When I'm teaching I have to become an extrovert, with the expression of 'I'. It is hard for me to say how 'I' as second person functions when I'm doing the *āsana*, whereas at the time of teaching, the "I" expresses and take it from me that my spiritual heart sees and feels that "I". Therefore if I say I have experienced, it becomes an expression of pride, and if I say no, I am telling the untruth. Hence, I leave it for others to comment as it pleases them.

To be precise, the *sādhanā* is that practice by which one unfolds one's body, mind and intelligence so that the soul reveals itself.

- So I suspect you have experienced that state... -

Yes!

- ...but you won't say so... -

Yes! By the grace of God, yes. With humility I would not like to say, because it sounds boastful.

- But you wouldn't be a realised person if you were not humble about it, would you? -

Yes. We are made up of five elements and those five elements have infrastructure, what you call *śabda, sparśa, rūpa, rasa, gandha;* that means, you know, sound, touch, shape, taste and smell. When we are doing the *āsana*, we have to create these five infra-atomic structures of the elements in each and every part. We have to create space, we have to give shape, we have to see that intelligence, in the form of the element of the air, moves everywhere without any impediments. This is how the *āsana* have to be done by balancing the five elements and their infrastructures with the power of the soul. On one side is the wall of the soul, on the other side is the wall of these five elements and we have to unite and balance evenly in each *āsana* these two powers. If this happens, you are in a state of divinity. In order to reach that state you need to be humble. Without humbleness, the mind, intelligence, ego, pride, consciousness and conscience interfere creating the partitions between self and Self.

Q.- And what is your view on meditation, do you think that is a valuable way of achieving something?

For me, bringing the complex mind to a tranquil state of simplicity is meditation. People often think that sitting in a corner, closing the eyes, is meditation. But meditation is an inward attention. For me, the moving intelligence of the heart and the moving intellect of the head are to be united together and held at the seat of the Self is meditation.

Q.- Your success in the West largely sprung from your meeting with Yehudi Menuhin.
Yes.

– How did you meet him? –

Well, I met Mr. Menuhin in 1952, when he visited India for the first time at the invitation of our first Prime Minister, Honourable Jawaharlal Nehru.

There was a Menuhin's reception committee in Mumbai and some of the committee members had seen my demonstrations. One of the committee members, Mrs. Mehra Vakil, was my student.

Mr. Menuhin had some problems with his nervous system. He was finding it difficult even to hold the violin, as he used to play hundreds of concerts for the army at the time of the Second World War. This caused in him not only physical exhaustion, but nervous exhaustion and mental fatigue. On account of that, I was told that he could not relax easily.

I was requested by Mrs. Mehra Vakil to come to Mumbai to meet him at Raj Bhavan. I met him and seeing his physical and mental state, I asked him whether he would like to experience relaxation. He said, "Yes". Though he had just got up from the bed, I made him do *Śavāsana*.

– That's lying on the bed? –

Yes! Lying straight on the back. With my fingers, I blocked his ears and eyes and created a gentle compression of the floor of the brain. I kept two fingers on the eyes, thumb plugged into ears, two fingers on the nostrils to control the regulation of breath and two fingers in order to separate the eyeballs from the contact of the brain. This is known as *Ṣaṇmukhī mudrā* in yoga. I kept him in *Ṣaṇmukhī mudrā* to still the movements of his eyeballs, thumbs on ears to cut the outer sound. In a minute or so he went into deep sleep. Believe me, he slept forty-five minutes. As his eyeballs started flickering, I released my fingers from his face and asked him how he felt. He said, "I never experienced this type of rest in my life".

Then I told him, "You have heard about yoga but you must not have seen what yoga is. I read in *Times of India* that you did head balance in front of our Prime Minister". He said, "Yes!" So I asked him whether he would like to show or see what I do. He said, "Lovingly, I would like to see you perform". I gave a forty-five minutes demonstration. He was much impressed and requested me to teach him for a few days as long as he stayed in Mumbai.

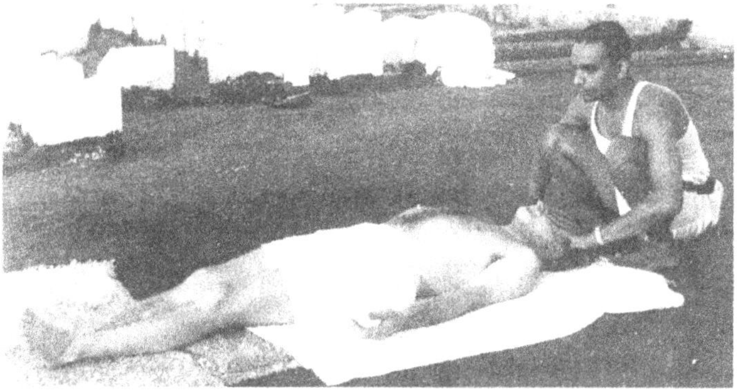

Plate n. 49 – *Sanmukhi Mudra* for Yehudi Menuhin

Next day I took him to *Śīrṣāsana* and kept him for five minutes. He said, "Mr. Iyengar, I have done *Śīrṣāsana* but I never had this experience". As he was very much impressed, I took him to *Sarvāṅgāsana* and *Halāsana* with a few more *āsana*, and he was delighted in feeling the goodness of these *āsana*.

Then Mr. Menuhin said, "Please, I want you to come tomorrow, will you come and teach me?" I said, "Yes". Thus, I taught him for four days, both morning and evening.

On the fourth day he gave his concert and he said, "After years, this is the first time I've played at a concert so well." And he was very much impressed and asked me to come to America. Then he realised that he had lots of commitments and had to postpone them.

He came again in 1954. Mrs. Mehra Vakil sent me the message that Mr. Menuhin wanted me to come and teach. I left for Mumbai immediately and I started teaching him. He stayed four-five days and whenever he played his concerts were successful. This made him invite me to Switzerland.

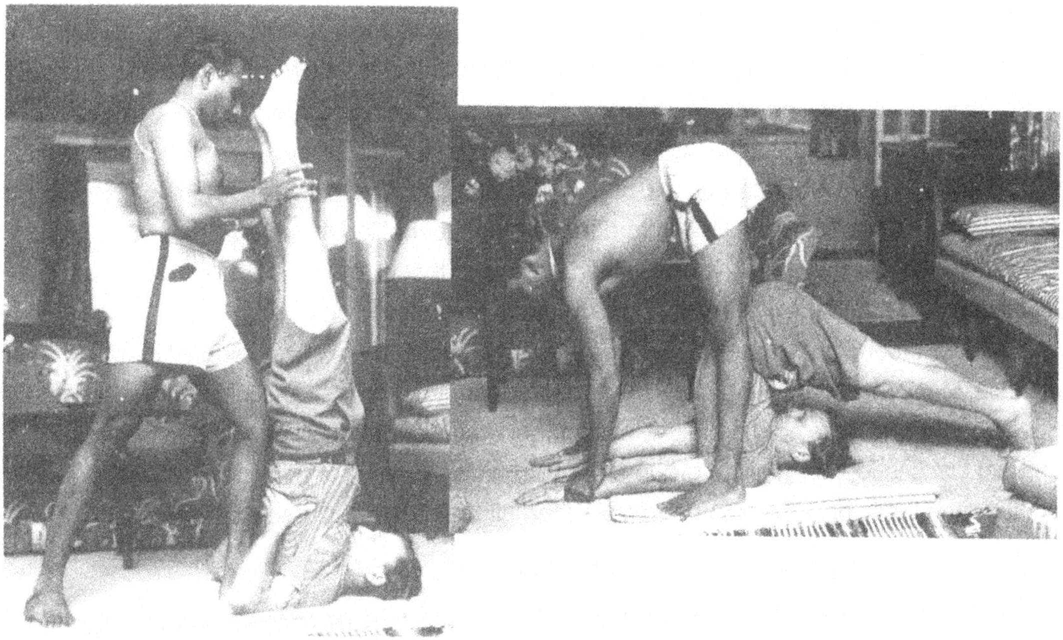

Plate n. 50 – Yehudi Menuhin taken for *Sarvāṅgāsana* and *Halāsana*

I went to Switzerland for two months to teach him and after the yogic session his first concert was in Zurich. He told me, "If I play very well in Zurich, the credit is yours. And the merit is also yours. If something happens, because this is the first concert I am playing after years in western countries, that means I may not get that positive mind". I told him, "Don't worry, you are going to play very well". Before the concert I took him through few *āsana* in order to enhance his confidence and he played so well that he received such an applause that even he couldn't control himself. Then he played two or three encores. As we were in the same hotel, I relaxed him after the concert, because he had in his mind that he can't sleep after the concert. I took him in some *āsana* which helped him to forget the event. After the last *āsana*, he came to my room and, to my surprise, he gave me an Omega watch with the inscription, "To my best violin teacher, Mr. B.K.S. Iyengar from Yehudi Menuhin. Gstaad, 29th Sept. 1954". And that's how our relationship grew closer and closer.

Q.- And had the expansion of the movement started as well in the West?

Yes, yes.

- Because the press reported a lot about him of this? -

Yes, the reviews were full of praise and the effect of yoga on him. Menuhin is really like a flower. When he began improving himself, he never kept quiet. He hadn't that selfish attitude. So he began telling his musical friends how he had improved greatly through yoga. This had a telling effect on all top class musicians who were in Gstaad and they also tried yoga and they too felt better improvements in their play. Musicians like Malkuzinski, Clifford Curzon, Gina Bachaiar, Lily Cross, Maurice Jonron and many others benefited from yoga.

I taught them and everybody started observing that there was something in yoga. They felt lightness, got better skilful movements in their fingers and voice.

The cream of the music world to whom I taught realised my way of teaching was valuable. Many musicians who were playing for Menuhin's orchestra, Berlin Orchestra, and all those people who were coming to Switzerland became interested in yoga. At that time I used to conduct classes for the musical group alone, en masse. Twenty to thirty people were learning together and that's how the yoga built up. When all the musicians started praising...

- Then it spread... -

It spread. I taught also Krishnamurthy and Aldous Huxley, as they were there. On one side there were intellectual people and on the other side artistic musicians. Because I was teaching all classes of people, it grew.

Then I taught the Queen Mother of Belgium. She wanted to stand on her head, you must have read she was 84 years old. Her ambition was to feel the sense of head-balance since young. Her joy was beyond words.

When I returned to India, the turning point was when the *Times of India* interviewed me at the airport. It wrote an article about my visit to foreign countries, "Yoga is the king amongst all exercises and Mr. Iyengar teaches queens and kings only". This upset me. Then when I was again invited to come to England in the following years, I told Mr. Menuhin that I would not only teach the intellectual cream, but I would like to help common people and that's how I started running classes for the average people in England in 1961. It spread like wildfire. If I only remained with the cream, probably I would have been a V.I.P throughout my life. I devoted more time in teaching the local average people, problematic people and remedial cases. As these classes proved successful, this caught the world in the field of yoga.

- Great. Well I think we should perhaps leave it there... -

Part TWO – THE EVOLUTION

Q.- *Guruji,* what is yoga? There are some confusing ideas about it.

Yoga has a lot of connotations, but according to the earliest texts, the union of the individual soul with the Universal SOUL is considered as yoga. Probably the intellectual standard was so high in those days that they had touched the subtlest of the subtle to start with. And later the terminologies changed. For example, Lord Krishna says, equanimity is yoga, and at the same time at other place he says, the skilfulness in thought or in action is yoga. Again he comes down to a common man's level telling that that which removes sorrows is yoga. Patañjali says, restraint of the consciousness is yoga.

Yoga is a word which has come from the root *yujir,* which means to join, to unite, to associate, to work with, to attain to. Yoga means *samādhi,* which is derived from *sam* and literally means "putting together". So union of the individual with God is possible through *samādhi.* Like that, it has several meanings but from understanding these things, I say that union of the body with the mind and mind with the soul is one meaning and the other is the union of the intellect of the head with the intelligence of the heart is yoga.

Q.- And you are always called *Guruji?* What is a *guru,* exactly?

Gu means heaviness or darkness, *ru* means lightness, light. The one who removes the darkness of the aspirants and uplifts them from nescience towards the light of wisdom is a *guru.*

Q.- Yoga has to be taught by a *guru* doesn't it? So who is a *guru?*

Guru is one who uplifts the pupils and builds up through developing their intelligence and enlightens them. As ignorance is heavy and intelligence is light, the word *guru* has come so that the heaviness or the ignorance in the student is removed and the light of wisdom is brought into its place, and one who does that is called a *guru.*

Q.- But the tradition of *guru* and disciple in India is quite different to the tradition of teacher and pupil in the West.

You are right. When we accept *guru*, according to Indian tradition, he is the father, he is the mother and he is the *ācārya* – meaning the teacher. As he takes the role of looking after students like parents and educates them, the reverence is built up and they do not consider him as an ordinary teacher but as a *guru*. Can I say "enlightened teacher"? He educates and cultures them towards spiritual knowledge.

– *But the* guru *also has to give a lot to his pupils.* –

Naturally, yes, yes, yes.

– *I remember once reading I think that you said that* guru *should put his body into the student's body in a way.*

Yes, to some extent. That means all his thoughts, all his actions have to be like the mother who looks after the child; becomes one with the child . The *guru* is like that. That he takes his *śiṣya*...

– *Śiṣya is his disciple...* –

Yes. So *guru* adopts the *śiṣya* as his own son or his own daughter, and takes the full responsibility of building him or her up to the level of his standard.

Q.- So there is in a way a loving relationship between the *guru* and his pupil?

Adoration, more than loving. It is adoration.

– *But the* guru *himself loves his pupils?* –

Naturally. But that love is without any attachment or expectation. Otherwise the education is not possible at all.

Q.- You must sometimes find it difficult to love some of your pupils when they're not very good or they don't learn.

No, no. You know, the way in which we have to understand love is the love without lust, which is quite different, and that love is the real love, which the *guru* throws because he has no lust for his pupil. And therefore that pure love builds up that reverence in the pupils to respect their master. *Guru* loves his pupils as his children, whether it is he or she.

Q.- You also, your sort of God almost in a way is Patañjali who wrote or is said to have written a great original treatise on yoga. Who was he?

According to the *purāṇic* texts – legendary books, Gauṇikā was a great *tapasvini,* a great yogini. She had full knowledge but she was unmarried, following an ascetic and celibate life. At an old age, she was feeling that she could not transfer the knowledge which she had gathered. So she praised the Sun God saying, "I developed this knowledge through your light and I am returning this knowledge to you". She had water in her hands just as we have when we pray to God, and she wanted to surrender her knowledge through that water to the Mother Earth for the Sun to accept it. At that time Ādiśeṣa, who is the couch of Lord Vishnu, appeared in the form of a worm, who was named by Gauṇikā as Patañjali.

– So Patañjali is a serpent, isn't he, the serpent on which Lord Vishnu rides? –

Yes, he is a serpent and he is the seat or couch, for Lord Vishnu. I will repeat the story for you. It so happened that when she had the water in her hand and closed her eyes, Patañjali in the form of small worm fell in her palms. When she opened her eyes, she saw something moving. At once, he took a human form and that's why she named him Patañjali. *Pata* means fallen and *añjali* means into the folded palms at the time of prayer. The snake fell on her palm at the time of prayer and evolved into a human being, so she called him Patañjali.

And this also has got a little background according to legendary stories, that once Lord Shiva invited Lord Vishnu to see his *Tāṇḍava nṛtya,* the famous dance, what you call the *Naṭarāja* dance. Lord Vishnu was sitting on Lord Ananta – Ādiśeṣa – the snake – and watching the dance. The body of Lord Vishnu became heavier and heavier as the dance was progressing, and Ādiśeṣa was feeling breathless. The moment the dance came to an end, he felt the lightness of Lord Vishnu: He addressed the Lord, "You were so heavy, I was not even able to breathe but now You have become light". The Lord answered, "When Lord Shiva was dancing, my body was vibrating in the same level, that's why you felt it". Then Ādiśeṣa thought, "My Lord is so fond of dance, I should learn and please him." He requested Lord Vishnu for permission to learn dance. Lord Vishnu told Ādiśeṣa to go to Lord Shiva, who will ask him to write the *Mahābhāsya* on grammar. At that time he can go to the planet Earth and learn the dance. That is how he took the birth in the palms of Gauṇikā and that is the story. It was about 500 BC, or even earlier.

Q.- And what is it about his *sūtra*, his treatise on yoga, which makes it so marvellous?

You see, according to the Indian way of thinking, he is the author of *āyurveda, vyākaraṇa* – grammar – and yoga. He wrote a commentary on grammar for right use of words. As I told you that he was learning dance, he understood the body movements to such an extent and wrote *āyurveda* in the name of Caraka with this background of body movements. Many classical dancers of India pay homage to Patañjali as he was considered as a great dancer.

Then he reflected, "I've spoken about the health of the body, I have spoken about the correct usage of words, but I've not said anything about the silence or the tranquillity of the mind". So he took the subject of yoga as his last work and started with the prescription, "*Atha yogānuśāsanam,* now I will explain to you what yoga is".

- After explaining all the other subjects? -

Yes. And that's why we consider him as the author of yoga, author of *āyurveda,* as well as the author of grammar.

Q.- And is your yoga as practised today basically the yoga of Patañjali?

Well, I say 100% it is based on Patañjali though there is... You see, the modern mind gives denominations to various aspects of yoga. God is one but He's called by different names. Truth is one but people define truth in different ways. Similarly yoga is one but unfortunately, say about a century ago or so as far as my study goes, the problem started when Swami Vivekananda wrote on *rāja yoga, karma yoga, jñāna yoga, bhakti yoga* and so on, divisions began to grow. In olden days these four were called paths, like *karma mārga, jñāna mārga, bhakti mārga* and *yoga mārga.* As Swamijī changed the name of path to yoga, he titled *Pātañjala Yoga Sūtra* as *rāja yoga.* This created divisions. Patañjali has said *aṣṭāṅga yoga* and not *rāja yoga.* Patañjali defines yoga as *cittavṛtti nirodhaḥ.* It means restraint of *citta* – the consciousness.

– Restraint of the movements of the consciousness. –

Yes, this is yoga according to Patañjali. *Citta* has three constituents: the mind, the intelligence and the I-consciousness. As the days grew, people naturally forgot about the word *citta*, the consciousness, and stuck to the mind. Svātmārāma, in *Haṭhavidyā Pradīpikā*, which is a treatise much later than Patañjali, used the word *rāja yoga* saying that the mind is the king of the body. Then later various authors of yoga texts used the word *rāja yoga, haṭha yoga, laya yoga, mantra yoga* and so on, giving different names.

The divisions came probably at that period in order to differentiate one yoga from the other yoga, but in the early days they were not called different yogas but were called paths – the ways.

Q.- I think we in the West find it very difficult not to categorise things, to describe them too accurately and then this leads to splits, new churches being formed and all that sort of thing. Do you think that?

Yes, that is what is happening. That's what I'm saying. If Mr. Iyengar is doing a lot of *āsana*, he is a *haṭha yogi*, that is "Iyengar Yoga". But *haṭha* has a very wonderful meaning and I would like those who are ignorant of its meaning to refer to its meaning. *Haṭha* means will power, and will power comes from the mental and intellectual levels. So what is *citta?* Citta is a compound word covering or encasing the mind, intelligence and "I" or "me". It is also will power. So *haṭha* is will power, wherein it has no bearing on physical movements.

You know, if you read *Haṭhavidyā Pradīpikā* or Patañjali's *Yoga Sūtra*, you find the eight aspects of yoga that are common in both, namely, *yama, niyama, āsana, prāṇāyāma, pratyāhāra, dhāraṇā, dhyāna* and *samādhi*. Patañjali expresses in depth these eight aspects of yoga while Svātmārāma emphasises on *āsana, prāṇāyāma* and *samādhi* more but touches the other aspects implicitly. Hence, *haṭha yoga* observes all the eight aspects of yoga. Just because he speaks on *āsana* as the first *aṅga*, people think that those who practise *āsana* are *haṭha yogis*. Though he expresses his views on *yama* and *niyama*, first, and then deals with *āsana* and calls *āsana* as the first aspect and proceeds with the techniques of *asana*, this wrong notion has prevailed. But I request those who have such notions to read this text once again, so that they realize how the author of *Haṭhavidyā Pradīpikā* takes one towards *samādhi*.

Svātmārāma and Patañjali both emphasise on *śarira śuddhi, sauca* of *niyama*. Both want internal and external cleanliness. As Svātmārāma emphasises body cleanliness adding *ṣaṭkarma* for internal cleansing, yet, he cautions that all should not perform these *ṣaṭkarma*, except those whose *doṣa* are greatly vitiated. Patañjali does not speak of *ṣaṭkarma*, therefore I do not teach them since the *doṣa* can be corrected with *āsana* and *prāṇāyāma*.

Q.- So for you Patañjali is *haṭha yoga* as well, really?

Well, as I said, Patañjalı is a yogi. His aim is to put the whole subject in front of his followers as complete yoga, so he curtails the details but puts aptly. He speaks of *āsana* as dealt in *haṭha* texts. Patañjali elaborates *yama* and *niyama* in depth, Svātmārāma elaborates *āsana* and *prāṇāyāma* in depth. Both deal with yoga as an evolutory method with moral practice, physical practice, vital practice, mental practice, intellectual practice.

Q.- Now some people in the West I think would think seeing you for instance doing your *yogāsana* ... that you are a man of extreme asceticism because they're used to see *sādhus*, people like that and in particular that you were a celibate. But you are not a celibate and you don't think it's necessary; you don't even think it's right to be a celibate, do you?

Well, I am a married man, yet a celibate in a certain way. There were also many yogis who were married.

- So you are a celibate in the way that your sexual life is fully under your control? -

Not only under control, but I crossed thaqt age of lust long back. This is a very small phase of life.

- And you believe, don't you, that semen has a particular power? To be preserved rather than wasted? -

It is. That's why Vasiṣṭha called himself as a celibate though he got married and he had a hundred children, because his semen was not wasted at all.

Q.- And you also said something to me which to me seemed very interesting, a bit like St Paul's famous saying "marry lest ye burn", and you somewhere have said marry lest you start looking lecherously at women.

Yes, you are right. Because a celibate naturally may be saying that he is physically a celibate, but what goes in his mind is unknown. At least married peoples' minds may be free from looking at other women or winking at them. To that extent, it is great.

Q.- Does yoga specifically help you to control your sexual desires?

Yes. You see, the practice of yogic discipline is such that it takes your mind away from these distorted attractions. The sex is such that it could be a physical demand, or it could be a mental demand. The physical demand is always at the early age but the memory of mental wants increases as one grows. Yoga helps one to restrain the demand both from physical as well as mental sides. There are certain *āsana* like *Mūlabandhāsana, Baddha Koṇāsana, Upaviṣtha Koṇāsana...*, where the genital organs are made to become passive and pensive for controlling the physical temptations, and certain *āsana* like inverted *āsana* and *Paschimottānāsana* and certain *prāṇāyāma* for controlling the mental demands. These two aspects of yoga help the practitioners to live a contented life and be free from temptations.

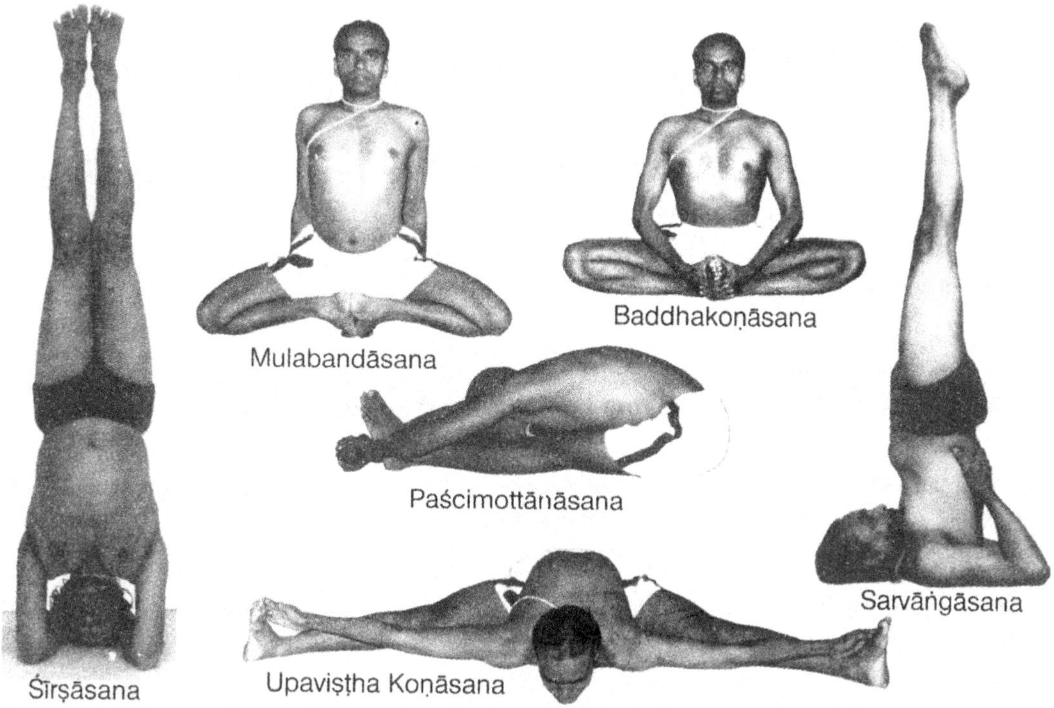

Plate n. 51(a) – Yogic discipline for sexual desire – *āsana*

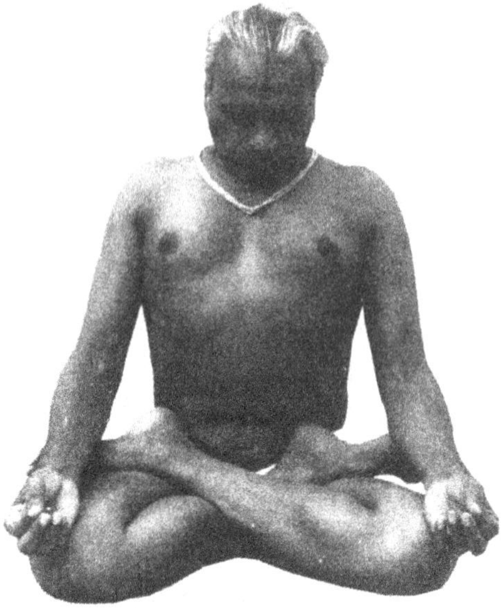

Plate n. 51(b) – Yogic discipline for sexual desire – *prāṇāyāma*

Q.- What about other things which are associated with asceticism, like for instance food and drink? You certainly are opposed to...

I'm not opposed, my friend. If I go on telling that you have to eat this food and that food, you have to have fruits, you have milk..., what about poor people in our country who cannot get food even for sustenance? Patañjali speaks of mind controi but he does not speak on diet. He speaks of mastery of body, of mind and of morals to live by, but does not speak of the food though it is hidden in the principles of *yama* and *niyama*. But one thing he says to us, to surrender all to God. I think that this may cover food habits also.

- So in a way it's controlling greed really rather than a specific diet? -

Coming from a poor family, I could not have a rice plate, which was then costing two *anna*, equal to twenty *paise* of today, and I practised yoga. Having undergone yoga practice without nourishment, how can I tell people about food? Secondly, yogic discipline controls the greed of the tongue.

Q.- You don't even insist, do you, that people should be vegetarian?

You know, I began teaching yoga when people were ignorant of the subject. I wanted to popularise yoga and not 'isms'. For example, if I insist that you should be a vegetarian, you should have nourishing food, then how do I know that actually yoga has changed the person or the induced words have changed the person? I wanted natural changes to take place in the given surroundings through yoga. One thing I was sure, that three to three-and-half hour classes in the West at a stretch kept them away from smoking or drinking. Having seen me living only on vegetables, they were impressed with the energy I had, and probably this changed their eating habits. And that acted as a turning point in their lives to change.

I think the *āsana* I teach filter the blood and increase the biochemical as well as psycho-chemical changes which make them change their food habits. But I never insist they become vegetarians.

Q.- What is your personal diet?

My personal diet is *chappati*, vegetables and yoghurt or milk, and if I take rice, I don't take *chappati*. Sometimes I may take a little fruit. And that's all my food. *(Laughs.)*

Q.- So you do cook food though?

Well, my daughters are there, they cook and I take it.

– Somebody like my friend Morarji Desai used to insist that you should only eat raw food. He used to eat nuts and salads and fruit. –

I answered that question already, that my life is for middle class people to give them health and happiness. I want them to assimilate of what they eat. This is my approach.

Q.- That's a very good way of looking at it. So you don't want to express, to advocate something, very expensive diet?

No, no, not at all.

Q.- Yoga has expanded remarkably. You yourself said somewhere in the 50s and 60s your job was to propagate yoga. Now you feel your job is to correct distortions.

See, when a specialised subject becomes very popular, you have to expect some distortions taking place in the art. Yoga was unknown in the 1950s. Very few people knew it. Even in India, in the nineteen thirties, there were only a few yoga teachers in the whole of India including Pakistan and Bangladesh. I am speaking of those days when one could count the number of yoga teachers on one's fingertips. Today we find yoga teachers at each corner of the road. As the yogic wind is blowing, everybody is taking advantage of this. That is why I want to give what is the right practice and what is distorted practice, so that the quality of it is maintained.

We have guides from the epics of *Mahābhārata.* Dharmarāja was there, who was a virtuous man, Duryodhana too was there, who was a vicious man, so virtue and vice both go together and live together in society. It is for a discriminative person to choose the method to progress. My duty, my job, is to bring as far as possible that virtue in the field of yoga.

Q.- What are the particular dangers you see, maybe perhaps in the West? Some people I think are very concerned about what's called Power Yoga, where people seem to be doing it specifically to get something out of it, to make themselves more powerful, strong, rather than what you're saying, which is completely the opposite.

My friend, as you said, this Power Yoga has come only very recently. As the word is fascinating and attracting, people are pulled towards that yoga. When I was teaching in the early days from 1936 to 1960, this so-called Power Yoga, both in the East as well as in the West, then the *Yoga and Health* magazine of London started condemning me that I am more on physical yoga. When I was labelled as a physical yogi, I refined and gave lots of new things. I said, "Let me work in each *āsana* to reach perfect alignment and how to attend to each and every part, every fibre, every cell, by going into these subtleties". However the same old system which I was doing and teaching has come back in the name of Power Yoga.

Patañjali explains this Power Yoga in a very different way. In the third chapter, he speaks on the effect of *āsana,* which many people do not refer to[1]. He does not speak of the health of the body. He speaks of the wealth of the body. What is the wealth? He enlists them as beauty, elegance, strength, compactness and various illuminative lights that the diamond reflects. These are the qualities of the *āsana* that Patañjali asks from the practitioner.

I realised that this wealth of *āsana* can be achieved by performing various *āsana* for a longer period with total attention with detailed corrections to gain strength, endurance, elegance, grace and form. The wealth that Patañjali speaks of is hidden in this *sūtra,* i.e., *sthira sukham āsanam.* It means that all reflections from the body mind and Self should reflect and re-reflect without distortions in the cells, fibres and so forth.

I thought that when one considers the three units body, mind and soul as one unit, every part of the body, every aspect of the mind and the total presence of the soul have to be felt while performing the *āsana.* I attended that way and that is what I felt as a spiritual practice

---

[1] *Rūpa lāvaṇya bala vajra saṁhananatvāni kāyasaṁpat.* Perfection of the body consists of beauty of form, grace, strength, compactness, and the hardness and brilliance of a diamond (*Y.S.,* III.47).

of *āsana*. I transformed the *āsana* from the physical level to the spiritual level, but people unfortunately want to go back on to the physical level, as power yoga is nothing but connative movement. Practice of āsana demands not only connative movements but cognitive, mental, intellectual and conscientious action balancing harmoniously in the connative movement. Then the 'Power Yoga' may be coined differently.

However, *āsana* practised with the frame of Power Yoga without any deliberation or without applying the mind and intelligence, for me are raw practices.

Q.- There seems to be something philosophically wrong with many people's attitude to yoga in the West. They seem to want to do it to achieve, to benefit themselves, to make themselves stronger or more beautiful. They forget that it is really in a way about dumbing down or reducing the path of ego. They do it the other way round. They want to boost their ego by doing it.

You want me to quote Patañjali again, sir? Patañjali knows the mentality of the human beings. In the second chapter he speaks, *prakāśa kriyā sthiti śīlaṁ bhūtendriyātmakaṁ bhogāpavargārtham dṛśyam (Y.S., II.18). Bhoga* means sensual pleasure, *apavarga* means spiritual upliftment or emancipation. The practice of yoga is like standing on a precipice. If you slip the right method, you may fall into the *bhoga*, the pleasure or temporal joys; if you cross over to the other side of the cliff, you may become liberated and emancipated. It is common that it's a precipice, but unfortunately as you said, in western countries this attitude is there to a very great extent, but I am sure this attitude will change as their practices get intensified.

Yet, I say with experience from 1954 onwards that with my contact with Western people, many have developed to go into the spiritual aspects. From this positive angle, I think that this Power Yoga may not survive too long, as I am certain that in the majority of the western people the spiritual attention has set in.

Q.- In some ways spiritual awakening that you talk about seems to be happening more in the West than in India. For instance you have many more schools abroad and many more foreign pupils than you have Indian pupils. Why is this?

In India we have taken it for granted that we are all the children prodigy of the *ṛṣi*, or sages, so it is in our blood. This has caused a kind of stagnation. Indians have not realised that they are in a stagnated state of spiritual life. But the Westerners have been doing the *sādhanā*, and a purificatory process is taking place in them. Their mind has touched the inner mind. Now the inner mind has to touch their innermost mind. In India a kind of ego, pride, has imbibed in their blood as if the impressions of our rich spiritual heritage run in them.

I hope my Indian brothers realise this weakness and come back to the *sādhanā* or spiritual attitude as followed by our sages and *ṛṣi*.

Q.- Do you think it's also partly to do with the fact that in the West people have almost got satiated, have had enough of wealth and all these sorts of things whereas in India people are still not wealthy.

That's also one of the reasons. In India we have yet to find means of economic satisfaction. Probably this has kept the Indians away from higher thinking. If the poverty is lessened, naturally the majority of the people with the background of philosophy may adopt the yogic way of living for spiritual growth. You can see the essence of spiritual life in the villagers even today. It is possible to transform them, but unfortunately they are stuck with poverty, which is affecting them in the field of spiritual life.

It is not wealth that comes in the way. Certainly money is required for the needs of life for it to run smoothly. In the West wealth brought dissatisfaction and spoiled the way of life. Obviously, this must have made them to turn to yoga. In India lack of basic requirements and poverty are keeping the yogic cup far away.

So as you point out, the material wealth undoubtedly did not satisfy them. Their inner urge inclined them towards yoga.

Q.- In your own life, when did you first realise that this was something much more important than just a job and being a teacher?

In 1966 the change took place in me, after thirty years of practice.

- As long as that? -

Yes. I could meet with comfort my family commitments and at that time my thoughts changed towards the interior world.

Q.- What was the change? Can you describe it?

As I told you, I was not able to maintain the load of family comforts, I was thinking of giving public performances to make extra earnings to fulfil the wants. Like a stage artist, I presented and satisfied the audience and thought that it was a wonderful work. I became an exhibitionist, which I don't deny. Without exhibitionism, people could not be attracted towards the subject, and I went on presenting with elegance each and every *āsana*, with grace, so that it would attract the people to see the rhythm of the body, and I won them.

I was in need of material needs as I had a big family to take care of. This I don't deny. Being a practical yogi, I knew the needs of the material world, as that was my want. Yet knowing people's weaknesses and what they came for to me, I used to work so that they are satisfied with their wants, and then to uplift them from that state of mere enjoyment to the practicality of touching divinity that lies hidden within.

When material satisfaction came, my life naturally changed to dive deep into the spiritual aspects.

Q.- Did anything special happen in 1966 to make you to do so or feel so?

That's what I said, my mind changed. The transformation took place in me to use the body as an instrument to penetrate that which exists beyond body and mind. People, when they are tired, they go for a holiday to hill resorts. For me a holiday resort is to stay in each *āsana* for a long time and to live in that *āsana* and feel the freshness in my body and mind ebbing and flowing. I can see that freshness moment to moment. The experiences of yesterday's *āsana* will not be the same in today's practice. I reflect on what I did today, watch what was I missing, and keep those points in mind to bring that in next day's practice. This is how I enjoy my holiday resort by remaining close to the Self. I am free from external thoughts in my practice and hence it is a change in thought from external to internal. A holiday to the mind and intelligence from the gravity of external thoughts.

– Get out of the heat in a different way? –

Yes! In away, it is a different approach of getting out of the mental environment so that my consciousness remains ever fresh in me.

Q.- Was there any dream or any vision or anything that led you to change your mind?

Yes, in 1946 I had a dream and that is the turning point in my life. Up to 1946 I was a mercenary in the field of yoga. Well, I tell the truth because if somebody said, "Come and teach me", I used to ask them, "Can you give me money for my meal, and I will come and teach you". Because nobody was interested in yoga, so I had to teach yoga just to make a living.

I went to Bangalore and got married in 1943. During that period, I was teaching a good number of people. Due to the marriage I had extended my holiday, which cost me to lose all my students.

At one stage my relatives, my *guru,* the people around me insisted that I should get married. You know, in India, way of living is quite different. You must have known as you are in India. If one doesn't get married, they suspect that one must be having some "clicks" and that's why he's not getting married. In those days this type of feeling was very strong. The social norms and ways of thinking were quite different. I never wanted to fall a prey for such twisted ways of gossip and so I got married. I lost my job. For three months I had no job. Then all of a sudden some School Authorities called me, "Can you come and teach children in school? You will be paid fifty rupees". I accepted the job and I told my wife, "Now I am having fifty rupees job, please come to Pune". Until then, she stayed in Bangalore with her mother.

I was teaching since 1936 as a mercenary and it went on till 1946. In that year I had a dream of my family Deity called Bālajī. You must have heard of Tirupati temple. The Deity there is our family God. One night I saw the Lord Śrī Veṅkaṭeśvara in the dream and the Lord blessed me with a grain of rice because I was cursing Him saying that I can't get even one meal per day to live and what yoga do I have to practise? Though I was practising, I was not getting smoothness or perfection in the *āsana.* I was crying, weeping if the *āsana* was not coming. But that grain of rice which the Lord gave me in a dream, the same night my wife also had the same dream... We narrated the dream to each other. I told her, "I saw Bālājī in my dream". She said, "I saw Lakṣmi, the goddess of wealth, in my dream. She gave me two *annas* which she said that she had borrowed from you years ago and she has returned that".

Whether you believe or not, the next day people came for therapeutic treatment and that's how my therapeutic treatment started in 1946. Patients started asking me, "I am suffering from such and such a problem, can you teach?" so I took the chance and since then I have never looked back. Poverty was not there, though money was not much, but I lived a life without a want: I think this is the first turning point in my life to take to yoga seriously and not for just mercenary purposes.

So, from '36 to '46, I too was caught in "Power Yoga". Then I shifted as a performing artist. In 1966 it was a true transformation from physical towards the philosophical. This transformation came not from the dream but on realisation. The dream freed me from the wants of necessity.

1965 was the period when I took the responsibility of completing my book *Light on Yoga* Mr. Gerald York, the reader for George Allen & Unwin, helped in the art of writing. It became a classic work in yoga.

This was the period when I had to teach intellectual people as well as the philosophers. This forced me to read *Yoga Sūtra* of Patañjali and conversing with intellectuals and philosophers helped me in forming the *Light on Yoga* book. All these things helped me to develop my intelligence to reach a sense of maturity in 1968.

Part THREE – UPS AND DOWNS

Q.- How do you see the future of your Institution? Even now it must be very difficult for you to control it because it's so widespread?

No sir, no sir, no, no, no. I am a *vedāntin*[1] from inside, though I do not appear so from outside. Yet I am a *sannyāsin*.[2] Through circumstances though I don't wear the saffron robes. People may not look at me as a philosopher because there is no outside sign. I came with an empty hand, I will go with an empty hand. Today the empire of yoga has grown by the grace of God and I have learnt also not to feel sorry if something happens. Time and circumstances played on me and I leave the future also to time.

The new things, new visions which I introduced in yoga must not fade. Yoga is a growing subject and I'm sure that it is going to grow for several centuries to come. I may be called a legendary figure, which matters nil for me. But I like that these new introductions to this yoga does not die as I have blown the cosmic life into it. As life is dynamic, I've changed the static yoga into a dynamic yoga, and I hope that it will always be ascending with a geometric progression.

I have got trained thousands of yoga teachers. Some teachers are not only direct pupils of mine but their pupils too have become yoga teachers. As all are my children, my great-grandchildren who practice my method are also yoga teachers. Generations after generations

---

[1] An adept in *vedāntic sādhanā*.

[2] One who has embraced the life of complete renunciation; one who neither hates nor desires anything and is above *dvandva* or the pair of opposites *(Bhagavad Gītā*, V.3).

are following it. You see here I have got students from four generations coming still. Even in London, if you make enquiries, there are three generations continuing since 1950s.

Probably the quality of the blood, the genes, what we speak of today, I think my yoga has changed the quality of the genes in each individual who practises since years and I think, I feel that my method of yoga can never have an easy death. And that's why I'm happy.

Q.- Do you feel you should nominate your successor?

No, no, I will not do that. My *guru* never nominated me and I've no right to nominate anybody. It's God's will. The nominator is God. It is for Him to choose, not me. For me all my pupils are equal.

Q.- One question about your institution. As you said it's very widespread. You've got thousands of yoga teachers. Now you are very insistent with your method, people should do the yoga precisely. How are you able to make sure this happens when you're not a jet set *guru*?

I worked a great deal. Some were using my name because it is of a great value to them. People know that if they say that they are the pupils of Iyengar, they get a firm foundation and respect as well. To some extent it has become a marketing business. Yet there are many who devotedly practise and teach. As such members are more, I say yoga is in safe hands. Now I have made it a point that those people who use my name, cannot mix other methods. Some were very honest in saying that they mix. And things are going on well as the dedicated ones have me that carry on as thought in Pune.

Q.- Do you have people in each institution whom you trust thoroughly?

Trust is Trust. Sometimes misuse of trust takes place. Yet nothing can move without trust. The National Associations are there in every country. They seem to be firm regarding the principles. There assessments are taking place, certificates are given, so there is a methodology which I have introduced like a university model.

Q.- Now in your 50s, you almost started to fade out didn't you in a way? You had an injury and you thought gosh I can't cope with this.

Yes. Well I told you in the beginning, I'm a little fanatic with my art. See, in 1950s I was giving a lot of demonstrations all over the world but my inner body was empty, though the outer body was presenting. I felt that something was missing, *āsana* were coming but the feel of the *āsana* was not there. I was not getting of what you call feedback from my practice. The moment I thought that I should watch by connecting the outer body to the inner body, the exhibitionism of doing well started fading. It's a very funny thing which happened to me that when I went to study each *āsana* mentally, I lost even control of those *āsana* because my inner body was not taking it or should I say was not receiving any imprint from my practice.

This was in 1958. It took me about three months to recover. I used to feel dizzy while practising. I asked my *guru* about these blackouts and asked him for guidance. My *guru* told me, "You are married, you have got children, now you should not do as you were doing in the early days". I turned the question to my *guru* whether he had such feelings after his marriage. As the answer was not coming, I talked to myself, that I should not heed to his advice and I should not stop my practice. If yoga is meant for the old, the aged and ripe old people, how can I stop? I said no, something must be wrong. I wanted to correct the wrong. But my *guru*'s advice was to stop practising. So he said, "Better don't do so much".

I wrote to Swami Shivananda of Rishikesh. He also told me, "You are married now, you should lessen your practices". I felt that this was a hypothetical advice. I was not convinced with such advices. All the *ṛṣī* were married. Yājñavalkya had two wives. Vasiṣtha had a hundred children. So how can marriage come in the way, I wanted to know. But as I could not get the reply. I determined to continue, irrespective of success or failure, gain or loss.

In the beginning I used to get blackout in every two three attempts. I continued enduring this blackout. I questioned myself to try one or two times more even though I had blackouts. This way I increased the practice a little more and I went on, then the blackouts started lessening and lessening as I continued and the time lap also increased between blackouts. Then I wrote to my *Gurujī* that from my continued practice I got back the confidence, without stopping or dropping any *āsana*. In 1958 I was almost on the threshold of failure as I had started fading but came out of it successfully.

Then again in 1979 I had a very severe accident. I had lost consciousness also. I was driving a scooter and I met with the accident. Somebody recognised me and brought me home. The next day I found out that my shoulders, my back, all got swirled. I could not sit or stand. When my father died I was eight and a half years old and my father had predicted to me that before I reach the age of nine, he would not be alive. This was his premonition. He had told me, which I remembered very well that I would be the only person in our house who may survive and make a name but not live beyond sixty. His premonition was sentimentally in my heart and as I crossed sixty, I thought I would be free from his premonition but the accident put me back. Even *Tāḍāsana* was a painful process. Once again, I lost everything. I became a raw beginner. I decided to re-tool myself.

I started practising with these injuries to recover as far as I could. In a month's time, I had a second scooter accident as well. I remembered Lord Krishna's words, *samatvaṁ yoga ucyate*[1], equanimity is yoga, so even in pains I get these equanimities. Both the shoulders had lost power. I could not lift my hand up or down but I started learning the methodology to come back. I found lots of means to come back. Now, what I do nobody can believe that I have injuries at the shoulders and knees, I have slipped disc, dislocated shoulder and so on. My *sādhanā* is still continuing.

- Yoga means? -

Equanimity. Yoga means equanimity – to have a balanced state of mind. In spite of all these ups and downs, I did not lose my equipoise. Throughout my life I had always that spirit of let me try. I could build up and recover to a very great extent. After I lost yoga practice, in 1979, I never had a haircut. I grew hair, I said people should forget that I am Iyengar because when I lost my control, people should not call me on the street, he's Mr. Iyengar, and so I grew the hair longer and longer. When I began getting control, I started cutting my hair according to the progresses. As I have not come to the original level, I have not cut it to my original hair cut. The moment I get back everything, probably I may have my hair cut like all others. *(Laughs.)*

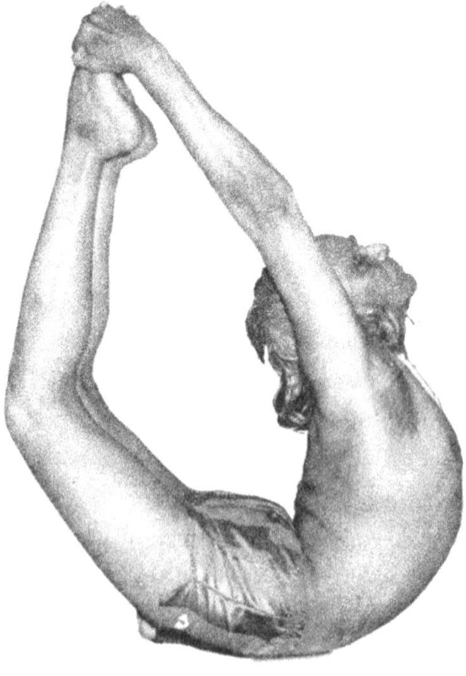

Plate n. 52 – *Pādāṅguṣṭha Dhanurāsana*

When we go to a temple, as the temple is kept clean, we too keep ourselves clean. We wash our feet and then go inside the

[1] *Bhagavad Gītā*, II.48.

sanctum sanctorum of the temple, so I thought that if I have to go to my body's sanctum sanctorum which is the Self, the body has to be completely clean and that made me to pursue my practice.

- Could you say that wonderful thing, "My body is my temple, āsana *are my prayers"?*

That's how I learned by study. For me the *āsana* are my prayers. Body is my temple and *āsana* are my *mantra*. As people do *mantra japa*, *āsana* is my *japa*, *āsana* is my *mantra*, *āsana* is everything for me. While practising I used to remember the story in *Māṇḍūkyopaniṣad*, where it says that *Āuṁ* is Brahman, *Sarvaṁ hy etad brahma* (*Māṇḍ. Up.* 2). See *Pādāṅguṣṭha Dhanurāsana*, which is a very difficult pose. That is in the form of *Āuṁ*. From that I used the body as the bow, *āsana* as the arrow and the target – the soul. Today I practise with this quotation of *Māṇḍūkyopaniṣad*.

- Wonderful! -

Q.- When I was talking to Prashant he emphasised the need for humility, accepting what you are as part of your destiny rather than thinking that you are a great person because you have achieved all this. But one of your pupils you were talking about the other day, Angela Marris, said that you lacked humility.

My friend, her reading of me was of the days when yoga had no respect. Unwanted questions and doubts of yoga was firing me to be tough and strong in answers, that maybe the reason for someone to brand me arrogant. I don't think if I had lacked humility in myself, I would have thousands and thousands of students. That humility alone has brought so many people to yoga. In my case I have got the nature where I can be more arrogant than any arrogant person and I can be humble to any humble person. How do you take it for granted that she is right? So definitely I say one person's reading does not merit much. If you had met Mr. Menuhin, or Krishnamurthy, they would have told you differently about me.

- You would regard humility as very important to you? -

Humility is the only ladder for learning. Humility should not be misunderstood to present day's sycophancy. Speaking sweet and good words is not humility. I may be rough if people cross with me for no reason. How can I remain humble at that time? In normal walk of life humility is perceived as soft speaking, sweet-speaking, consoling, which has not got much sense.

Q.- But you are doing that not with any sense of pride?

How can it be pride? If there's pride, I should be an intoxicated yogi, thank God, I am not. These days when teachers make mistakes in their practices, I do not correct them at once. Because I want them to undergo suffering so that they understand what humbleness means. If I correct them immediately, the arrogance and pride may set in. This delay in correcting them helps them in learning without pride. Secondly I want them to learn that humility is the key for success.

But if you see me in the class, I jump at once to correct students who are not teachers but remain as learners.

For anyone, a new adventure and enthusiasm traps in the net of ego. Any violinist in the beginning may think of becoming another Mr. Menuhin. It is fine to have a good aim to start with. But as one proceeds with practice, one has to come down to earth. The need for a good aim is faith, vigour, enthusiasm, cheerfulness and will power. Firmness and decision are also required. All these sprout from the 'I'. But as one goes on progressing, the ambitions from the 'I' have to be dropped to become a true practitioner or a true teacher. Humility alone makes one reach the goal.

Q.- Could you talk a little bit about the beginning of yoga in Britain, how you brought it into Britain?

In 1954, I visited London for the first time because my pupil Malkuzinski's concert was there and he told me, "You come with me, I will show you London after the concert". Mr. Menuhin had made arrangements for me to stay in Hotel De Vere. Being an Indian, they did not allow me to come to the breakfast table or to have lunch with whites and supplied food to my room. That was my first bitter experience of apartheid in London. It was not there officially, but it was there unofficially. At that time some of my Mumbai students were staying in London. So I wrote to them to ask whether they could arrange a talk or a demonstration. They tried but could not succeed. Nobody in London was interested in yoga then.

In 1954, when I got down at the Victoria Station, the customs officials asked me what my profession was. As I said yoga, they questioned me spontaneously whether I could walk on fire, chew glasses or swallow blades. I was shocked and surprised by these questions, because these things I knew only in India where the street performers do them. It pained me to hear such things on yoga. I replied that I am sorry, I don't know anything. I do various *asana* similar to callisthenics, as they were not aware of what yoga is like.

When I could not succeed in London, I returned to Switzerland to teach Mr. Menuhin. It so happened that on my return journey the customs again asked me what my profession was. I said yoga. I was shocked when they asked me, "How many currencies have you swallowed?" This upset me a great deal. Yet, I said mischievously, "If I can swallow currency, I could have swallowed Indian currency also. Then there was no need for me to come here to swallow currency". *(Laughs.)*

So this can give you some idea that how yoga was unknown in the West and what were their ideas regarding yoga.

In 1956 I visited America, Switzerland, and wanted to visit London. Fortunately at that time the deputy commissioner of Indian Commission was from Pune, whom I had known, called Mr. Gundevia. I wrote to Mr. Gundevia asking whether he could arrange a demonstration in the India House. He said that he could not do it in a short time, but asked me for a television show for two minutes. As it was not worth the trip, I dropped visiting London.

Then in 1960 Menuhin invited me to London. I started teaching the musicians. I suggested that I should have a class for the local people. He contacted Mr. Anya Deva Angadi of Asian Music Circle whether he could arrange general classes for me. There were only four students when I opened yoga for the public. Out of that four, one was Mrs. Silva Mehta who was my student while she was in India.

In 1961 the members increased to twelve. So, I was hiring a place for three hours at various halls. From mouth to mouth it spread and classes began at various places.

In 1971 I started classes for the Adult Educational Scheme, both in Greater London and Inner London and it caught on all over England.

– *What a story.* –

So I am grateful to Mr. Mc'Intosh, the Physical Director of Adult Education Authorities.

Q.- Did you live in London for some years then?

No, I never lived anywhere for years except in India. I used to come by invitation for two months a year visiting the continent.

Q.- And you never lived there for a long period?

No. I used to stay in London, Switzerland, France, Italy and other places of Europe. If I had to go to America, the Continent, Africa, I used to finish within three months and stay nine months at home.

– You're not a natural traveller then, are you? –

No, I am not a natural traveller.

– But you are not a person who loves travelling? –

I enjoyed in the early days.

– I don't either. Less and less do I like it. Airlines are so appalling. –

Part FOUR – INNOVATION

Q.- *Gurujī*, the props which I've seen people using when they do their exercises, benches, blocks and bars and other things like that... they're an innovation in yoga by you, aren't they?

To a great extent, though my *Gurujī* started with ropes, a few *āsana*, then I built up a great deal, afterwards.

– And did you invent these? –

Yes, many of the things are my own inventions.

Q.- And you got local carpenters to come and make them, did you?

Yes! I got them made from local carpenters. But it was not as simple as it looks. The guidance came from within. Realising that the patients cannot manage to do independently to get the effect, I factualised the imagination through props. I pictured the props and gave designs to the carpenters who designed with rough wooden material. I had to do on those shapes to try and then bring changes according to the body requirements and for the performance of various *āsana*. This way I built up and now it's easy for anybody to get and do the *āsana*.

Q.- And are these props now a standard part of your yoga really?

It's not a part of yoga. See, what happened is when Patañjali used the word *samādhi*, he uses the word 'with seed or supported' and 'without seed or non-supported', i.e., *sabīja* and *nirbīja samādhi*. This made me to think why not find ways to do *āsana* with support. Support means *ālambana*. In various *sūtra* Patañjali refers 'support'. I began thinking on his ideas and innovated props as "support" for good performance of *āsana* with ease but without risk.

If you see the book *Light on Yoga*, all the classical *āsana* are done without any support.

No doubt it has has become an authoratitive book for practitioners. But I realised later that all cannot master the *āsana* easily. So I began tracing supports to perfect the *āsana* without difficulties.

Q.- Yes, I was going to ask you about that. With all the pictures of you here as well, you don't have any support at all.

For years I was teaching without using any support, but realised later that these classical *āsana* cannot be done by one and all. When this Institute came into existence, people with various ailments started attending. In order to build up confidence in them, I thought that unless and until I innovate props for support to do the *āsana* with ease and also to keep their mental frame stable. I felt quick recovery from ailments may not be possible without innovating props.

In order to find props, the idea of *sabīja* and *nirbīja samādhi* came into my mind. If *samādhi* has support as well as non-support, why could not *āsana* too be *sabīja* and *nirbīja āsana*? Thus props like *sabīja* benefited in two ways; one is extension and the other is relaxation, taking place at the same time.

Q.- And is the intention that eventually, like a lame person who is cured, they should throw these away as crutches?

Yes, you can call it crutches. Once the *āsana* comes, they need not use them. These props take care of monitoring the *āsana* like intensive care units...

- Intensive care units, no, yeah... -

There were only general wards and special wards. Intense care units came later. Science has advanced. Intense care means everything is monitored and made available quickly and urgently on the spot. Wherever the doctor is, he looks at the chart and runs if the patient is in need, as the machines give alarming sounds. This idea struck me in yoga too. If they had to do the *āsana* independently, they have to strain a great deal and these props help them in monitoring and directing the right way to do the *āsana*. These props give a perfect direction to the patients and they cannot go wrong at all.

- You were telling of a particular bench, the Viparīta Daṇḍāsana *bench.*

Yes...

- And if you explain what the bench... -

You know, this is a slanting one, where the top of the chest is held up, head down and legs go downwards. This is a very exhilarating *āsana*, but when you do independently, it takes life out of each individual. You need to train the spine to get the concave curvature. Now everybody wants to do it, to get restfulness in their brains.

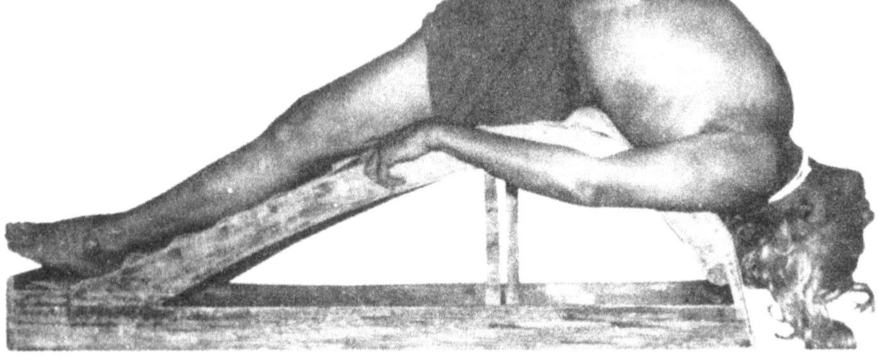

Plate n. 53 – *Dwi Pāda Viparīta Daṇḍāsana* on a bench

Now the world is in stress, strain and speed. The stress is so much, the nerves get blocked, the brain gets blocked. If a cup is full, you search for another cup; if the cup is empty, it is useful. I have to make the brain empty every now and then, so that the stress is not felt. On this *Viparīta Daṇḍāsana* bench, the head is kept down, so naturally it becomes passive on its own.

I tried this method. Now, each and everyone wants to do it. The conscious intelligence is in the head, the subconscious intelligence is in the heart, when one is in that *āsana*, it so happens that the conscious intelligence becomes subconscious and subconscious intelligence becomes conscious. I reverse the intelligence, so one lives in the heart and not in the head. At other times they live in their heads. That is how I found out.

- I must try lying on one then... -

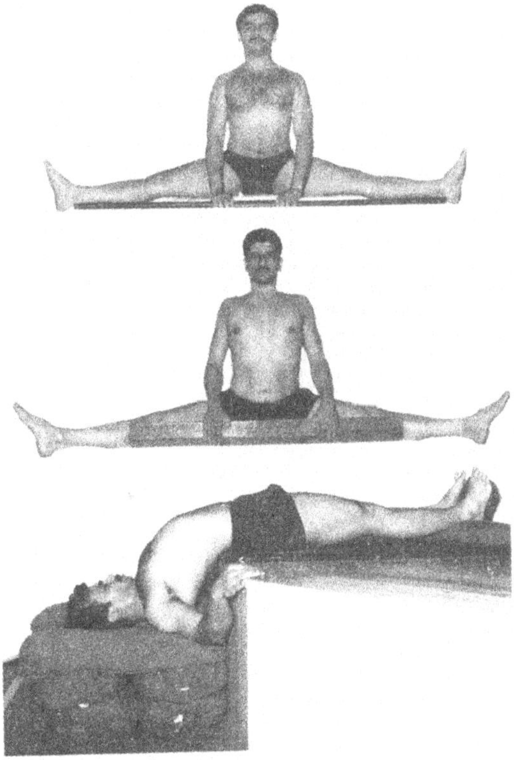

Plate n. 54 - *Upaviṣṭha Koṇāsana* with a stick between the legs, and *Setubandha Sarvaṇgāsana* off a bed

You can try, within ten minutes you will say my brain is quiet.

For example, one of the difficult *āsana* is *Kapotāsana*. One day I tried it curving myself on the ropes, resting my thighs on the trestler and feet on the pipe[1] and now even the beginners love to do it, saying, "No back ache". When the doctors say, "Don't bend backwards, it is painful", I make them do on the prop. Slipped disc people, who could not even turn this way or that way, enjoy this *āsana* five to ten minutes with ease. Hence, I say that these crutches make them stay longer, whereas independently they cannot stay even five seconds. As it gives a good feeling for them to be in a good thought by staying in those *āsana* on the prop, I am happy.

- Brought in the equipment, really? What other things did you use, did you use any domestic things in the house? -

[1] See plate n. 40(a).

In the beginning, I started using household things. For example in my early days I could not get *Baddha Koṇāsana*. So I was picking stones, cement blocks and what are all good to learn the *āsana*, and bringing them home. People used to laugh at me. If you were there, you too would have called me a madcap! I used to keep these stones on my thighs to get *Baddha Koṇāsana* – cobblers' pose.[2]

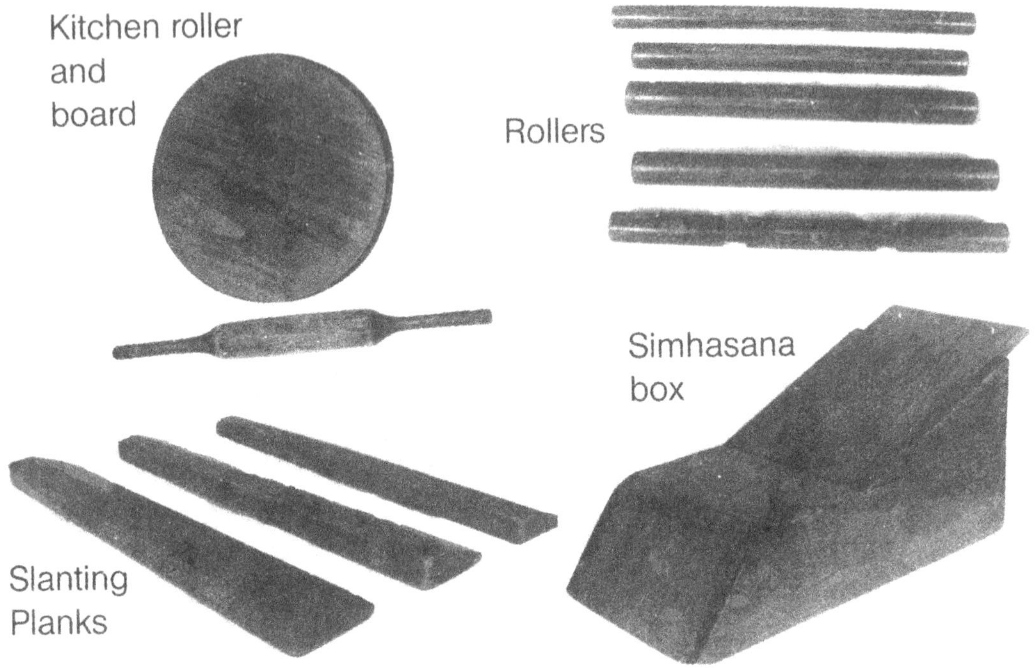

Plate n. 55 – Kitchen rolling pin; roller, slanting plank and Simhāsana bench – used for lumbar, cervical and chest

I used to use a walking stick between my knees for *Upaviṣṭha Koṇāsana*. As I could not spread my legs apart, I used the walking stick between the knees to spread my legs sideways. Similarly, I tried *āsana* on chair, bed and so on. People lie on the bed with head up, I used to lie with the head down, keeping the trunk on the bed. I started in a crude way and from this crude method, I refined them as props now.

Q.- And hasn't one of your props come from a rolling pin and plank for rolling out *chappatis*...

---

[2] See *Aṣṭadaḷa Yogamālā*, vol 4, plate n. 3.

...yes, same...

... what prop is that?

You know, when they do the *chappatis*, they use a roller to roll out the paste for it to become flat. I used that for the curvature of the neck, and for the tailbone for it to roll in. In the Institute you can see small rollers of different sizes, which I use for lumbar and cervical pains.

– You roll out the chappatis with a rolling pin on rolling plank... –

Yes, I use for the back and for some to get better breathing. We call it *Simhāsana* bench. The king and queens used to sit on a throne and I found that *āsana* throne for the heart, so that the chest may open in cases of emphysema, asthma. Like this I am inventing more and more.

Q.- Are you still inventing?

Yes, if a patient with a new problem comes, I have to find something that works. I try first and then help others to tell me what and how they feel. Then I improve on it to fit to all. Yesterday Susan was in the class, there was a spastic child. I was trying so many things, but suddenly I thought of a square foam and used it on the knees and made him stand independently, when he could not stretch the leg. I made him sit on two stools and made his legs straight and put weight on the back of the knee for the kneecaps to get contraction and relaxation. I think like that and I go on. *(Laughs.)*

Q.- What do you mean by the organic body, some people may be confused by this?

Muscles are not called organs. The liver is an organ, the spleen is an organ, and that is why yoga works on the organic system more than on the skeletal system, though there is an effect on the skeletal system. These vital organs are liver, spleen, pancreas, lungs, respiratory system, circulatory system, digestive system, glandular system and so forth. The yogis call it *prāṇamaya kośa*.

– Right... –

Q.- How did it come that a star's named after you?

Well, I do not know how it came, but one of my students sent me a note saying that a star in my name is registered in Washington. Probably, if God calls me I have an abode there to maintain my practices. *(Laughter)*

- So when the time comes we'll... (More laughter) think of you up there... -

Yes, yes, I maybe then be on my head...

- ...doing your yoga, yes we may all come up there, we'll do yoga with you. Lovely. -

Q.- Tell us about your eyebrows, *Gurujī*.

What? *(Laughter)* You know, somewhere people said that I've got double eyebrows. You can see there are two, one above the other, giving an impression that it is a double eyebrow. These eyebrows create a sort of fear in people and that's why they attribute that I am harsh, arrogant, rough and so on. My eyebrows created more comments than me! And I say that it has saved my character to a very great extent.

- How's that? -

Well, it is a very subjective matter. You have heard people saying that some God-men have the power of attracting lots of women, but in my case it worked quite the opposite way. My eyebrows kept people away from me.

- And the power lies in your eyebrows?

Maybe! Secondly, the heat in my body vibrates one inch away from the skin. The moment somebody comes closer, the magnet tells me about the character of the person.

- That is very interesting... -

If you keep your hand here *(he shows the distance with hand at the distance of one foot and half)*, you frequently feel the heat up to this level. Now for example, you feel nothing. now...

– Yes, yes, yes, just let me do it again, would you? –

Now do you feel anything?

– Nothing. –

Now see...

– Yes, I do... definitely, definitely, yes... –

... and that is my yogic practice and that keeps people away from me. Probably this is one reason why people say I am arrogant.

(Question from the producer)
– What did it tell you about his character? (Laughter)

Huh?

(The producer again)
– You said you could tell people's character...

(The interviewer)
– No, no, no that's not the matter now... –

No, that I won't say, it is close to attachment.

– This is something you've acquired, not from the beginning? –

No, never. This came only late. My *āsana* practice taught me a great deal. That's why I say *āsana* are my Deity *(Iṣṭadevatā)* and are my prayers.

Q.- But interestingly, your *āsana* are your God but at the same time you go to the Tirupati temple and you talk of the God there as your deity...

That is the God of Gods. He is our family Deity.

– *So we have two Gods, one is on individual's choice* (Iṣṭa devatā) *and the other, universal God...* –

Yes, when they unite in someone, he becomes a Universal Human Being.

Outside my skin is cosmic consciousness but inside the skin is the individual consciousness. The dialogue between the universal consciousness and the individual consciousness goes on, and that's why I practise *āsana*, so that they mingle together.

Q.- Could you run through your day for us *Guruji*, what time do you get up in the morning?

Previously I used to get up at three-thirty or four in the morning for years at a stretch. I used to practise like a fanatic sometimes even at three o'clock in the mornings. But now as I am semi-retired, I take it easy.

– *Certainly not...* –

...I'm semi-retired and in a semi-retirement I just want to remain in studentship. Now I get up at five-thirty or so. Though I am awake I may only be tossing on my bed, as I do not like to disturb others. I have a cup of coffee, finish my morning chores and do *prāṇāyāma* for one hour.

After doing *prāṇāyāma* for one hour, I glance through the morning papers.

– *You read a newspaper?* –

Yes.

– *I can't imagine you being very interested in newspaper.* –

Well, one should be in contact with the world at the same time in order to know what is happening around the world.

Q.- Do you take any interest in India's favourite subject, politics?

I'm interested in politics but I don't get involved in politics. I see the right and the wrong of the politicians and society. In politics, power has become important and not the humility to serve the poor in helping them in education, health, and to meet their daily needs. That is a pity, for me.

Q.- I was going to say... When you finish your newspaper reading, what time of day is it?

After *prāṇāyāma*, I glance through, but I read the editorials.

- How many newspapers... -

I get three-four newspapers. *(Laughs)* After reading the papers, I have another cup of coffee...

- Haven't we got to about nine o'clock then... -

Yes, the classes end at nine. So, I adjust the timings for my practice after the class and not earlier.

- Not to disturb them... -

Who knows... they may feel. So I am there at nine-fifteen to eleven-fifteen or eleven-thirty and I'll be practising. Sometimes students who come to practise ask me questions and I answer them as I practise. Then I go home, take bath, pray and have a little food and then relax for half an hour.

Q.- How long do you pray for?

Pray my God, that's all.

- How long for? -

About fifteen, twenty minutes.

- Do you have a little pūja... -

Yes, I've got in my room... my family deity...

- ...a shrine... -

... I've installed it in my room and I sit there. Incidentally my bed is also there. I do *Gayatri japa* also.

- Then after that, that takes... -

I relax for about half an hour or so, and I come to the library, reply to letters, read some books, write on the subject, up to six in the evening...

Q.- By this time, you have only had one very light snack in the whole day?

Yes.

- And aren't you hungry? -

No, I'm not. It was built up from the childhood and now it has become a natural thing for me.

- People like us are spoiled, huh? (Laughter.) -

In the mornings I do advanced difficult *āsana* and in the evenings, as I get tired, I do recuperative *āsana* so that I am fit for the next morning.

Q.- So when is your main meal of the day?

Only in the night, at about eight-thirty or nine.

- And what would that meal consist of, vegetables? -

Vegetables, rice, curds and sometimes the *rasam*. That's all. Very mild, light food. I can take food with anyone, in any party, anywhere though I'm a practitioner of yoga.

Q.- And television?

Yes! I see. There is a news item at nine o'clock and if there are good things, I see. Sports, because I'm fond of all sports. Then there are serials, dramas, which I see, and then I go to bed.

Q.- And what time would it be when you go to bed?

Say, it would be about ten-thirty or eleven o'clock. And sometimes I play with my grandchildren in the evening, have fun with them...

Q.- How many grandchildren do you have?

I have five grandchildren. Four of them are here just now, studying. One is in Bangalore.

– Good. –

Q.- When you do your *puja,* you are reciting the traditional Sanskrit prayers...

...which has been taught to us in our childhood...

– And is this a seven day a week routine for you? –

It is not a routine but reverence to the Universal Spirit.

– Perhaps we just ask... –

Hundred per cent, I say I work like the sunrise and sunset.

– It's as regular as that, seven days a week? –

So regular...

Q.- You never take a holiday?

Well, very rarely. Previously I used to work all three hundred and sixty-five days, including Saturdays and Sundays. I used to conduct classes in Mumbai on weekends. Only recently I have stopped. I have told my pupils, "Unless there is a good place where I can come and teach, do not expect me". Very often we have to vacate places and search for new places. Now, the Mumbai students are searching for a permanent place, 'til then I've got a little freedom. *(Laughter.)*

Secondly, I don't feel the subject boring at all.

– I wish I could say that journalism was never boring. I certainly can't say that. (Laughter.) –

I feel if I don't do, I may miss something that might have flashed to me. This expectation of illumination keeps me going in yoga.

Q.- Which is the most recent book you wrote?

Aṣṭadaḷa Yogamālā, volume one.

Now... I'm showing you a photo.

– Yes... –

Now I've covered a part of the portrait. Now, what face do you see sir?

– Quite a severe face. –

Which one does it represent?

–In what sense? –

I say... which animal does it represent.

- Oh, animal! oh definitely yes, well it... it could be Hanumān? (Laughter.) -

Very good, very good.

- Really is, yeah....yeah. -

See! Often people say that I look like Lord Hanumān.

Q.- But your movements are not like Hanumān's. Your movements are like... I suppose like Narasimha's movements must have been, or something like that...

Yes, yes...

- ...your movements are more like a lion... -

....lion, ...yes...

- ... stride around the place, you know? And with your long hair... -

Yes, yes, I think you're right...

- ... you look like a lion. A lion amongst yogis, perhaps. -

...you are right, you are right. I am a lion. *(Laughter.)*

- Thank you, Sir.

www.ingramcontent.com/pod-product-compliance
Lightning Source LLC
Chambersburg PA
CBHW080412270326
41929CB00018B/2999
* 9 7 8 8 1 7 7 6 4 9 7 6 5 *